PRAISE FOR

From Fatigued to Fantastic!

"*From Fatigued to Fantastic!* is not just a title, it's a promise. And this is one promise backed by an empathetic, innovative practitioner whose focus is always on getting his patients well. Jacob Teitelbaum has single-handedly revolutionized the way fibromyalgia, chronic fatigue syndrome, and thyroid disease are diagnosed and treated."

—MARY SHOMON,
author of *The Thyroid Diet* and *Living Well with Hypothyroidism*

"First published in 1995, *From Fatigued to Fantastic!* has continued to be at the top of the fibromyalgia patient's 'favorite books' list. . . . Dr. Teitelbaum's book will provide you with practical information and new and easy-to-understand insights on how to better manage and improve how you feel despite fibromyalgia."

—LYNNE MATALLANA,
founder of the National Fibromyalgia Association

"Jacob Teitelbaum's *From Fatigued to Fantastic!* is a must-read for all those suffering from chronic illness, as well as those treating patients with chronic illness. I use the information presented in this book every day in my practice with great success. I highly recommend this book for all to read and learn."

—DAVID BROWNSTEIN, MD,
author of *The Miracle of Natural Hormones*, 3rd edition

"An absolute classic in the field. . . . As a practicing doctor-nurse team, we encourage *all* people with fatigue to read this book thoroughly. It is a timeless contribution and provides crucial information for everyone."

—RICHARD L. SHAMES, MD, AND KARILEE H. SHAMES, PHD, RN,
creators of the health education website www.feelingfff.com and authors of
Feeling Fat, Fuzzy, or Frazzled?

"Jacob Teitelbaum is an outstanding and compassionate patient advocate. If you read just one book on CFS and fibromyalgia, this is absolutely the one I'd recommend!"

—HYLA CASS, MD,
author of *8 Weeks to Vibrant Health*

From
Fatigued to
Fantastic!

*A Clinically Proven Program to Regain Vibrant Health
and Overcome Chronic Fatigue and Fibromyalgia*

FOURTH EDITION

Jacob Teitelbaum, MD

AVERY   *an imprint of Penguin Random House*   *New York*

AVERY

An imprint of Penguin Random House LLC
penguinrandomhouse.com

Most Avery books are available at special quantity discounts for bulk purchase for sales promotions, premiums, fund-raising, and educational needs. Special books or book excerpts also can be created to fit specific needs. For details, write SpecialMarkets@penguinrandomhouse.com.

Library of Congress Cataloging-in-Publication Data
Teitelbaum, Jacob.
From fatigued to fantastic! : a clinically proven program to regain vibrant health and overcome chronic fatigue and fibromyalgia / Jacob Teitelbaum.
p. cm.
Includes index.
ISBN 978-1-58333-289-4
1. Chronic fatigue syndrome—Popular works. 2. Fibromyalgia—Popular works. I. Title.
RB150.F37T45 2007 2007028118
616'.0478—dc22

Printed in the United States of America

ISBN 9780593421505

2nd Printing

To Laurie, my beautiful lady, my best friend, my wife,
my coconspirator, and the love of my life,
who always continues to inspire me;
my children, David, Amy, Shannon, Brittany, and Kelly,
who already seem to know so much of what I'm trying to learn;
my ten beautiful grandchildren; my mother, Sabina, and father, David,
whose unconditional love made this book possible;
the memories of Drs. Janet Travell, Hugh Riordan, and Billie Crook,
who were the pioneers in this field; and to my patients,
who have taught me more than I can ever hope to teach them.

Contents

Introduction: *Start Here*

BFF (Brain Fog–Friendly) Summary

Whether you simply have day-to-day fatigue, pain, or even if these have cascaded into the worst forms of the human energy crisis called chronic fatigue syndrome (CFS) and fibromyalgia syndrome (FMS), this book is for you.

Many of you will find that the cognitive dysfunction (which we call "brain fog") can make even reading more than a single page daunting. No worries. We will have the BFF (Brain Fog–Friendly) summaries through the book. You will get the information you need if you simply skip from summary to summary.

For those of you who have mild to moderate day-to-day fatigue, simply read Part One.

Is your energy fine but you have pain? Look at the introduction to Part One, and then read Part Two.

Have chronic fatigue syndrome or fibromyalgia syndrome (CFS/FMS)? If you have widespread pain, along with the paradox of inability to sleep despite being exhausted, you have CFS/FMS unless proven otherwise. For you, I recommend reading the whole book, or at least simply skimming through the BFF Summaries.

Some of you will want more detail, so I've included lots of information in the chapters but without the heavy technical stuff. We have put together a detailed resources section for those of you who want the latter. You can get everything you need even if you skip that section.

Want to keep it even simpler? If you have day-to-day fatigue, simply do the free quiz at www.tuneupdocs.com.

Have CFS or FMS? Do the free quiz at www.energyanalysisprogram.com.

Both of these will determine the underlying energy drains and tailor a protocol to optimize energy and overall well-being.

I remember 1975. I was in my third year of medical school, doing my pediatrics rotation. I had always excelled, having finished college in three years. Now I was the second youngest in a class of more than two hundred students, and I was continuing to perform well.

My approach to life was to move quickly—"full speed ahead." But then, a nasty viral illness hit me and made it hard for me to even get out of bed for my morning pediatrics lecture. I remember walking into an auditorium full of medical students, the professor saying, "Teitelbaum, why are you . . ." As he said "late?" I just about collapsed on the steps.

Because I had to drop out of medical school and was too ill to work, I was also homeless and sleeping in parks. I was to meet many teachers on my journey. Most important, I was taking time to get to know myself.

It was as if the universe put a "holistic homeless medical school" sign on my park bench. Herbalists, energy workers, holistic physicians, naturopaths, and countless others all seemed to wander by. Sometimes they even had pizza with them, and I ate. With what I learned, I was able to recover my energy and strength, and I went on to finish medical school and my residency.

My experiences with chronic fatigue syndrome and fibromyalgia left me with an appreciation of the impact of these afflictions and drove me to learn how to help others recover.

ABOVE ARE THE OPENING WORDS I USED FOR THE 1995 FIRST edition of this book—which started out as a pamphlet. All the CFS and FMS research at the time filled less than 20 percent of the size of this book. Since then, both the research and our understanding of CFS and fibromyalgia has skyrocketed.

The 2007 edition became more of a textbook. It was long and complex because I needed to lay the scientific foundation for these conditions. But this made it a challenge for those people reading the book who suffered with brain fog.

Now there's so much outstanding information available that my work here is to distill it and make it easy to understand. This is a wonderful thing. Whether you have day-to-day fatigue, pain, or even the incredibly crippling and devastating conditions of CFS and fibromyalgia, it means that we know enough for you to get well. *Now!*

Experiencing my own pain, treating thousands of people with CFS and FMS, and reading tens of thousands of studies has given me a much different understanding of the human energy crisis than I gained in medical school. Which, sadly, wasn't much. Most medical schools still teach almost nothing about treating fatigue effectively. This is not surprising, as most of our education is done in university hospitals, where we are addressing life-threatening conditions.

Why Include Day-to-Day Fatigue and Pain in a Book on CFS and FMS?

Even the basic key concept of pain management is still not even on most physicians' radar: that most pain involves an energy crisis in the muscles and nerves. This is why I am including pain in this book.

Sadly, and simply put, most physicians are taught almost nothing about pain management. In fact, I can summarize most of it in thirty-nine sad words: Give them acetaminophen (Tylenol), ibuprofen, or epilepsy- or depression-related medications. Don't give them narcotics unless the person has cancer. And look for things that are operable or expensive to treat, like compression syndromes, cancer, and autoimmune and disc disease.

We were also taught that any other specialists (e.g., chiropractors or herbalists) who knew anything we didn't were quacks. Basically, this means anybody who knew how to treat pain effectively.

So, it is no surprise that one-third of Americans suffer needlessly with pain. And over sixty-five thousand people die needlessly from pain medications each year. Fortunately, this is slowly changing, as physicians are becoming more and more open to research-proven complementary therapies.

Meanwhile, most adults wish they had more energy, while 31 percent suffer with severe ongoing fatigue. The lessons I learned in developing effective treatment for CFS in fibromyalgia also turned out to be powerfully effective for fatigue and day-to-day pain. So this is all included in one book.

This Book Is About the Energy Crisis Caused by Modern Life

Whether you simply have fatigue or pain from one or two of the dozens of conditions we will discuss, or it has cascaded into full-blown CFS/FMS, this book will give you your life back.

Most of you have not been able to fully recover by treating just one piece of the puzzle, because most people have a mix of these processes. That is why we have integrated all the key known components involved in the human energy crisis. This book makes it simple for you to understand each process and determine if you have it, and then teaches you how to treat it. So you can recover. *Now.*

How to Use This Book

For those with fatigue without CFS or FMS, Part One will show you how to do an energy tune-up so you feel great.

Got pain? Part Two will show you how to get pain-free. I would also suggest scanning through the quick Brain Fog–Friendly (BFF) summaries in Part One to see which areas apply to you. This is important, as these frequently contribute to or are the main causes of your pain. These can include poor sleep, low hormones, infections, and nutritional deficiencies.

You can then scan through the rest of the book for things that catch your eye.

Got CFS/FMS? Parts One and Two lay the foundations for recovery, so read these; but you'll also need the "intensive care" discussed in Part Three, along with the mind-body-spirit tools in Part Four.

Why do we include mind-body issues? You know how when you call computer tech support, the first thing they do is tell you to reboot? Part Four will show you how to reset your psyche and brain circuitry.

One more key thing that will help you get the most out of this book. It's written to be very user-friendly, whether you have brain fog and can't get through a single page or you are a science geek like me who wants all the details. Here's how:

1. Got brain fog? It's okay to simply look at the Brain Fog–Friendly (BFF) Summaries as you page through the book. This will make the information short and sweet. The free online quizzes we offer below can then analyze your symptoms, and even pertinent lab tests, to tell you what *your* underlying problems are. It will then tailor a protocol to optimize your energy. This way, it can be really easy.
2. Want more detail without being technical? Then look at the BFF Summaries, and read the full chapters that apply to you.
3. More of a science geek? Want more in-depth detail on what is going on with the immune system? Then read the more technical areas in the resources section.

We have put together two free online tools to make it very simple for everybody. These are fifteen-minute quizzes that can analyze your symptoms and even lab tests if available.

If you have day-to-day fatigue, simply do the free quiz at www.tuneup docs.com.

Have CFS or FMS? Do the free quiz at www.energyanalysisprogram .com.

Both of these will determine the underlying energy drains, and tailor a protocol to optimize energy and overall well-being.

I will also give you information on how to optimally navigate your way to picking the best supplements and treatments. When the brand does not matter, I will simply give the name of the herb or nutrient. When the brand does matter, which is often the case, I will specify the supplements by name, as well as any medications or other treatment modalities.

So, now that you understand the layout of the book, are you ready to feel great? Then read on . . .

PART ONE

Optimizing Energy with SHINE

BFF Summary

1. The keys for optimizing energy production can be summarized with the acronym SHINE:
   Sleep
   Hormones
   Infections
   Nutrition
   Exercise as able
2. In Part One, we will lay the foundations for optimizing these aspects of your life with one chapter dedicated to each letter of SHINE.

*I*f there was an owner's manual for your body, would you read it? Judging by how many of us read our car's owner's manual, the answer is likely no, at least not until a light starts flashing or things stop working. That's when I pull out my car manual.

If you have fatigue or pain, these are the red flashing lights on your body's dashboard. Things still work . . . for now . . . but something needs attention.

In Part One, we will discuss simple troubleshooting and basic maintenance. For most people, this is enough to not only make your fatigue go away, but also leave you feeling, well, fantastic!

Addressing these basics will also lay the foundation for recovering from CFS and FMS. They also will often be surprisingly effective at eliminating pain. For specific types of pain, you may then choose to work your way through Part Two and begin with those instructions.

Don't want to read all of Part One and would rather just go right to the things that are most important for you? The simple questions below will tell you what sections to look at:

1. Insomnia? Trouble falling or staying asleep? Fall asleep easily during the day? Read Chapters 1 and 13.
2. Tired, achy, gaining excessive weight, intolerant of cold temperatures, constipated, or having trouble getting pregnant? If you have any two of these, read Chapters 2 and 14.
3. Do you get "hangry," or irritable when hungry? Are you anxious? Do you "crash" with stress? Do you have relationship problems? Read the section on adrenal fatigue (page 25).
4. Read about reproductive hormones (page 34) if you are over forty-five years of age and:
   A. If female, do you feel worse around your menses, including irritability, fatigue, headaches, or insomnia? Vaginal dryness? Hot flashes?
   B. If male, do you have any two of these: high cholesterol, hypertension, diabetes or prediabetes, a spare tire around your abdomen, decreased libido, erectile dysfunction, depression, or decreased motivation?
5. Nasal congestion, sinusitis, or postnasal drip? Gas, bloating, diarrhea, and/or constipation? Read about candida in Chapters 3 and 15.
6. I recommend that everybody read Chapters 4 and 17 on nutrition, as this is the foundation of optimal energy and health. In these chapters, we'll also talk about digestive problems.

But what about those of you with crippling fatigue and pain? Especially if you have the paradox of insomnia and exhaustion (most people who are exhausted sleep long and easily), which is the hallmark that tells you that you have CFS or FMS? For you, I recommend reading this whole book. I understand that brain fog can make this a daunting task, so for each section we have a Brain Fog–Friendly (BFF) Summary.

Just how well does the treatment protocol we will be discussing work in the real world? Well, some of you may have seen me on TV with Dr. Mehmet Oz, a remarkable man who challenged me to "prove it" with regard to my fibromyalgia protocol. He then sent me a woman with disabling fibromyalgia and said, "Get her well."

One month later, she was dramatically improved. That's when he invited me to be on his show.

It was that woman who looked at my protocol and gave me the acronym SHINE. This stands for addressing and optimizing:

Sleep
Hormones and hypotension
Infections and immunity
Nutrition
Exercise as able

I would note that exercise is a small part of recovery, but important for maintaining conditioning.

Remembering this acronym as you go through the book will help tie everything together.

Ready for the foundations needed to make your energy level soar? Read on . . .

The Perfect Storm for Human Energy Crisis

Wondering why 31 percent of Americans experience severe fatigue, and 2 to 4 percent deal with CFS/FMS, the worst form of the human energy crisis? Here are just a few reasons:

1. With 18 percent of our calories coming from added sugar and another 18 percent from white flour, the modern American diet has lost about 50 percent of its vitamins and minerals.

2. The average night's sleep in America until 140 years ago when lightbulbs were invented was nine hours a night. We are now down to an average of six and three-quarter hours—a 30 percent pay cut for our bodies.

3. The speed of life has dramatically accelerated.

4. There are over eighty-five thousand new chemicals in the environment, which stress both our immune and hormonal systems.

5. Many medications have fatigue as a side effect.

1

Sleep: Recharge Your Batteries

BFF Summary

1. One of the most effective ways to improve energy, mental clarity, and immune function while decreasing pain and weight gain is to simply get your eight hours of sleep a night.
2. Begin by making time for sleep. Do this by cutting out things that don't feel good.
3. Create a restful bedtime routine.
4. If your mind is wide awake and racing at bedtime, consider phosphatidylserine, a natural phospholipid (100 to 200 milligrams), or an herbal mix called Sleep Tonight taken an hour before bedtime.
5. Wake frequently in the middle of the night? This suggests low blood sugar. Have a high-protein snack (1 to 2 ounces) before bedtime. A hard-boiled egg works well.
6. Take a mix of six herbs called the Revitalizing Sleep Formula. You can also add a mix of four essential oils called Terrific Zzzz. If using melatonin, use the Dual Spectrum Melatonin 5 Mg by Nature's Bounty. All three of these can be used together.
7. Anyone who has high blood pressure, snores, falls asleep easily during the day (especially while driving), has a shirt collar size of 17 inches or larger, or is overweight should consider testing getting tested for sleep apnea.

8. If you tend to scatter your sheets and blankets, and especially if you tend to kick your bed partner or if you note that your legs tend to feel jumpy and uncomfortable at rest at night, you may have restless leg syndrome (RLS).

9. Most people with CFS/FMS will need to add medications as well. These are discussed in Chapter 13, "Sleep Intensive Care."

O ne of the most effective ways to improve energy and mental clarity is to simply get your eight hours of sleep a night.

But is it really that simple? Like so many other things in life, the answer is yes . . . and no. Let's put things into perspective.

Until 140 years ago, when lightbulbs were invented, the average night's sleep in the United States was nine hours a night. Average. That means as many people got ten hours a night as eight. Going back further in time, to most of human history, anthropologists tell us that the average night's sleep was eleven hours. Most nights, when the sun went down it was too dark, boring, and dangerous to be outside. So people went to sleep. Then they woke up with the sunrise, an average of eleven hours later. Now we are down to an average of about six and three-quarters hours of sleep a night, compliments of lightbulbs, radio, TV, the internet, social media, and so on. This means the average person has lost 30 percent of their sleep in the last century.

In addition to simply not having time to get your eight hours of sleep a night, you may also find that the stress of modern life is causing insomnia. In this chapter, I will teach you how to treat day-to-day insomnia with natural therapies and sleep hygiene. In Chapter 13, "Sleep Intensive Care," we will discuss sleep medications for those with CFS and FMS.

Why Is Sleep So Important?

Beyond giving us energy, sleep has a number of critical functions. For example, sleep:

- Is when tissue repair occurs, which is why poor sleep causes pain.
- Is also critical for proper growth hormone production. Growth hormone has also been called the "fountain of youth hormone" and is associated with looking young as well as increasing muscle and decreasing fat.

- Has been shown to be critical for immune function.
- Is important for weight regulation because appetite-suppressing hormones such as leptin are produced during sleep. Studies have shown that poor sleep was associated with an average six-pound weight gain. In a study of 68,183 women, followed over sixteen years, those sleeping five or fewer hours per night had a 32 percent increased risk of gaining thirty-three pounds relative to those who slept seven hours per night.

So, it pays to make time for your eight hours of shut-eye. Not only will you have more energy and less pain, but you'll lose weight and look younger as well.

Finding Time for Sleep

With life going haywire, you may wonder where to even find that extra two hours to get the shut-eye you need. Here are some thoughts to make it easier.

STEP 1: YOU'LL NEVER GET IT ALL DONE

Realize that you will never get it all done, no matter how fast you run. In fact, you may have noticed that the faster you run and more efficiently you do things, the more life puts on your plate. Here's a secret: If you slow down and take the time to sleep, you'll find that fewer things find their way to your to-do list, and a lot of things and problems seem to simply drift away. Mostly, things that you didn't really want to do anyway. Then you'll find getting your eight hours of sleep a night will make you more efficient and effective, and you'll be enjoying the things you do more.

STEP 2: KEEP WHAT FEELS GOOD AND DITCH THE REST

Make a list of most of the things you spend time doing in life, both at home and at work. Put these in two columns. Column 1 contains the things that feel good to do, or at least feel better to do than not to do. In column 2 put those things you *think* you should do but that feel awful. These include things like many committee meetings, school meetings, and other things that you don't really like but think you *should* do. This has been called "shoulding on yourself," thinking "I *should* do this; I *should* do that." Here's your chance to stop that. I am giving you doctor's orders to cut out the things in your life that don't feel good and won't leave you fired or arrested if you cut them loose. So, tell the chairwoman of the "committee of a thousand ways to waste everybody's time" that you would love to help, but the doctor said absolutely no more commitments.

Column 2 can also include things like watching the news. If you enjoy it, watch it. But when it starts making you feel bad, turn it off.

Once you start making these lists, you will find it is fun to take more and more things and put them in column 2. Then start tendering your resignations (I am not talking about to the job that pays your bills—yet). When I first realized this, I resigned from almost ten committees within a week, and I have never missed them for a second. Happily, I have avoided committees that I don't enjoy ever since then. It's been great—and has freed up the time needed for me to get my eight hours of sleep a night.

So, now that you've learned how to make the time for sleep, here's how to handle insomnia and poor sleep quality.

The Basics: Good Sleep Hygiene

The following are some things to consider:

- Limit alcohol to one or two drinks before bedtime.
- Do not consume caffeine after 4:00 p.m.
- Do not use your bed for problem-solving or doing work. If you are in the habit of using your bed for doing work, it is best to change your work area to another part of the house. If it helps you to fall asleep, you can watch relaxing television (perhaps on a timer that turns the television off if you fall asleep while watching) or read a relaxing book in bed until you can no longer stay awake.
- Take a hot bath before bed if it's cold outside. Adding 2 cups of Epsom salts (magnesium) can result in powerful muscle relaxation and pain relief as well.
- Keep your room cool.
- If your mind races because your brain thinks it is daytime when it is nighttime, continually focus your thoughts on things that feel good and do not require much "thinking energy." If you find that you

cannot help but continue to problem-solve, get out of bed and write down all your problems on a piece of paper until you can't think of any more—then set them aside and go back to bed. Do this as often as you need to. It may be helpful to schedule thirty minutes of "worry time" early in the afternoon or evening when you can update a checklist of your concerns. In addition, the herbal mix Sleep Tonight by Enzymatic Therapy can be very helpful in this situation.

What to Do with Your To-Do List

We seem to think that we're responsible for making everything happen. That kind of stress and anxiety can make a good night's sleep difficult to come by. I certainly struggled with this and have adopted a simple strategy that works for me. You may find a similar approach to be useful as well.

When I feel overcome by details, I list my problems and projects on the left side of a page, and what I eventually plan to do about them (if anything) in another column down the middle of the page. I consider these two columns to be what I leave in the hands of God, the universe, or whatever name you wish to use. Every so often, I move a problem to a third column on the right side. The items in the third column are the one or two things that I want to work on right now. I am constantly amazed at how the things that I leave in the universe's hands (on their own) progress as quickly as the things that I've put in my third column.

Simpler yet? Do what feels good in the moment and leave the rest for later.

I also have a separate list for day-to-day errands. I put a star by those items that must get done soon. I do other items if and when I feel like it.

It is helpful to remember that neither you nor anyone else will ever get everything done. Just do those things that feel good to do on any given day, even if it's nothing. It will usually feel good to do the things that really have to get done. When I was doing general hospital internal medicine, I never heard a dying patient bemoan not having worked enough or not having completed all the errands on their checklist.

- If your partner snores, get a good pair of earplugs or noise-canceling headphones and use them. The wax plugs that mold to the shape of the ear are often the best ones. It may also be useful to have either a sound generator that makes nature sounds or, better yet, a tape that induces the deep-sleep (REM) stage. Spouses of people with sleep apnea or snoring often also have severely disturbed sleep. You may need to sleep in a separate bedroom (after tucking in or being tucked in by your partner) until you find a way to sleep soundly through the snoring.

- If you frequently wake up to urinate during the night, do not drink a lot of fluids near bedtime. Also gravity can cause water to pool in your legs during the day. This water redistributes when we're lying down and it's like drinking several glasses of water at night. The solution? While sitting around in the evening, simply prop your legs up so gravity can drain them before you go to sleep.

- When you wake up during the night and notice your bladder is full, just talk to it (in your mind, so your spouse doesn't think you're nuts) and tell it, "Nighttime is for sleeping. We will go to the bathroom in the morning when it is time to wake up." Then roll over and go back to sleep. If you still have to urinate five minutes later, then you can go to the bathroom. More often than not your bladder will happily go back to sleep, and when you wake up in the morning, you won't even have to urinate as badly as you thought you did when you woke up in the middle of the night. If your bladder wakes you once per night, don't worry about it; but if it happens more often, then it's time to retrain your bladder.

- Put the bedroom clock out of arm's reach and facing away from you so you can't see it. Frequently looking at the clock aggravates sleep problems and is frustrating.

- Have a high-protein snack (1 to 2 ounces) before bedtime. Hunger causes insomnia in all animals, and humans are no exception. In addition, low adrenal (see Chapter 2) can cause low blood sugar during the night, which will wake you up between 2:00 a.m. and 4:00 a.m. A high-protein snack such as a hard-boiled egg at bedtime can help. If this is the problem, you will know the first night or two that you have the high-protein bedtime snack, as you will sleep through the night without waking as often.

Getting Started

For almost all of the treatments I recommend, you will know most of the effects (both positive and negative) that the treatment is going to have by the next morning. In rare cases, some of these treatments have the opposite of their intended effect, activating you instead of putting you to sleep. If this happens, don't use that treatment.

HERBAL SLEEP REMEDIES

Most of the natural sleep remedies discussed here are not sedating, yet they help you fall asleep and stay in deep sleep. The good news is that many natural remedies that are effective for sleep also directly help pain because they are muscle relaxants. *The first six herbs listed below are my favorites. They are available in an excellent combination formula called the Revitalizing Sleep Formula.*

SUNTHEANINE

Theanine, an amino acid (protein) that is found in green tea, has been shown not only to improve deep sleep but also to help people maintain a calm alertness during the day.

Take 50 to 200 milligrams at bedtime, although you can also use it several times a day for anxiety.

LEMON BALM

Lemon balm makes it easier to fall and stay asleep. Try 20 to 80 milligrams of lemon balm (also known as melissa). This has the side benefit of supporting immune function, which keeps viral infections in check.

5-HYDROXY-L-TRYPTOPHAN (5-HTP)

Your body uses 5-HTP to make serotonin, a happiness molecule neurotransmitter that helps improve the quality of sleep. It also can help pain, mood, and anxiety and can even help some people lose weight. The dose is 50 to 200 milligrams at night. You can take as much as 400 milligrams, if you are not taking other serotonin medications such as antidepressants. It takes six weeks to see the full benefits of 5-HTP.

HOPS

The hops plant is a member of the hemp family, and the female flowers are used in beer making. Take 30 to 120 milligrams of a hops extract at bedtime.

PASSIONFLOWER (PASSIFLORA)

This herb is commonly used throughout South America as a calming agent, even present as an ingredient in sodas. Passionflower has other pain-management benefits as well. Take 90 to 360 milligrams of the extract at bedtime.

VALERIAN

Commonly used as a sleep remedy for insomnia, valerian has many benefits, as shown in a number of studies, including an improvement in deep sleep, speed of falling asleep, and quality of sleep without next-day sedation. The benefits were most pronounced when people used valerian for extended periods of time, as opposed to simply taking it for one night. Take 200 to 800 milligrams of the extract at bedtime.

Clinical experience shows that, for around 5 percent of people, valerian is energizing and may keep them awake. If this happens to you, you can use valerian during the day instead of at night, as valerian does have a calming effect and can be used for daytime anxiety.

To keep it simple, all six of these herbs can be found in combination in the Revitalizing Sleep Formula. The dose is two to four capsules at bedtime if you just need them to help you stay asleep, or one to two hours before bedtime to also help you fall asleep. This formula can also be used during the day for anxiety and pain.

ESSENTIAL OILS FOR SLEEP

There is an excellent new mix of essential oils that works well with the Revitalizing Sleep Formula. It contains a combination of Ravensara (*Ravensara aromatica*), lemon balm (*Melissa officinalis*), lavender (*Lavandula angustifolia*), and mandarin (*Citrus reticulata*).

You can find this combination in a product called Terrific Zzzz by Terry Naturally. Essential oils add a whole new dimension to natural therapies. When it comes to sleep, these have the benefits of decreasing brain fog and pain, while improving energy and immune function.

LEMON BALM (*MELISSA OFFICINALIS*)

A lemon-scented herb, lemon balm is both an effective calming agent and mild sedative. It is synergistic to take the essential oil along with the whole herb in the Revitalizing Sleep Formula. Recent research suggests that it optimizes function of the gamma-aminobutyric acid (GABA) receptors in the brain, which helps our nervous system calm down.

These receptors also have the benefit of decreasing pain. Another benefit? In a placebo-controlled study done in England, lemon balm significantly improved both cognitive function and calmness.

LAVENDER (*LAVANDULA ANGUSTIFOLIA*)

Long recognized in France for improving people's sense of well-being, lavender flowers were commonly placed in pillows to help promote sleep. Even the smell of lavender is calming. Research suggests that lavender oil is sedating, relieving anxiety and improving deep sleep. The effect? People who use lavender also experience more energy and alertness in the morning. Research also suggests that lavender supports your body's own endorphin molecules. These are the same neurotransmitters that your body stimulates to decrease pain, and which triggers the "runner's high" in athletes. So, it is no wonder that this herb is so prized.

MANDARIN (*CITRUS RETICULATA*)

In traditional Chinese medicine, the mandarin herb has been used to calm the nervous system and induce sleep. In fact, mandarin oranges get their name from the Chinese Mandarins, who traditionally received this fruit as a gift.

RAVENSARA (*RAVENSARA AROMATICA*)

The fragrant leaves, bark, and nuts of this rainforest tree have a long history of being used by the indigenous population of Madagascar for their powerful effects in supporting sleep, improving mood, and calming anxiety.

All four of these essential oils can be found in combination in Terrific Zzzz. This and the Revitalizing Sleep Formula herbal mix are synergistic with the natural products below, and the sleep medications that we will discuss in Part Three. Most people find that one, or if needed both, of these products will leave them sleeping like a kitten. The third thing I add is the sleep hormone melatonin; however, I find that most melatonin products are not very effective. The exception is the brand Dual Spectrum Melatonin 5 Mg made by Nature's Bounty. This contains both immediate release and sustained release melatonin, and people have found it to be uniquely effective. It is available at Walgreens or on Amazon.

Simply try each of these individually, and then they can be combined as needed.

If you find that your mind is wide awake and racing at bedtime, this is a different problem. It suggests that your cortisol stress hormone levels are too high at night. This is discussed in more detail in Chapter 2 on adrenal problems. A simple herbal mix called Sleep Tonight, taken an hour or two before bedtime, can resolve this problem and may be all you need. If you tend to wake in the middle of the night, especially when using this herbal mix, it is also a good idea to have a 1- or 2-ounce protein snack at bedtime (such as meat, cheese, or a hard-boiled egg) to keep blood sugar from dropping too low during the night.

MAGNESIUM

There is one other natural remedy that helps sleep. Taking 75 to 200 milligrams of magnesium at night may be helpful. Lower the dose if it causes diarrhea. This can be avoided by taking Jigsaw brand MagSRT.

For those who have CFS or FMS, or persistent problems with sleep, it is necessary to add medications to help sleep (more on this in Chapter 13, "Sleep Intensive Care"). But the herbals are an excellent way to begin on your own, and I then add medications to these as needed.

Earthing: Humans Are Disconnected

by Martin Zucker

Past cultures honored connectedness to the earth and described the energy of the earth in different ways. They went barefoot routinely or used hides and leather for footwear, allowing them to feel and conduct the earth's energy into their bodies.

Many aspects of our modern language can lead to a disconnect from our planet's healing energy. Except on rare occasions, we don't make skin contact with the "skin" of the earth.

Today, we wear insulating rubber- or plastic-soled shoes that separate us from the earth's energy. And of course, we no longer sleep on the ground. We sleep in elevated beds. We often live and work in high-rises.

We are disconnected, a separation from the earth that research suggests may be an overlooked cause of abnormal physiology contributing to inflammation, pain, fatigue, stress, and poor sleep. By reconnecting to the earth's energy—popularly known as earthing or grounding—many common symptoms are relieved and sometimes even eliminated. People are more energized. They sleep better.

They feel better.

For additional information on earthing research, observations from clinicians and patients, and medical advisories, please read my book *Earthing* and visit the Earthing Institute website (www.earthinginstitute.net). You can also find earthing products at www.earthing.com.

Sleep-Related Disorders

In addition to poor sleep caused by stress (which we'll discuss later after hypothalamic dysfunction), let's look at two other common sleep problems: sleep apnea and restless leg syndrome (RLS).

SLEEP APNEA

Sleep apnea is a condition in which a person repeatedly stops breathing during the night. There are two main types of sleep apnea. Obstructive sleep apnea (OSA) involves intermittent blockage of the upper airway, while central sleep apnea (CSA) occurs when there is a problem in the brain. Obstructive sleep apnea is most common.

In OSA, the pharynx (throat) repeatedly collapses during sleep. The person with OSA fights to breathe against a blocked airway, resulting in dropping blood oxygen levels. Eventually, the sense of suffocation wakes the person, their throat muscles contract, the airway opens, and air rushes in under high pressure. When the airway is opened, the rushing air allows the patient to once again drift back to sleep, but it creates a loud, gasping sound.

People with OSA are generally not aware that this is happening, although their bed partners often have severely disrupted sleep from the snoring and gasping. This cycle may repeat itself many times throughout the night. This constant waking from deep sleep, as well as the loss of oxygen in the blood, can cause next-day sleepiness, brain fog, poor concentration, and mood changes.

Another side effect of OSA is high blood pressure. I generally recommend testing for sleep apnea for anyone who has high blood pressure, snores, falls asleep easily during the day (especially while driving), has a shirt collar size of 17 inches or larger, or is overweight. The screening test is best done at home, so ask your physician if it can be arranged that way. If it needs to be done in a sleep lab, ask them to do a split night study where they look for sleep apnea during the first half of the night and, if needed, check the CPAP (continuous positive airway pressure) measurements during the second half of the night. This way, it can all be done in one night instead of two. You'll be glad you did.

Although some doctors do not consider OSA to be significant until there are fifteen or more apneic episodes per hour of sleep, evidence suggests that even five or more episodes per hour are associated with increased risk of auto accidents and high blood pressure. Basically, if you tend to fall asleep easily during the day, the sleep apnea is likely to be significant. This is also a common problem in CFS/FMS.

For sleep testing, the lab will often recommend that you be off all sleep medications for several nights before doing the test. If you have not yet started sleep medications, this is reasonable. However, I recommend that people with CFS/FMS who have been on sleep medications stay on them during the test, because most CFS/FMS patients need the sleep medications. As a doctor, I need to know whether they are developing sleep apnea from the medication.

The Poor Man's Sleep Study

Doing a sleep study (called a polysomnogram) in the sleep lab can cost upward of $2,000—and sometimes your insurance company will make your life miserable trying to get them to pay for it. Be sure to have them preauthorize the test. The diagnoses fatigue, daytime somnolence, snoring, and high blood pressure should be enough to get them to cover the study.

Another alternative? Set up a video camera at the foot of your bed to record yourself while you're sleeping. Position it so that you can see both your feet and your face. Then hit record and go to bed with only a sheet over you (you'll pull the blanket on later when you're sleeping, so don't worry). The next day, watch the tape. Do you have periods where you snore and stop breathing? If yes, is it only when you're lying on your back, or does it occur in any position? About how many times during the hour does it happen? If more than a few times during the hour, get the sleep study done doing a split night study. Also check to see if your legs are jumpy and if it seems like this leg jumpiness disturbs your sleep. If yes, ask your physician to treat for restless leg syndrome (see below).

In addition, watching the tape is a good way to help you fall asleep.

CAUSES OF SLEEP APNEA

The primary cause of sleep apnea is excess body weight. Just as fat deposits are present elsewhere in the body, they occur in the tissue surrounding the throat. When a person is lying down, the angle of the head can cause compression of the trachea, the pipe that carries air into the lungs. As noted above, because of the often-large weight gain associated with the metabolic disturbances in CFS/FMS, OSA is a common occurrence in these individuals.

TREATING SLEEP APNEA

The standard medical treatment for sleep apnea is to wear a CPAP (continuous positive airway pressure) mask over your nose or face while sleeping. This maintains increased pressure, keeping the upper airway from obstructing. During the sleep study, the lab does a CPAP titration. This is where they see how much pressure is needed in the mask to keep your sleep apnea from happening. CPAP is an excellent treatment for sleep apnea and is very helpful.

Many people are not willing to continue with the CPAP treatment because of the noise of the machine, the discomfort of wearing the mask, and the cost. However, patients who can tolerate the CPAP for at least three months become adapted to the treatment and eventually begin sleeping comfortably through the night. Fortunately, the newer CPAP machines have become much more user-friendly and are better tolerated. Be sure to get one that also has a humidifier; otherwise it can dry out your mouth and lungs.

The Tennis Ball Cure for Sleep Apnea and Snoring

Avoid sleeping on your back if the video shows that this is usually the position where you snore and have sleep apnea. Do this by taking a tennis ball, putting it into a cloth pocket, and then sewing or pinning it to the midback of your pajama shirt or a tight T-shirt. The tennis ball makes lying on your back uncomfortable, forcing you to roll onto your side or stomach without waking you. This works a lot better than having your spouse repeatedly jab you in the side during the night.

RESTLESS LEG SYNDROME AND PERIODIC LEG MOVEMENT DISORDER

People with restless leg syndrome (RLS) have the sensation that they need to continually move their legs. When that happens predominantly at night, it is called periodic leg movement disorder of sleep (PLMD). Most people are talking about PLMD when they talk about restless leg syndrome.

It is not uncommon for your bed partner to be aware that your legs are kicking much of the night or are constantly moving. You may or may not be aware of your own movements. It has been estimated that as many as one-third or more of FMS patients have RLS/PLMD, and it is also common in the population in general. Although the cause of RLS is not clear, experts suspect it comes from a deficiency of the brain chemical dopamine (a neurotransmitter). It can also be aggravated by iron deficiency (having blood ferritin levels less than 60), nerve injuries, vitamin B12 and folic acid deficiency, hypothyroidism, and other problems. In some people, RLS may be associated with the drops in blood sugar during the night (from adrenal fatigue; see Chapter 2). Some medications, especially amitriptyline (Elavil), can also aggravate RLS.

DIAGNOSING RLS/PLMD

If you tend to scatter your sheets and blankets, and especially if you tend to kick your bed partner or if you note that your legs tend to feel jumpy and uncomfortable at rest at night, you probably have RLS/PLMD. You can also have a sleep study done to look for periodic leg movements. In most cases, however, it is usually not necessary to perform a sleep study as the history usually gives enough information, and nighttime video recording is adequate confirmation.

TREATING RLS

There are both natural and prescription approaches to treating RLS. Following are summaries of those that have been found to be most successful.

Natural Treatments

Natural remedies focus on diet and nutritional supplementation. Avoiding caffeine helps, as does a high-protein snack at bedtime, which can decrease the tendency to have a drop in blood sugar (a drop in blood sugar can aggravate RLS).

Often, the most important means of keeping your legs calm while you sleep is keeping your serum ferritin level over 60 ng/mL. Technically, ferritin levels are considered to be in the normal range if they are over 12. I have found this to be not only misleading but also, in many cases, outright wrong as it labels approximately 90 percent of those with severe iron deficiency as being normal (see page 24). I recommend taking an iron supplement that has 25 to 50 milligrams of iron and 60 to 120 milligrams of vitamin C, which helps the iron to be absorbed. I like a brand called Iron Complex by Integrative Therapeutics. Take iron supplements on an empty stomach, and if it causes upset stomach or constipation, it's okay to take it every other day. It is normal for iron supplements to turn your stool black. Aim to get your ferritin level to over 60 but under 120 ng/mL.

Taking 200 milligrams of magnesium at bedtime can also be very helpful.

Prescription Treatments

The medications zolpidem (Ambien), clonazepam (Klonopin), and gabapentin (Neurontin) usually do a superb job in suppressing RLS, especially once the ferritin level is optimized. I tell patients to adjust the dose not only to get adequate sleep but also to keep the bedcovers in place and to avoid kicking their partners. As clonazepam can be addictive, like diazepam (Valium), I am more likely to use the other medications. Clonazepam does have the added benefit of helping pain, so there are times that it may be helpful.

Although it is heavily marketed, I rarely use ropinirole (Requip). I find the other medications to be more effective and to have fewer side effects, while being low cost.

2 Hormones: Your Body's Communication System

BFF Summary

1. Hormones are a critical part of our body's communication system. It is best to use bioidentical hormones. The reason synthetic hormones are routinely used is because they are patentable and therefore profitable. So, physicians are trained to recommend these. The science, however, suggests that bioidentical hormones are much safer and more effective.

2. Blood testing is unreliable. All it means when the blood test is abnormal is that you are not in the highest or lowest 2 percent of the population. Most doctors don't realize this, and they think "normal" means okay. But this would be like saying that any shoe between size 5 and 13 (the normal range) should fit everybody.

3. The thyroid is our body's gas pedal, determining how much energy we make. If you have any two of the following symptoms, you may warrant a trial of thyroid hormone to see if it helps: tired, achy, weight gain, cold intolerance, constipation, or unexplained infertility. For most people, I begin with a trial of desiccated thyroid (Armour Thyroid), as I find this often works much better than levothyroxine (Synthroid). Supplementing with 6.25 milligrams of Tri-Iodine for three months can also help.

4. The adrenal glands help us handle stress. Because of the stress of modern life, about a quarter of the population has adrenal fatigue. Most doctors don't recognize that this exists and will only treat when the adrenals have failed to the point of being

life-threatening. If you get irritability when hungry (aka "hangry"), especially if you tend toward low blood pressure, consider adrenal support by cutting back sugar, increasing salt, eliminating unnecessary stress (like watching the news), and taking Adrenaplex.

5. The ovaries are important for much more than just reproduction. For example, progesterone is our natural diazepam (Valium), helping us sleep and stay calm. Because of this, progesterone is critical even if somebody has had a hysterectomy. If your symptoms of fatigue, brain fog, insomnia or headache are worse around your menses, this suggests that you may benefit from bioidentical (not synthetic) hormone replacement. This can be prescribed by a holistic physician. If you simply have PMS (irritability around your menses), then the bioidentical prescription progesterone (Prometrium) taken around your menses can help. Estrogen and progesterone deficiency begin five to twelve years before blood tests become abnormal and one's menses stop. So, I treat based on symptoms much more than the blood testing.

6. Testosterone deficiency is very important in men. It is suggested by low libido, decreased erectile function, depression, low motivation, increasing waist size, high cholesterol, high blood pressure, and/or diabetes. Again, the normal range for the blood test is not helpful. If several of the above are present, and the testosterone level in an adult male is under 540 ng/dL, I consider addressing this. Testosterone deficiency is also important in women who need estrogen and progesterone replacement. Research shows that these help decrease fibromyalgia pain.

---

*O*ur body's metabolism is controlled by a series of glands that create chemical messengers called hormones. These hormones are controlled by feedback mechanisms in the hypothalamic/pituitary master gland, which is the "circuit breaker" that malfunctions in CFS and fibromyalgia.

Hormonal problems are becoming very common in the general population, in part because of the increasing number of chemicals found in modern life. For example, a World Health Organization report looked at just some of these "endocrine disruptor chemicals." There were so many that the report was 296 pages long.

Whether you have day-to-day fatigue or CFS/FMS, there is a very good chance that hormonal problems are contributing—*even if your blood tests are normal.*

The Problem with Blood Testing

Before we begin discussing each of the individual hormones, it is important to understand why we cannot rely on blood tests to tell us if there is a hormone-function problem. Many people with fatigue, and most people with CFS/FMS, have had the experience of going to the doctor convinced that their thyroid was low, only to experience the frustration of having the tests come back normal. Most often, it turns out you are right and hormonal deficiencies were present. The problem? Most physicians have no clue that the testing is not reliable.

Why is this happening? By definition, the normal range for most blood tests is created by doing a large number of tests and defining only the highest and lowest 2.5 percent of the population as being abnormal (called two standard deviations). This does not work well if more than 2.5 percent of the population has a problem.

To show how absurd it is to use a 2.5 percent cutoff, research has found that despite "normal" thyroid hormone levels, antibodies attacking the thyroid gland were present in 34 percent of FMS patients and as many as 19 percent of "healthy" controls. In addition, people whose thyroid tests were "normal" but in the low end of the normal range are a whopping 69 percent more likely to have a heart attack than those who are high normal.

I gave my friend Dr. Oz a simple analogy he likes, which makes this easy to understand.

Pretend your lab test uses two standard deviations to diagnose a "shoe problem." One hundred people go to the mall and their shoe sizes are measured. From these one hundred people, a normal shoe size range of 5 to 13 would be established. As far as the shoe doctor is concerned, they could randomly give you any shoe between size 5 and size 13, and they would consider it totally normal for you. No matter what size *your* foot is. Of course, you would insist that the shoes did not fit because they didn't feel right on your feet. And the physician would then imply to you that you're crazy—because the shoe's size is in the normal range.

Sound familiar?

Like shoes, hormone levels are not one-size-fits-all. Because of this, treatment needs to be based predominantly on symptoms, using the blood tests only as one more piece of information. The goal is to restore *optimal* function while keeping lab results in the normal range for safety. Using this information, let's look at each gland and determine how to tell if there is a malfunction. Then we will discuss how to optimize function.

Let's begin with the adrenal gland—your "stress handler."

The Adrenal Glands: Your Body's Stress Handler

The adrenal glands, which sit on top of your kidneys, are actually two different glands in one. The center of the gland makes epinephrine (also known as adrenaline) and is under the control of the autonomic nervous system. Malfunction of the inner adrenal contributes to such symptoms as hot and cold sweats, neurally mediated hypotension (NMH), POTS (postural orthostatic tachycardia syndrome), and panic attacks.

The outer part of the adrenal gland, called the adrenal cortex, makes hormones that allow you to handle stress, regulate immune function, and maintain your blood pressure. The key hormone is called cortisol.

The adrenal glands increase their production of cortisol in response to stress. Cortisol raises blood sugar and blood pressure levels and moderates immune function, in addition to playing numerous other roles.

SYMPTOMS OF ADRENAL FATIGUE

If your adrenal glands are underactive, what might you be experiencing?

The adrenal glands' responsibilities include maintaining blood sugar and blood pressure during stress. Sugar is the only fuel that the brain can use. When a person's blood sugar level drops, he or she feels anxious, irritable, and then tired.

Low adrenal function can cause, among other symptoms:

- Fatigue
- Recurrent infections that take a long time to go away
- "Crashing" during stress
- Hypoglycemia (low blood sugar with marked irritability when hungry, sometimes called "hangry")
- Anxiety
- Low blood pressure and dizziness upon first standing

Sound familiar?

Hypoglycemia deserves special mention. To me, the single best test to tell if somebody needs adrenal support is to simply ask them if they get irritable when hungry. And we're not talking about normal day-to-day irritability, but rather the "feed me now or I'll kill you" type of irritability. If you're not sure if you have this, just ask the people around you.

People with adrenal fatigue have repeated episodes during the day where they become shaky, nervous, and irritable. When this occurs and they don't eat, after about an hour, they may find themselves yawning and fatigued.

They often feel better after they eat sweets, which improve their energy and mood for a short period of time. This causes sugar craving. Sweets make their blood sugar level initially shoot back up to normal, which is what makes them feel better, but then their blood sugar continues shooting up beyond normal. The body responds to this by driving the sugar level back down below normal again. The effect, mood- and energy-wise, is like an emotional roller coaster. It can also be very stressful for your relationships.

Don't bother doing the standard tests for low blood sugar or low adrenal, as these tests are geared to picking up the one in one hundred thousand people who have complete and life-threatening adrenal failure or insulin-producing tumors—not the problem we're looking at here.

PROBLEMS WITH ADRENAL TESTING

Although the adrenal glands make several kinds of hormones, the lab tests for these glands use the production of cortisol as their marker. However, unlike other lab tests, where you are considered low if you're in the bottom 2 percent of the population, cortisol levels are only considered low when your adrenals have largely been destroyed and the condition becomes life-threatening—in other words, in approximately 1 out of 100,000 people. So, it is either so low that they have to put you in the hospital, and it can kill you, or it is considered *totally* healthy. At least this is the current medical viewpoint.

Let's look at this a bit more closely. Most people have morning cortisol levels of approximately 16 to 20 mcg/dL. However, a cortisol level of 10, half of what most people run, or 8, or even 6.1 mcg/dL is considered *totally* normal. To technically have adrenal insufficiency, your morning cortisol needs to be less than 6 mcg/dL. Shockingly, a cortisol level of

6.1 mcg/dL is considered totally normal and no problem. But a level of 5.9 mcg/dL is considered life-threatening. This method of evaluation goes from normal to deadly in just .01 mcg/dL. Unfortunately, the testing equipment is not all that reliable. I've frequently seen as much an 8 mcg/dL variation on two cortisol levels accidentally done on the *same* tube of blood. Simply put, this rigid interpretation of test results doesn't make sense. Salivary cortisol levels can supply helpful information, but they have their own problems as well.

Instead of relying only on testing, if symptoms suggest low adrenal in anybody without high blood pressure, I consider a treatment trial of adrenal support.

WHY WE ARE SEEING MORE ADRENAL FATIGUE

If you think back to your biology classes in high school, you may remember something called the fight-or-flight response. This is a physical reaction that occurs during times of stress. During the Stone Age, when a caveman met an animal that wanted to eat him, the caveman's adrenal glands activated multiple systems in his body that prompted him to either fight or run. This reaction helped the caveman survive. In those days, however, people probably had a couple of weeks or months to recover before facing the next major stress.

Today, people often experience stress reactions every few minutes. For example, when driving to work, a woman is delayed because of heavy traffic. While sitting behind the wheel, she frets about the consequences of her walking into the office late. Every time she hits a red light or pulls up behind a car that has slowed down, her adrenal glands' fight-or-flight reaction goes off again.

In addition, the speed of modern life is rapidly accelerating. Whereas it used to take six months to send a letter and receive the answer by ship or Pony Express, it now takes minutes by email. Meanwhile, and perhaps most important, our news media seems to confuse drama and news.

A quote often attributed to Mark Twain puts it very well: "If you don't read the newspaper, you are uninformed. If you do read the newspaper, you are misinformed." A hundred years before that, Thomas Jefferson said, "Nothing can now be believed which is seen in a newspaper . . . I will add, that the man who never looks into a newspaper is better informed than he who reads them."

Sadly, things haven't improved much in this regard in the last two hundred years.

A simple recommendation? If watching the news makes you feel bad, turn it off. You won't be any worse for doing so. If enough people start doing this, perhaps the media will change its reporting style.

Because of these problems, adrenal "stress handler" fatigue is very common—even in the overall healthy population.

Optimizing Adrenal Function

Begin by cutting sugar and *excess* caffeine out of your diet; having frequent, small meals; and increasing your intake of protein while decreasing carbohydrates. It's best to cut way back on white flour and sugar and to substitute whole grains and vegetables. Fruit—not fruit juices, which contain concentrated sugar—can be eaten in moderation, so enjoy one to two pieces a day. If you get irritable, eat something with protein.

I would note that everyone is different, and some people will need a higher carbohydrate diet to avoid depression. Although these can be helpful guidelines, eat what leaves you feeling the best overall.

For quick relief of low blood sugar irritability, put ¼ to ½ teaspoon of sugar (a sugar packet is about 1 teaspoon) under your tongue and let it dissolve. This is enough to quickly raise your blood sugar level, but not enough to put you on a sugar emotional roller-coaster ride.

The next step is to give your adrenal glands the natural support that they need to heal.

Natural Adrenal Support

Below are several things that can help your adrenal glands recover:

1. Adrenal glandulars supply the raw materials that your adrenal glands need to heal. It is critical, however, that you get them from reputable companies, so that the purity and potency are guaranteed.
2. Vitamin C is crucial for adrenal and immune function. A dose of 100 to 500 milligrams is optimal.
3. Pantothenic acid, known as vitamin B5, also supports adrenal function. Take 50 to 150 milligrams daily.
4. Licorice slows the breakdown of adrenal hormones in your body, helping to maintain optimal levels. There is no licorice in licorice candies in

the United States because of this, as too much licorice can raise cortisol levels and blood pressure too high.

Another beneficial effect of licorice is that it helps in the treatment of indigestion, being as effective as heartburn medications. Do not take licorice if you have high blood pressure, as too much licorice can cause excess adrenal function and worsen high blood pressure. I like to give 100 to 400 milligrams a day of a licorice extract standardized to contain 5 percent glycyrrhizin.

5. Taking 450 milligrams of tyrosine supplies the raw materials to make a form of adrenaline (another key adrenal hormone).

6. Two key adrenal hormones, pregnenolone and DHEA, supply your adrenals with the raw materials they need and take the strain off them as well. Take 15 milligrams of pregnenolone and 10 milligrams of DHEA.

7. Taking 75 milligrams of rehmannia is also used for adrenal support in traditional Chinese medicine.

As usual, to decrease the number of pills people need to take, I like to give well-made combinations. For adrenal support, I recommend people use a product called Adrenaplex by Terry Naturally, which contains all of the above. For women with diabetes, hormonally sensitive cancers, or PCOS (polycystic ovary syndrome), I use Adrenal Stress End by Enzymatic Therapy instead, as it does not contain DHEA or pregnenolone.

Take one to two capsules of either in the morning. If symptoms recur in the afternoon, you can add another capsule at lunch.

These simple measures can stabilize most people's adrenal function within a few weeks. If you have fibromyalgia, adrenal intensive care is often needed, and discussed in Chapter 15. But I begin with the recommendations in this chapter first, and I then add the hydrocortisone (Cortef) discussed in that chapter to these.

The Thyroid Gland: Your Body's Gas Pedal

Thyroid problems are common in both day-to-day fatigue and CFS/FMS. Because of this, the discussion below applies to both. Those with CFS/FMS, however, will often need to add thyroid intensive care as discussed in Chapter 14.

The thyroid gland, located in the neck, is the body's gas pedal. It regulates the body's metabolic speed. If the thyroid gland produces insufficient amounts of thyroid hormones, the metabolism decreases. Symptoms of hypothyroidism (low thyroid) include:

- Intolerance to cold
- Fatigue
- Achiness
- Constipation (though diarrhea from bowel infections is common in CFS/FMS)
- Unexplained infertility, despite normal tests

The thyroid makes two primary hormones. They are:

- **Thyroxine (T4).** T4 is the storage form of thyroid hormone, which is tyrosine attached to four iodine molecules. This is where the name T4 comes from. It has very little activity on its own until the body removes one of the iodine molecules to turn it into triiodothyronine (T3). T3 is the active form of thyroid hormone.

  Most synthetic thyroid medications, such as Synthroid and Levothroid, are pure T4. These synthetics are fine if your body can properly turn them into T3. Unfortunately, many people, especially those with CFS/FMS, have trouble doing this.
- **Triiodothyronine (T3).** T3 is the active form of thyroid hormone. It can be found in prescription liothyronine (Cytomel), combined with T4 in desiccated thyroid (Armour Thyroid), or made by compounding pharmacies.

TESTING

The tests that I routinely recommend for thyroid screening are:

1. **Free T4.** This measures the level of the thyroxine hormone made by your thyroid gland. It says nothing about how well your body can use the hormone. If symptoms are suggestive, I am more likely to treat if it is 1.1 ng/dL or less. Anything over 0.9 ng/dL is considered normal.
2. **TSH.** This is a messenger made by your hypothalamus/pituitary control center in the brain that indicates if your brain thinks you're

getting enough thyroid. In concept, it is not a bad test. In real life, it is horrible.

Most doctors consider your thyroid normal if the TSH result is under 5.4 mIU/L. Higher levels suggest inadequate thyroid. But many researchers consider a level over 2.5 to be suggestive of low thyroid. And if your hypothalamus/pituitary is being stressed and therefore malfunctioning, especially as occurs in fibromyalgia, the test has been shown by the research to be very unreliable. So, it can be helpful, but only if interpreted properly and in the context of the entire person's symptoms and situation. Yet, some doctors use *only* this and ignore everything else.

3. **Anti-TPO antibody test.** This looks to see if your body's immune system is accidentally attacking your own thyroid (most commonly, a form called Hashimoto's thyroiditis). This is the main cause of low thyroid in day-to-day fatigue. This is one of the very few thyroid blood tests that gives a straightforward and reliable yes or no answer. If this is elevated, it makes me even more likely to give a trial of thyroid treatment.

Pregnancy and Hypothyroidism

We discussed how undiagnosed and untreated hypothyroidism can result in infertility. But research is also showing that it can dramatically increase miscarriage risk, being responsible for 6 percent of miscarriages. Untreated low thyroid is also associated with learning disabilities.

This is all easily preventable, if doctors would bother to read the research and do simple testing.

Treating a low thyroid is both safe and easy during pregnancy. The earlier it is treated the better. As soon as you know you're pregnant (or trying to get pregnant), get a TSH blood test to check your thyroid. Most doctors do not yet know that the TSH has to be less than 3 or you need treatment, so see the result for yourself. (Many still use the dangerous and outdated criteria that says a TSH must be over 5.4 to be abnormal.)

In addition, check an anti-TPO antibody blood test (positive in 1 out of every 8 pregnant women). If positive (showing thyroid inflammation), taking Synthroid thyroid hormone (even if the other thyroid tests are okay) decreases the risk of miscarriage from 13.8 to 2.4 percent, as well as drops the risk of premature birth from 22 percent to normal.

What to do if your physician won't order the tests? No problem. Mary Shomon's website below will show you how to get the tests on your own.

The Best Thyroid Support Group Leader in the World

For those of you looking for the most helpful, reliable, and up-to-date thyroid information available, I happily and strongly recommend Mary Shomon. Her website is www.thyroid-info .com, where you can access a wealth of resources and sign up for her free email newsletter. More good news? She does thyroid coaching, offering personal guidance for you and your physician on how to optimize *your* thyroid treatment. And you can get thyroid testing on your own through the website, if your physician will not order the tests for you.

Treating an Underactive Thyroid

Though I use the guidelines above to decide when to give someone with day-to-day fatigue thyroid hormone, almost everybody with fibromyalgia deserves a treatment trial with thyroid (more on this in Chapter 14).

We are constantly learning powerful new tricks for treating hypothyroidism, and there are many reasonable treatment approaches. In fact, as is true of trying on shoes, it is not unusual for people to need to try several different thyroid protocols to see what works the best for them.

Here is how I usually begin:

1. **Prescription desiccated thyroid.** This is simply ground-up thyroid gland. I begin with desiccated thyroid; Armour Thyroid is the easiest to get at a regular pharmacy, but if your pharmacy is willing to order in, as many are, I would use Nature-Throid instead. These forms of thyroid work much better in many cases than levothyroxine (Synthroid), because they also include the active T3 hormone. Most physicians use only levothyroxine.

   Each grain (60 milligrams) of desiccated thyroid contains approximately 38 µg of T4 and 9 µg of T3. I begin with 30 milligrams and slowly adjust the dose to what *feels best* to the person I am treating. When they find the dose that *feels best*, I check the free T4 to make sure it is not high or high normal for safety. It is okay if the free T4 is low, as it may simply be being suppressed by the T3 component of the treatment.

When switching somebody from levothyroxine, I consider 60 milligrams of desiccated thyroid to be about equal to 50 to 75 µg of Synthroid.

2. If the thyroid forms above, which also contain active T3, make people shaky or hyper, I am likely to simply use the plain T4 (levothyroxine) from a regular pharmacy. Again, I adjust it to the dose that *feels best*, making sure the free T4 test is in the normal range for safety.

To determine optimal dosing, most physicians ignore everything except the TSH test. Once that's in the normal range, they will leave you on that dose. Sadly, that works about as well as putting everybody in a size 5 shoe (which again is in the normal range). So, it is no shock that most people are dissatisfied with their thyroid treatment, as they are getting both the wrong form and incorrect dose.

Put simply, it is critical to treat the person, and not just the blood tests.

I know I am repeating myself, but this is important enough for me to do so. Like trying on shoes, seeing what treatment form and dose *feels best* to you is much more reliable than trying to chase blood tests. If you feel like you've had too much caffeine or coffee, the thyroid dose is likely too high. Tired, achy, weight gain, or cold intolerant without feeling like you had too much coffee, then the dose is often too low.

Also, do not take thyroid hormone within six hours of taking iron or calcium supplements, or you won't absorb the thyroid. Thyroid treatment is best taken on an empty stomach.

All thyroid treatments must be prescribed and monitored by a physician. Holistic physicians are more likely to be familiar with optimizing thyroid support.

A Money-Saving Tip

For most medications, and thyroid is no exception, you largely pay by the pill and not by the dose. So, if you get a pill twice as strong as your daily dose and break it in half, you can often cut your cost in half as well. For example, if your physician prescribes 90 milligrams of desiccated thyroid a day, ask them to prescribe 180-milligram pills, with a dose of a half pill per day instead, which can cut your cost in half.

POTENTIAL SIDE EFFECTS OF THYROID HORMONE

All treatments carry some risk. Here are the key ones to be aware of for thyroid treatment.

If someone has blockages in the arteries that feed the heart and is on the verge of a heart attack, taking thyroid hormone can trigger a heart attack or angina. Thyroid treatment can also trigger heart palpitations as well. These are usually benign and very common in CFS/FMS. But if chest pain or increasing palpitations occur, stop the thyroid supplementation and call your doctor at once, just to be on the safe side. Because of this concern, I may recommend that patients at significant risk of angina have an exercise treadmill test done before treatment, even if they can't complete the test.

To put the risk in perspective, of the many thousands of people I have treated with the thyroid treatments above, none experienced heart attacks from taking it. But just like exercise, thyroid treatment is more likely overall to decrease heart attack risk.

Excessive levels of thyroid hormone can also increase the risk of bone density loss (osteopenia). But the studies I have read did not show this happening unless the free T4 level was in the top 10 to 15 percent of the normal range, regardless of the TSH levels.

If the dose is too high, you may feel too stimulated, like you had too many cups of coffee. Lower the dose. A small percentage of people who are hypothyroid are unable to tolerate even tiny dosing of thyroid. In these cases, taking 500 milligrams of vitamin B1 (thiamine) three times a day sometimes allows them to take the needed thyroid comfortably, after they've been on the thiamine for at least six weeks.

Reproductive Hormones

Many people going through midlife develop fatigue, poor libido, or depression after age forty-five. This includes men and women alike. Just as your car needs a tune-up when it hits forty-five thousand miles, so does your body.

Both research and clinical experience have found that if the estrogen and testosterone levels in females or the testosterone level in males is suboptimal, natural support including bioidentical hormones can result in dramatic improvements.

ANDROPAUSE (TESTOSTERONE DEFICIENCY)

Testosterone is practically synonymous with manhood. Unfortunately, testosterone levels in men often decline by the time they're in their mid-forties, causing andropause (or "male menopause") and producing symptoms such as:

- Loss of libido
- Erectile dysfunction
- A combination of high blood pressure, prediabetes or even overt diabetes, and elevated cholesterol (metabolic syndrome)
- A large waist size
- Fatigue, low motivation, poor concentration and memory, or depression
- Achiness
- CFS/FMS

If the testosterone level is in the lower 30 percent of the normal range (under about 540 ng/dL), *and* the person has one or two of the symptoms above, I consider treatment. I'm especially likely to recommend testosterone if deficiencies are contributing to health problems such as high blood pressure, high cholesterol, or diabetes (a very common combination called metabolic syndrome).

Know the Difference

It is important that we not confuse giving safe levels of healthy *bioidentical* natural testosterone with the high-dose, synthetic, and toxic testosterone that can be misused in sports. The latter is what you will hear discussed as "steroids" in the news and can be quite toxic.

TREATING LOW TESTOSTERONE IN MEN

If your testosterone level is low, I recommend talking to a holistic doctor. These practitioners specialize in giving men and women over forty-five years of age regular "tune-ups" to keep their health and vitality optimized.

These are much different than the checkups people get at their family doctor, which primarily look for signs of disease. See more info on this in Chapter 7.

For men under fifty years of age, it is often preferable to stimulate your body's own production of testosterone, using a medication called clomiphene (25 milligrams by mouth) at bedtime each Monday, Wednesday, and Friday. If needed, the dose can be increased to 25 or even 50 milligrams nightly. Simply recheck the testosterone levels after at least a week on the treatment to see if it is working.

If clomiphene doesn't work, one can use HCG (human chorionic gonadotropin) hormone. Unfortunately, HCG is expensive and requires injections, so I rarely use it.

For those over fifty, I am more likely to recommend a topical bioidentical testosterone cream or gel, applying 25 to 100 milligrams to the skin daily. You can get the testosterone cream by prescription (e.g., Androgel) from a regular pharmacy. It is obscenely expensive but is often covered by prescription insurance.

The good news: You can also get prescription testosterone cream from almost any compounding pharmacy. A compounded version of the drug is *much* less expensive and quite effective. This is an excellent option for those without prescription insurance that covers testosterone. For reproductive hormones, I recommend Women's International Pharmacy (www .womensinternational.com).

Caution: Wash your hands after applying the gel or cream to your skin and apply it to a part of the skin that doesn't come in contact with other people. Otherwise, women—such as your spouse—can develop a high, unsafe blood level of testosterone. This increases the risk of her getting diabetes.

It's best to apply the testosterone on your thighs or other areas that people don't often touch, so the cream does not get on anyone else. Rotate the area you put the cream on, or less may be absorbed over time.

Most men feel best with a blood level around the 70th percentile of normal range, and that's what I aim for in my patients. Especially if it can be achieved with a dose no higher than 50 to 100 milligrams a day. Follow-up blood testing is best drawn two to three hours after applying the testosterone. Otherwise, the blood levels can be falsely low.

I generally do not recommend testosterone injections or oral testosterone.

Don't Chase a Testosterone High

Caution: Too high a dose can initially cause a bit of a "libido high." Sometimes men then try to "chase the feeling" by pushing the dose higher and higher—not a good idea. Your body adapts to the extra testosterone by converting it to estrogen or hormones that can cause hair loss.

Make sure your blood levels don't exceed the upper limit of normal, which can cause problems such as acne or too high of a blood count. Fifty may be the new thirty, but I don't think you want to be a teenager again.

The best way to get testosterone? Once the man is clear that he feels better on the testosterone, I recommend getting testosterone pellets. These are inserted every three to six months in a very simple in-office procedure. The main downside is the cost, if they are not covered by insurance. But they have the benefits of:

- Guaranteed absorption (sometimes the skin stops absorbing the cream after a year or so)
- Decreased conversion to other hormones that we don't want
- Convenience
- Steady blood levels
- Not getting the cream on other people

To find practitioners near you who insert them, see www.biotemedical .com.

Natural Help for Male Libido and Sexual Function

A special new form of ginseng called HRG-80 can do wonders for energy. Also have erectile dysfunction? The research is showing that this ginseng can also stimulate the hormones in your body that make testosterone. Because of this it is now being combined with a number of other herbs in a second product. This combination not only helps you feel better overall but can leave parts of you standing up and taking notice.

The latter product is called HRG80 Red Ginseng Male Sexual Enhancement. Give it six weeks to show its full effect.

MENOPAUSE (ESTROGEN AND PROGESTERONE DEFICIENCY)

In women, estrogen and progesterone levels start dropping in their mid-forties, but the blood tests will miss the deficiency for the first five to twelve years that your body is missing the estrogen. So once again, the tests are not reliable.

How do you know if bioidentical estrogen and progesterone may help you?

Although estrogen and progesterone deficiency can cause a host of problems, including fatigue, brain fog, headaches, and insomnia, these symptoms can also be caused by many other conditions. They are more likely to be caused by low estrogen/progesterone if you also have:

- Worsening of insomnia, fatigue, and headache around your period (menses)
- Decreased vaginal lubrication
- Loss of libido
- Hot flashes

Remember, however, that menopause is not an illness any more than puberty is. If you feel comfortable weathering the change, it's fine to simply ignore the symptoms or live with them. Unlike low testosterone in men, which can be associated with high cholesterol and hypertension and greater risk of heart disease, low estrogen or progesterone does not cause these problems in women.

The time to consider addressing perimenopause or menopausal symptoms is when a woman becomes uncomfortable or has any of the symptoms described above. Many women also find that they feel and look younger on the bioidentical hormones and prefer them for this reason. If I were a menopausal woman, I would absolutely be on the bioidentical hormones, starting with the cream and then switching to the pellets (more info at www.biotemedical.com).

But whether you prefer to simply add more edamame to your diet (as discussed below), take an herb, take bioidentical hormones, or simply weather the changes, it's always a personal preference that depends on you. There is no right or wrong answer for how to approach the natural process of menopause. Choose the options that *feel best* to you. It is especially important to learn to trust your intuition/feelings and what your body is telling you.

Fifty Can Be the New Thirty for Women, Too

As you can tell, I strongly believe that both men and women deserve to get a major tune-up once they turn forty-five years of age, and then every one to three years. Just like your car would feel like it was on its last legs (or perhaps I should say tires) if it had never had a tune-up or oil change by the time it hit forty-five thousand miles, many people complain of symptoms they (or their physician) attribute to age by the time they hit forty-five. Most often, it is not simply the aging process. You may be in need of a tune-up.

This tune-up should address not only hormone deficiencies but also other factors such as optimizing bone density; addressing skin and hair health; and addressing sleep and many of the other factors discussed in this book.

These tune-ups are not the same as getting an annual physical. The purpose of the latter is to screen for illnesses, whereas the tune-up is to *optimize* your function and vitality. See Chapter 7 for information on how you can get one. They can even be done for free online (www .TuneUpDocs.com).

You deserve to look and feel great!

NONHORMONAL THERAPEUTIC OPTIONS FOR MENOPAUSAL PROBLEMS

Eat More Edamame

More commonly known as soybean pods, this tasty food is a standard appetizer in Japanese restaurants. You can find edamame in the frozen food section of most supermarkets and health-food stores.

Edamame is rich in phytoestrogens, a weaker, plant-based version of estrogen. Eating a handful a day raises your estrogen levels naturally—the dietary approach traditionally used by Japanese women for centuries to manage menopause symptoms. Eat the pea-like beans inside the pod, not the pod itself.

Take Black Cohosh for Hot Flashes and Night Sweats

Along with edamame, you may want to take the herb black cohosh, which my patients find very helpful. Black cohosh stabilizes the functioning of the autonomic nervous system, which can decrease hot flashes and night sweats.

I prefer Remifemin by Nature's Way. This is a black cohosh product that has been proven effective in dozens of studies. Take two capsules two times daily for two months (it takes two months to see the full effect). After that, you can usually lower the dose to one capsule a day.

New Research on Fish Oil for Menopause

Although I would begin supporting your body through perimenopause with edamame and Remifemin, consider fish oil essential fatty acids if more support is needed for hot flashes. Canadian researchers studied ninety-one women with hot flashes (an average of 2.8 hot flashes a day). Those given fish oil had an average decline of 1.6 hot flashes a day; there was an average decline of 0.5 in the placebo group. I recommend one to two tablets a day of Vectomega by EuroPharma. This replaces seven to fourteen fish oil pills.

BIOIDENTICAL HORMONES

As I've noted above, if I were a menopausal woman, I would be on bioidentical estrogen, progesterone, and likely a small bit of testosterone.

If symptoms of estrogen/progesterone deficiency are still problematic despite the above, especially in those with CFS/FMS, I consider bioidentical estrogens and progesterone to be healthy. These are not to be confused with the synthetic or horse estrogens such as Premarin and conjugated estrogens, or synthetic progestins like Provera. I consider the synthetic hormones to be horribly toxic, in contrast to the bioidenticals, which I consider to be health promoting.

Using the bioidentical estrogen and progesterone is especially important:

- In women who have had a hysterectomy or had their ovaries removed before age forty-five. Even if the ovaries are left in, a hysterectomy will routinely cause estrogen deficiency within two years. I have found that younger women are much less able to tolerate low estrogen than women in their fifties, and the younger women will need the bioidentical hormones. However, if the hysterectomy was because of endometriosis, one needs to be cautious with the estrogen.

- In women with CFS/FMS. Low estrogen and progesterone often are occurring because of hypothalamic control center dysfunction and not simply because of perimenopause.

The main treatment I use in my perimenopausal and menopausal patients is the bioidentical estrogen Bi-Est, along with natural progesterone. These hormones can be compounded into a vaginal cream by any compounding pharmacy. I use Women's International Pharmacy, as they have low pricing and excellent quality. For most women, I start with a 2.5-milligram dose of Bi-Est and 30 milligrams of progesterone. If the testosterone level is suboptimal, and they are not diabetic, I add 0.5 to 2 milligrams of testosterone.

The main problem is that compounded medications are generally not covered by health insurance. An alternative is to simply use an estrogen patch, all of which now have bioidentical estradiol. In addition, bioidentical progesterone is available in the prescription Prometrium (100 milligrams at bedtime). This is equal to 30 milligrams of the topical cream. This combination will not include the testosterone, but generally works well (except for the patches not sticking) and tends to be covered by insurance.

More good news? Although a Women's Health Initiative (WHI) study raised the concern of breast cancer from using Premarin (a strong and potentially toxic estrogen derived from pregnant horses) when started in women in their sixties, new research using a lower dose, starting at a younger age, or using bioidentical estrogens is not showing increased cancer risk. So, women taking these hormones can feel much safer.

When treating with estrogen and progesterone, I also adjust the hormone dose based on symptoms rather than on blood testing.

Consider Testosterone, Too

I've found that a deficiency of testosterone in women can cause some of the problems that occur with low levels of testosterone in middle-aged men: fatigue, depression, osteoporosis, weight gain, muscle achiness, and low libido.

As with men, I test for low free testosterone levels (not only total testosterone, which measures the inactive, storage form of the hormone).

If levels are in the lower quarter of the normal range, I treat with a testosterone cream made by a compounding pharmacy. The usual dose is 0.5 to 2 milligrams a day. With this dosing, most menopausal women notice they have more energy, thicker hair, younger skin, and an improved libido. Testosterone supplementation is especially important in women with chronic pain, as both the pain and pain medications can cause testosterone deficiency, and testosterone deficiency (even with normal blood tests) will amplify pain.

If you also are taking estrogen and progesterone, the compounding pharmacy can combine the three hormones in one cream, for ease of application and lower cost. Many women find the vaginal cream works much better for overall health improvement than taking the estrogen by mouth or simply applying the cream to the skin. It also avoids the loss of hormone absorption by the skin, which commonly occurs over time.

A Few Other Treatment Tips

1. In women, simply optimizing DHEA hormone levels can often adequately increase testosterone levels. This will not help in men because men need much higher levels.

2. Acne suggests that the testosterone dose is too high, as does increased facial hair in women.

3. With hormone creams in general (for both men and women), rotate the skin area you apply it to; otherwise, absorption drops over time.

4. Wash your hands after putting on the estrogen. Apply it to an area where it won't rub off on your gentleman. I know you may want to bring out a bit of his understanding feminine side, but you don't want him growing breasts.

Side Effects

The more common side effects of bioidentical estrogen and progesterone (as opposed to the very toxic synthetics, whose side effects could fill a book) are fluid retention, moodiness, spotting, and breast tenderness.

Fantastic Help for New Moms!

Since we are talking about reproductive hormones, I thought I would mention an excellent new resource for women called Pebble.

There are real physiological implications from pregnancy and birth on a woman's hormones, pelvis, abdomen, back, urogenital systems, and nutrient stores. Becoming a mother also impacts a woman's relationships, self-image, and overall world view.

When new mothers focus only on the baby and deprioritize their own rehabilitation, they can send themselves on a path of long and slow recovery. But if women honor their postpartum needs, they have the opportunity to emerge even stronger, empowered to enter motherhood with more energy to tend to themselves and their growing family. Fortunately, there is a wonderful resource that can help you throughout your recovery journey.

Pebble is an online community of postpartum specialists committed to reimagining postpartum care. The platform enables you to easily connect with a personalized postpartum care team through video chat, without needing to leave home with your baby. You can book with top-rated therapists, lactation consultants, nurse-midwives, women's health physical therapists, sleep coaches, and more. Visit www.pebbleparents.com to learn more.

3

Infections and Immunity: Our Body's Defense System

BFF Summary

1. The most common chronic infection we see is from candida (yeast or fungal) overgrowth.
2. There is no test for candida.
3. Suspect candida if you have chronic nasal congestion, sinusitis, or irritable bowel syndrome.
4. Fungal overgrowth may suppress the body's immune system while also triggering food sensitivities.
5. The most important part of eliminating yeast overgrowth is avoiding sugar and other sweets, although I will add the three magic words: "except for chocolate."
6. Treatment is with:
   A. Probiotics
   B. Natural antifungals. There are many natural or nonprescription products that fight candida. I recommend one called Lufenuron; take 9 grams each day for two weeks until symptoms are controlled and then once each month for three to five months. Then it can be used as needed. I also recommend Caprylex.
   C. Most important is the medication fluconazole (Diflucan). I give 200 milligrams a day for six weeks. You will need a holistic physician to get this prescription.
   D. For chronic sinusitis, I add a compounded nose spray called the Sinusitis Nose Spray (from ITC Pharmacy). This should be taken along with the fluconazole.

7. Killing off candida may initially flare your symptoms. So, start slowly and ease back on any treatments you're taking.
8. Bladder infections can often be prevented or eliminated with a supplement called D-mannose.
9. Autoimmune illness is becoming more common because of excessive chemicals in the environment along with changes brought about by food processing.

We like to think that we are at the top of the food chain. But for most of human history, our main battle has not been against dinosaurs (extinct when we showed up), or even bears or other humans. Rather, it has been against microscopic organisms. This has been an ongoing arms race. In recent history, we have had antibiotics, antivirals, and even vaccines. So, we've largely forgotten about this war, but the microorganisms haven't. They have been developing resistance to our antibiotics. Frankly, this poses a much bigger threat to our existence than invasion by other countries. This is a problem that we are ignoring much to our peril, as we are seeing with COVID-19. The obvious and simple solution would be for the government to develop several new classes of antibiotics and antivirals, and grant them a permanent patent based on national security. They would then only be able to be used under the direction of the Centers for Disease Control and Prevention (CDC).

But for now at least, this is not the key problem. Doctors do know how to treat most routine infections, so we do not need to discuss those here. Rather, my focus will be on a very common infection that many doctors don't know how to diagnose or treat—or simply deny the existence of.

Candida: The Yeasty Beasties

For this discussion, I will use the terms "yeast," "candida," and "fungal infections" interchangeably for simplicity's sake.

Most people are familiar with the concept of vaginal yeast overgrowth occurring after taking antibiotics. That can be hard for people (and physicians) to ignore, because there's an obvious and uncomfortable discharge.

In addition, because there is a test for vaginal yeast overgrowth, physicians are quick to treat it.

Unfortunately, the big problem with candida overgrowth is not in the 4 to 6 inches of vagina, but rather in the sinuses and the 25 to 28 feet of large and small intestine. But because it does not cause an obvious discharge, and there is no test that distinguishes normal growth from overgrowth, most physicians make believe that bowel candida overgrowth doesn't exist.

This is common in medicine, where it seems that "if there is no test for a medical condition, the problem doesn't exist." It reminds me of small children covering their eyes and thinking that they're invisible.

Unfortunately, antibiotics kill off the healthy bacteria that normally live in the colon and allow overgrowth of candida. The body is often able to rebalance itself after one or several courses of antibiotics, but after repeated or long-term courses—and especially if the body has an underlying immune dysfunction—the yeast can get the upper hand.

The second major factor? The 140 pounds of sugar per person added to our diet in food processing each year. Yeast grows by fermenting sugar, and if you pour a 16-ounce soda, which contains a massive twelve spoonfuls of sugar, down your throat, you're turning your gut into a fermentation tank—and creating trillions of little baby yeasties. This contributes to a spastic colon (also called irritable bowel syndrome), which is a hallmark of candida overgrowth. Candida overgrowth is also the major cause of nasal congestion and chronic sinusitis. We will discuss both below.

Let's start by looking at why candida overgrowth can cause widespread food allergies and other immune problems.

CANDIDA AND IMMUNE FUNCTION

Fungal overgrowth may suppress the body's immune system. It is suspected that this occurs in part because the bowel yeast infection causes what is called leaky gut syndrome or, to use more research-based jargon, increased intestinal membrane permeability. Why? Because during part of the organism's life cycle, it grows in threads that can spread into the bowel wall, making it "leaky." This contributes to food proteins getting absorbed into the blood system before they are fully digested. These partially digested proteins may be treated as outside invaders by your immune system. This results in:

- A marked increase in food allergies
- Immune system overactivity (as occurs in autoimmune diseases) combined with immune fatigue

In addition, as the yeast organism is massive in size compared to viruses or bacteria, it is a difficult bug for your immune system to kill without help once it overgrows. Because of this, once the yeast gets the upper hand, it can trigger a cycle that further disrupts the body's defenses.

Fortunately, once again knowledge is power. So, let's look at the information you need to take care of this problem.

Yeast is a normal member of the body's "zoo." It lives in balance with bowel bacteria. Some bowel bacteria are helpful, and others are detrimental. The problems begin when this harmonious balance shifts and the yeast begins to overgrow.

PROBLEMS CAUSED BY CANDIDA

Candida can cause a vast variety of symptoms, in both healthy people and those with CFS/FMS. There are several conditions, however, that leave me presuming candida overgrowth until proven otherwise. These are:

- Chronic nasal congestion or sinusitis
- Spastic colon, also known as irritable bowel syndrome (This basically means that you have gas, bloating, diarrhea, and/or constipation and your physician doesn't know why. Although there are several causes, most often when we treat for candida, the spastic colon goes away.)
- Recurrent small painful mouth sores that last for about ten days

---

Getting Rid of Chronic Sinusitis

Research done at the Mayo Clinic showed that over 90 percent of chronic sinusitis is caused by immune reactivity to fungal growth in the sinuses. The result is a stuffy nose, eventually leading to nasal passages swelling shut. In the body, any time something gets blocked (e.g., an appendix or gallbladder), it results in a secondary bacterial infection—and the sinuses are no exception. When this happens, your nasal mucous turns yellow-green and you go to the doctor in pain. They give you an antibiotic, which knocks out the bacterial infection and leaves you feeling better. Unfortunately, the antibiotic worsens the underlying yeast/fungal infection in your nose, causing more swelling and blockages and therefore more attacks of bacterial infections. Treating sinusitis with antibiotics is why sinusitis in the United States usually becomes chronic.

In my experience, sinusitis (even chronic) usually responds dramatically to the yeast treatments discussed below, especially a combination of six weeks of oral fluconazole (Diflucan) and a special sinusitis nose spray. The spray contains Bactroban and xylitol, which kill the bacterial infections; low-dose cortisol to shrink the swelling; bismuth to strip away the infection's protective armor (called biofilms); and antifungals. This combination will often knock out the sinusitis, and some patients like to stay on the nose spray for the long term or use it intermittently for recurrent infections. Your physician can call in a prescription for the Sinusitis Nose Spray to ITC Compounding Pharmacy (888-349-5453), which will mail it to you, and fluconazole is available by prescription at any pharmacy.

TREATING YEAST/CANDIDA OVERGROWTH

A number of effective treatments can be used to eliminate yeast overgrowth. I find that the best approach is to combine dietary changes, natural remedies, and prescription medications.

DIETARY CHANGES AND NATURAL REMEDIES

The most important part of treating yeast overgrowth is avoiding sugar and other sweets, although I will add the three magic words: "except for chocolate." Chocolate has been associated with numerous health benefits, including a 45 percent lower risk of heart attack death. You can also enjoy one or two pieces of fruit a day, but don't consume concentrated sugars like fruit juices, corn syrup, jellies, pastry, candy, or honey. Stay far away from soft drinks, which may have up to 9 teaspoons of sugar in every 12 ounces. This amount of sugar has been shown to markedly suppress immune function for several hours. If you simply decide to stop sugar cold turkey, prepared to go through severe withdrawal for about one week. This can be avoided by first treating the candida and addressing adrenal and reproductive hormone deficiencies. My book *The Complete Guide to Beating Sugar Addiction* can help you become a recovered sugar addict—easily.

Using stevia as a sweetener is a wonderful alternative to sugar. Despite some misconceptions, stevia is safe and natural, and you can use all you want. The brand of stevia that you choose is important, however. Some brands of stevia are not filtered and therefore are bitter. The plain stevia that I use is called BetterStevia by NOW. Stevia Select has a superb line of flavored stevias, which I also love. My morning coffee is sugar-free and all natural, and tastes like an ice cream sundae!

There are now even several good sugar- and chemical-free sodas. I like Zevia sodas (sweetened with stevia), which can be found at most health-food stores and even at Safeway.

Several books have been written on the yeast controversy and offer additional dietary methods to try. One of the best is an old classic called *The Yeast Connection and Women's Health* by the late Dr. William Crook, a remarkable physician who introduced and advanced our understanding of candida overgrowth. His work is so important that he is one of the three physicians to whom this book is dedicated.

Many books on yeast overgrowth, including Dr. Crook's, advise readers to avoid all yeast. This information is based on the theory that an allergic reaction to yeast is the cause of the problem. However, the yeast that is found in most foods (except beer and cheese) is not closely related to candida, the predominant yeast that seems to be involved in yeast overgrowth.

In my experience, trying to avoid all yeast in foods results in a nutritionally inadequate diet and does not substantially help most people. Although a few people do appear to have true allergies to the yeast in their food, they account for a small percentage of those with yeast overgrowth. These people may benefit from the stricter diet recommended in Dr. Crook's books.

Interestingly, once adrenal insufficiency and yeast overgrowth are treated, most people find that their allergies and sensitivities to yeast and other food products seem to improve and often disappear.

SUPPLEMENTS
Probiotics

Healthy gut bacteria compete with candida. This is why probiotics are so helpful. Unfortunately, over 99 percent of these healthy bacteria are usually killed by stomach acid, so they don't put up much of a fight. Because of this, I recommend that the probiotics be taken in an enteric-coated form, such as the Pearls Elite form by Nature's Way. These pearls act like tanks that carry the probiotics past the stomach acid safely and then dissolve in the alkaline environment of the intestines, releasing your healthy bacteria "troops" to fight the candida. Take one a day for five months, and then every other day as needed to maintain bowel health.

Lufenuron

There are many natural or nonprescription products that fight candida. The one I prefer is Lufenuron.

This is available in 800-milligam capsules. I recommend taking one a day for twenty-four days, then skipping six days. After that, you can either take one capsule every Monday, Wednesday, and Friday, or twelve capsules (9 grams, if you get the powder) the first day of each month for six months.

This regimen can be continued long term, especially if you get recurrent nasal congestion or irritable bowel syndrome when you stop it. It is best taken with an oily meal to increase absorption.

This is the only nonprescription antifungal that I know of that is absorbed into the body. Because of this, it can kill candida in the gut lining and the sinuses. The capsules can be ordered online from Canada at www .shop4lufe.com. The cost is very reasonable, at about $28 for twelve 800-milligram capsules.

As an aside, Lufenuron is sold to kill fleas in pets. Don't let this frighten you. It is not a toxic chemical like most insecticides, but rather it is a safe compound that simply dissolves the candida.

Caprylex

My next favorite natural antifungal is a special form of buffered caprylic acid called Caprylex by Douglas Labs. Take two tablets twice a day for three to five months. This is also excellent and will not upset the stomach like other forms of caprylic acid.

Other Antifungals

There are literally dozens of natural antifungals that can be helpful. These include 500 milligrams of berberine (I like the EuroMedica brand, Berberine MetX), Tanalbit, liquid grapefruit seed extract, and oregano oil (in that order).

Prescription Treatments
Diflucan

It is critical to add a prescription antifungal, because most of the natural products only kill yeast in the gut and are often not strong enough on their own. I routinely recommend that those with chronic sinusitis, spastic colon, or CFS/FMS take the medication fluconazole (Diflucan) at a dose of 200 milligrams a day for six to twelve weeks. You will need a holistic physician to prescribe this.

Herxheimer Reactions: Symptom Flaring When Infections Are Killed Off

For virtually every treatment, I recommend people stop it if they feel worse on it. This is your body's way of saying that it does not want that treatment. The exception is when you kill off a chronic infection or remove toxins.

When this happens, your body is flooded with the broken-up parts of the dead organisms. It can sometimes react to these, worsening the symptoms transiently. But do not play macho and try to treat through this worsening. It will only take you longer to get better. Rather, stop the treatment until symptoms settle down. Then resume at a tiny dose and work up slowly as is comfortable.

Those with a severe Herxheimer reaction may want to consider also trying a yeast-free diet for six to twelve weeks to see if this helps.

To decrease the risk of the Herxheimer reaction, I start the natural treatment with probiotics, and a few days later I add in the Lufenuron, Berberine MetX, or Caprylex. I do this for three to four weeks before starting the fluconazole (Diflucan). If symptoms flare on the fluconazole, I stop the medication until the reaction subsides and then lower the dose to 25 to 100 milligrams each morning (or even less) for the first three to fourteen days. I then raise the dose as is well tolerated until the person is on 200 milligrams a day, or whatever dose is comfortable.

If symptoms recur after stopping the Diflucan, I may continue the medication for an additional six weeks at 200 milligrams a day, or prescribe 200 milligrams twice a day *one day a week* over the long term to keep the candida suppressed. This is especially helpful if the person is on long-term treatment with antibiotics.

For irritable bowel syndrome, this is all that most people need. The probiotic alone can often maintain the benefit.

Sinusitis Nose Spray

For people with chronic nasal congestion or sinusitis, I add prescription Sinusitis Nose Spray. This should be taken while on the fluconazole. Most people can avoid sinus surgery with this combination, as their sinusitis goes away.

The best thing you can do to combat yeast overgrowth is to try to avoid it in the first place. When you get an infection, immediately begin treating it naturally (see "Treating Infections Without Antibiotics" below). Hopefully, you will be able to prevent it from turning into a bacterial infection that might require an antibiotic.

If you find, however, that you must take an antibiotic, all is not lost. You can still lessen the severity of yeast overgrowth by avoiding sweets and by taking Caprylex plus a probiotic.

Treating Infections Without Antibiotics

Many people do not realize how many things they can do before resorting to using an antibiotic to clear an infection. If you feel you are coming down with a respiratory infection such as a cold or the flu, I recommend that you try the following:

- Take natural thymic hormone. This is available as a product called ProBoost, and it is an outstanding immune stimulant. Dissolve the contents of one packet under your tongue three times a day and let it get absorbed there (any that is swallowed will be destroyed by your stomach acid). I recommend that this be in everyone's medicine cabinet and should be begun immediately at the start of any infection.
- Take 1,000 milligrams of vitamin C a day.
- If you have a sore throat, suck on a 20-milligram zinc acetate lozenge (or other zinc if acetate is not available) four times a day.
- Drink plenty of water and hot caffeine-free tea (or hot water with lemon) and rest.
- If you have a sinus infection, try nasal rinses. Dissolve ½ teaspoon of salt in 1 cup of lukewarm water. Add ¼ teaspoon of baking soda to make it more soothing. Inhale some of the solution about 1 inch up into your nose, one nostril at a time. Do this either

by using a baby nose bulb or an eyedropper while lying down, or by sniffing the solution out of the palm of your hand while standing by a sink. A neti pot (available in health-food stores) can be especially helpful for nasal rinses. Then gently blow your nose, being careful not to hurt your ears. Repeat the same process with the other nostril. Continue to repeat with each nostril until the nose is clear. Rinse your nasal passages at least twice a day until the infection improves. Each rinsing will wash away about 90 percent of the infection and make it much easier for your body to heal.

- Gargle with salt water, mixed as described above for the nasal rinse, to help a sore throat.
- Bladder infections can often be prevented or eliminated with the supplement mannose. See "Chronic Urinary Tract/Bladder Infections" on page 55 for more information.

What If the Yeast Comes Back?

The best markers that I have found for recurrent yeast overgrowth are a return of bowel symptoms, with gas, bloating, and/or diarrhea or constipation; vaginal yeast; mouth sores; and/or recurring nasal congestion or sinusitis. If these symptoms persist for more than two weeks, especially if there is also even a mild worsening of the CFS/FMS symptoms, it is reasonable to treat again. This is especially common after the holidays, when people are eating more sugar.

It is normal for yeast symptoms to resolve after treatment. After six weeks on fluconazole (Diflucan), most people feel a lot better. If not, you may have fluconazole-resistant candida, and a trial of terbinafine (Lamisil) may be helpful: I give 250 milligrams a day for six weeks.

If symptoms recur soon after stopping the antifungal, I often recommend taking the antifungal for another six weeks or for as long as is needed to keep the symptoms at bay. Alternatively, I will often give maintenance treatment with Lufenuron the first day of each month plus Berberine MetX or Caprylex. If needed, I add 400 milligrams of fluconazole each Sunday (or just one day a week).

Although I have never seen this be a worrisome problem, fluconazole can cause liver inflammation. But I see acetaminophen causing this more than fluconazole does.

Usually the people feel better after treatment and stay feeling fairly well for a year or two. Although many people never need to treat again for yeast, others need to repeat a course of antifungals after six to twenty-four months, especially after eating too much sugar or taking antibiotics.

The Human Biome

There are more bacteria in the human colon than there are cells in the whole rest of the body. As many as one hundred trillion. These are very important for health. Historically our gut bacteria developed growing on breast milk while we were nursing. When we were weaned, our stomach started producing acid, killing any other bacteria that tried to get in.

So these healthy bacteria that grew off our mother's milk reproduced and, for most of human history, would live in happy harmony with us for the rest of our lives. They would serve a critical role in our nutrition, offer protection from unhealthy bacterial invaders, and support our immune system.

Fast-forward thousands of years, and suddenly humans faced the benefits and pitfalls of antibiotics. Though overall a major plus, they started to kill off healthy bacteria and allow unhealthy ones to get in. Especially when people took acid blockers for indigestion. This knocked out the acid bath in the stomach, which was our major line of defense against unhealthy bacteria getting in.

Then food processors started adding 140 pounds of sugar per person each year to our diets. This supports the growth of unhealthy bacteria and fungi as well.

Modern medicine is just starting to realize the health costs of this microbial imbalance, which is called dysbiosis. As is usual, drug manufacturers are looking for the magic bullet. Preferably one that is very expensive and profitable.

In the natural health industry, we are also seeing the "probiotic wars." Stronger and stronger probiotics are being made. Unfortunately, any probiotic containing over twenty billion bacteria can actually cause small intestinal bacterial overgrowth (SIBO; see page 235), worsening symptoms.

So, which bacteria should we use?

Over the next decade, expect a flurry of both research and marketing claims. The research will eventually point us toward more effective treatments.

For now, I have found that using a product called Pearls Elite, with five billion milk-based bacteria, works best. The pearl coating acts like a little tank, carrying the healthy bacteria safely through the acid war zone of the stomach. When it gets to the alkaline environment, the pearl dissolves and the healthy bacteria are released to do the job. I have people take one Pearl Elite a day for three to six months. Then they can take one every other day to maintain benefits.

If you're looking for a stronger probiotic, which has strains that are stomach-acid resistant, then I recommend Colon & Bowel Probiotic by Terry Naturally, which has twenty billion bacteria per capsule.

I suspect that there is no single strain of bacteria that is important. So far, research in FMS and elsewhere is suggesting that it is the *diversity* of strains, along with having healthy forms, that is most important.

Especially important is to cut down on excess sugar (see Chapter 4), and increase the amount of fermented foods in your diet. Kefir can be especially helpful, having over sixty strains of healthy bacteria in high amounts. Many people have noted dramatic improvement using this.

CHRONIC URINARY TRACT/BLADDER INFECTIONS (UTIS)

The main symptoms of a UTI/bladder infection are dysuria (discomfort—for example, a burning sensation—when urinating), urgency (the feeling that you have to go very badly and right away when there is not much urine there), and frequent urination with low urine volume.

This group of symptoms is also common in CFS/FMS patients in the absence of bladder infections and, when very severe, is called interstitial cystitis (IC). However, I would not say that a person has interstitial cystitis unless this is one of the major symptoms of their CFS/FMS, because almost everyone with this illness has some urinary urgency and frequency. The few people who have IC need to be careful, as many vitamin supplements can cause bladder symptoms to flare up, and they should begin with very low doses to be sure they are tolerated. For more information on treating the disorder, see my book *Pain Free 1-2-3* and/or contact the Interstitial Cystitis Association (www.ichelp.org).

Taking antibiotics will kill a bladder infection but, as we noted, will also kill the healthy bacteria in the bowel. This sets you up for yeast overgrowth and other problems. So unless you have a fever, blood in the urine, back pain over the kidneys, or a toxic feeling, it is reasonable to try natural remedies for one to two days with a doctor's okay before going with the antibiotics.

Because bladder symptoms can be seen in both UTIs and CFS/FMS, it is important to have a urine culture done before initiating treatment with antibiotics to make sure it is an infection, and not just muscle spasms in the bladder, that is causing these symptoms. If there is an infection, more than 90 percent of the time it will involve *Escherichia coli* (*E. coli*), a bacterium normally found in the intestines and, except for a few rare, dangerous forms, a healthy part of normal bowel bacteria. The problem occurs when the *E. coli* gets out of the bowel, where it belongs, and into the bladder. Unlike most other infectious organisms, *E. coli* has little Velcro-like projections that stick to the bladder wall, so they cannot be washed out by urination.

My favorite natural way to clear bacteria in the bladder is called D-mannose. In addition, taking high doses of vitamin C (500 to 5,000 milligrams a day) can help. Drinking a lot of water also helps wash out the infection.

D-MANNOSE

Mannose is a natural sugar (not the kind that causes symptoms of yeast overgrowth) that is excreted promptly into the urine. Unfortunately for the *E. coli* bacteria, the "fingers" that stick to the bladder wall stick to the D-mannose even better. When you ingest a large amount of D-mannose, it spills into the urine, coating all the *E. coli* so that the *E. coli* are literally washed away with the next urination.

Meanwhile, D-mannose does not kill healthy bacteria, so it does not disturb the important balance of bacteria in the bowel. In addition, D-mannose is absorbed in the upper gut before it gets to the friendly *E. coli* that are normally present in the colon. Because of this, it helps clear the bladder without causing any other problems.

D-mannose is quite safe, even for long-term use, although most people need it for only a few days. People who have frequent recurrent bladder infections may, however, choose to take it every day to suppress the infections. The usual dose of D-mannose is ½ to 1 teaspoon every two to three waking hours to treat an acute bladder infection or ½ to 1 teaspoon a day to prevent chronic bladder infections. It is best taken dissolved in water. If you get bladder infections associated with sexual intercourse, you can take a teaspoon of D-mannose one hour before and/or just after intercourse to help prevent an infection.

You should feel much better within twenty-four to forty-eight hours on D-mannose. If you don't, see a doctor for a urine culture (you may want to get the culture at the first sign of infection) and consider antibiotic treatment after two days if the culture is positive. Some evidence exists that the antibiotic nitrofurantoin (also sold under the brand name Macrobid) causes less yeast overgrowth than do other antibiotics. Even with other antibiotics, most bladder infections are knocked out by one to three days of antibiotic use, instead of the old seven-day regimen.

In women over forty-five years of age who get recurrent bladder infections, this most often occurs because of thinning of the vaginal wall from dropping estrogen levels. Several months of using a bioidentical vaginal estrogen and progesterone cream can resolve this problem (see page 40). Be sure to apply some of the cream around the urinary opening.

Autoimmune Illness

In addition to new infections arriving on the scene (e.g., COVID-19, AIDS, swine flu, Lyme disease, and a host of others), we are also seeing a rising epidemic of autoimmune diseases. Autoimmune illness occurs when part of the person's own body is mistaken for an outside invader, and it is attacked by its own immune system. There are literally hundreds of autoimmune conditions, including multiple sclerosis, lupus, rheumatoid arthritis, and Hashimoto's thyroiditis—and they are becoming markedly more common.

Is It Lupus, or Really Fibromyalgia?

Systemic lupus erythematosus (SLE), or lupus, is an autoimmune illness where the body's immune system confuses our body with an outside invader and attacks itself. It can be mild, or severe and life-threatening.

A key problem is that lupus, and many other autoimmune illnesses like rheumatoid arthritis and Sjögren's syndrome, cause a secondary fibromyalgia in about 30 percent of cases, which is most often missed. Many if not most of the symptoms may then be caused by the secondary fibromyalgia and do not respond to the standard autoimmune medications, so the doctor gives higher and higher doses of prednisone and other toxic treatments.

So how can you tell? If you have widespread pain and fatigue, and also insomnia, you likely have a secondary fibromyalgia that should be treated with SHINE.

In addition, for those with lupus, several studies have shown that 200 milligrams a day (a large dose for women) of DHEA improves outcomes in lupus. Though this high a dose may cause acne or darkening of facial hair in other women, for reasons we don't yet understand, this was uncommon in women with lupus in the studies.

WHY THE AUTOIMMUNE EPIDEMIC?

It is important to step back and once again look at some of the root causes. Especially, why are so many people's immune systems becoming overwhelmed? In addition to sleep deprivation and nutritional deficiencies (especially zinc and vitamin D) contributing to immune dysfunction, there are several other major underlying factors that are becoming very common in the population as a whole:

1. Severe dysbiosis (unhealthy gut infections) caused by antibiotics, excess sugar intake, and acid blockers.
2. Incomplete digestion of proteins caused by the rapidly increasing and chronic use of acid-blocker medication, combined with the routine destruction of the enzymes present in food during food processing to prolong shelf life. These enzymes are what digest food completely, and deficiencies result in incompletely digested proteins.
3. Increased gut membrane permeability, often called leaky gut, allowing dramatic increases in absorption of these partially digested proteins, which, as discussed on page 274, are treated by your immune system as outside invaders, triggering food sensitivities and stressing our immune systems.

This trio of modern-day gut changes not only contributes to a marked increase in food allergies, and likely autoimmune disease, but can also overwhelm and exhaust the immune system. Why? If you consider that the total body burden of many infections may be measured in under 1 milligram, and that people may eat upward of 100,000 milligrams of protein a day, the concern is raised that even modest decreases in protein digestion, and the absorption of a small percent of partially digested amino acid chains, may increase the immune system's work dramatically.

Our Modern Digestive Disaster

Unfortunately, food processors learned that by destroying the digestive enzymes in food they could prolong the food's shelf life. This is because the enzymes in the food cause the food to ripen. The same enzymes, however, are necessary for you to properly digest your food. So the food looks good on the shelf, but it is difficult to digest, causing indigestion.

Instead of treating the poor digestion by giving people digestive enzymes, physicians turn off stomach acid—the other major factor needed for digestion. This is like going to your physician saying that you have a flat tire and having them shoot out the other tires to restore balance. Not a good idea.

So if you have indigestion, take some plant-based digestive enzymes with your meals (e.g., CompleteGest from Nature's Way) and improve stomach acidity.

To again put this in perspective and help you understand the stress that poor digestion puts on your immune system, consider this thought: It would take over twenty thousand trillion viruses to equal the weight of the amount of protein in a hamburger. You really want to improve your digestion, so that your stomach digests the burger. And everything else you eat. Otherwise, the partially digested proteins will have to be eliminated by your immune system, sometimes exhausting and overwhelming it, and triggering food sensitivities.

To give you an idea of the impact of these food sensitivities, a published study (*Integrative Medicine*, October 2011), which I ran and which was funded by my foundation, showed that twenty-three out of thirty children with autism were able to return to regular schools after one year of food allergy desensitization treatments with NAET (Nambudripad's Allergy Elimination Technique) versus zero out of thirty in the untreated control group. Interestingly, many researchers in the field are seeing overlaps in the pathophysiology of autism and fibromyalgia.

Another Major Cause of Autoimmune Disease

We now have over eighty-five thousand chemicals added to our environment that were not there one hundred years ago. To get a chemical approved as a medication, it has to go through a safety evaluation process that costs over $400 million. On the other hand, if you want to throw the chemical wildly into the environment, it is okay to do so without much real safety testing.

An example gaining more attention is bisphenol A (BPA), a chemical found in plastic and metal food containers. More than one hundred studies are showing that it can be very toxic and, like DDT (dichlorodiphenyltrichloroethane), acts as a hormone disrupter. Those of you old enough to remember DDT may also remember that it nearly drove our national symbol, the bald eagle, to extinction before it was outlawed. I suspect the universe has a sense of humor and sent us this metaphor as a warning. Which, because it affects financial interests, we have of course ignored. Though BPA has been banned in Canada, it is still allowed to be used in the United States.

Meanwhile, numerous chemicals can wreak havoc on our hormonal systems as well.

It is likely that this chemical load is one more major contributing factor that can result in the immune system confusing its own body's parts with outside invaders. It is neither possible nor recommended that all chemicals be avoided. Rather, simply trim back your overall exposure using common sense. For those with severe autoimmune illness, I recommend an excellent book called *The Autoimmune Epidemic* by Donna Jackson Nakazawa.

SUPPORTING YOUR IMMUNE SYSTEM

Fortunately, our bodies (including our immune systems) are built with a remarkable ability to adapt, especially if they are given a bit of help. Let's start with a few key things that are critical in helping your immune function.

1. Take a good multivitamin with zinc, such as the Energy Revitalization System vitamin powder or Clinical Essentials. Zinc is one of the most important nutrients for immune function.
2. Cut back excess sugar. The amount of sugar in a 12-ounce can of soda will suppress immune function by 30 percent for three hours.

3. Get adequate sleep.
4. Optimize adrenal function.
5. Improve digestion with a plant-based digestive enzyme.

All of these take a major load off your immune system, so it can get back to its real job of getting rid of the bad guys.

4 Nutrition: "Garbage In, Garbage Out"

BFF Summary

1. Foods you enjoy are usually actually healthy, until food processors get ahold of them.
2. This includes foods like eggs, coffee, tea, and chocolate. These are quite healthy. Unless people have high blood pressure, a high salt intake is very good to help adrenal fatigue and CFS/FMS.
3. What is most important is to cut out excess sugar and processed foods. Sodas and fruit juices have a whopping ¾ teaspoon of sugar per ounce. Eat an apple or orange instead.
4. In general, aim for a diet that tends to have whole foods without a lot of chemicals. Divide the grams of sugar in the nutrition box on the food label by four, and that will tell you how many teaspoons of sugar there are per portion.
5. Drink the Energy Revitalization System vitamin powder each morning. This replaces up to fifty supplement pills, containing almost all of the vitamins, minerals, and other key nutrients lost in food processing.
6. Take the Smart Energy System ribose plus herbal mix.
7. Combining the Energy Revitalization System and Smart Energy System often doubles energy levels after one month.
8. Consider adding one HRG80 Red Ginseng, one Vectomega, and 200 milligrams of coenzyme Q10 a day.
9. This one drink and five capsules can change your life.

For those of you who watch what you eat, here's the final word on nutrition and health. It's a relief to know the truth after all those conflicting medical studies:

1. The Japanese eat very little fat and drink very little red wine, and they suffer fewer heart attacks than Americans.
2. The French eat lots of fatty cheese and rich food and drink lots of wine, and they suffer fewer heart attacks than Americans.
3. The Italians drink a lot of red wine and eat lots of carbohydrate-rich pasta, and they suffer fewer heart attacks than Americans.
4. The Germans drink a lot of beer and eat lots of sausages and fats, and they suffer fewer heart attacks than Americans.

Conclusion: Eat and drink what you like. Speaking English is apparently what kills you.

*A*re you ready to give up everything you enjoy and switch to a diet of raw groats?

If so, you are reading the wrong book.

If you think about it, the concept that things you hate are good for you, and things that feel good are bad, is utterly insane. Whether you believe your body was made by God, evolution, or a mix of both, it makes sense that what feels good is good for us.

The problem is when food processors mess with our food to fool our bodies. This chapter will teach you how to enjoy what you eat, even given the problems with the modern diet, and thrive.

Myth Busting 101

There are so many medical myths floating around that it's a wonder anybody can enjoy their food anymore. Here are today's nutrition "myth busters":

1. **Myth:** *Eggs are bad for you and raise cholesterol.* Busted. Numerous studies have shown that eating six eggs a day for six weeks has no effect on cholesterol. In fact, eggs are the healthiest protein you can get short of eating another human being. So enjoy.

2. **Myth:** *Salt is bad for you.* Busted. Some studies even show that people who eat the so-called recommended amount of salt die younger than those who eat more. Especially for those with adrenal fatigue, salt restriction is a good way to crash and burn. Enjoy adding salt to your food as your taste directs you. This is especially important for people with adrenal fatigue or CFS/FMS.

   Studies show that severe salt restriction only lowers blood pressure 1 to 3 mm Hg. I don't restrict the salt intake of people with high blood pressure. Instead I have them increase their potassium (avocados, bananas, tomato juice, etc.).

3. **Myth:** *Coffee and tea are bad for you.* Busted. These are both natural compounds that are chock-full of healthy antioxidants. Coffee and tea have been associated with a wide array of health benefits, such as lowering the risk of heart attack, lowering the risk of diabetes, and even decreasing the risk of cancer, multiple sclerosis, and liver disease. The trick is to enjoy these in moderation. After your second cup each day, switch to decaf.

4. **Myth:** *Alcohol is bad for you.* Busted. Those who drink up to two drinks a day live longer than teetotalers.

5. **Myth:** *Chocolate is unhealthy.* Busted. Dark chocolate is one of my favorite health foods. A recent study showed it to be associated with a 70 percent lower risk of depression. It is also associated with a 45 percent lower risk of dying from heart disease (compared to perhaps 5 to 10 percent for cholesterol medications). It helps energy and cognitive function, even in CFS/FMS.

   But have it in moderation, as it is not low calorie. Go for quality and great taste versus quantity. Better yet, get sugar-free chocolates. Russell Stover and Lily's have excellent lines. And I recently came across an amazing sugar-free dark chocolate ginger bar called The Good Chocolate, available on Amazon. Chocolate is one of the best medicines in the world.

The list goes on and on. In general, the best way to tell what is good for you is by how it makes you feel in the long term. If overall you feel great, then your diet is working. If it gives you great pleasure at the same time, that's an even better sign that it is good for you.

What is it that's best avoided? Basically, those things that make you feel bad overall. I say *overall* because some things, such as heroin, make you feel better right away but much worse overall. The food equivalent of this is excess sugar.

This doesn't mean you can't have any sugar. In fact, as I noted, eating fruits and dark chocolate is actually very healthy. Simply avoid processed foods that have been loaded with sugar to cover the taste of "food-like materials" that are rancid or gross. Save your sugar budget for dessert, where it belongs.

Especially important? Cut out sodas and fruit juices. These have ¾ teaspoon of sugar per ounce. This means that 48-ounce Big Burp soda at your local Quickie Mart contains a whopping 36 teaspoons of sugar. (That's equivalent to 12 tablespoons or ¾ cup!) It will give you a quick high but leave you crashing overall.

Moderation in all things—including moderation.

—Mark Twain

So my nutrition advice?

1. Eat what makes you feel good.
2. Avoid excess sugar and sweets in processed foods.
3. When convenient, choose whole foods over processed junk. When looking at the ingredients (which is a very good idea), I recommend this simple guideline: "If you can't read it, don't eat it!" Anyway, do you really want to stuff your body with a chemical soup?
4. Drink plenty of water. If your mouth and lips are dry, it means you're thirsty.
5. If you have CFS/FMS or adrenal fatigue, enjoy your saltshaker or grinder and add as much salt as your body and taste buds are asking for.

Start with the Basics: A Healthy Diet

Although I strongly recommend taking nutritional supplements to ensure obtaining the necessary nutrients, I want to begin by stressing that a healthy diet is most important. Eat a lot of whole grains, fresh fruits (whole fruit, not fruit juice), and fresh vegetables. Raw vegetables also have enzymes that help boost energy levels.

You do not have to cut out all foods that might be "bad" or eat a diet that is impossible to follow. All you need to do is consume a diet that is reasonably healthy and low in added sugar. The more unprocessed your diet is, the healthier you will be. Your body will tell you what's good for you by making you feel good.

THE PROBLEM WITH SUGAR

I am not concerned with the sugar normally found in food, as in an apple or orange. It is the 140 pounds per person added each year in food processing that is dangerous. In addition to causing people to lose 18 percent of their vitamins and minerals with empty calories, the excess sugar also:

1. Suppresses the immune system. The amount of sugar in one can of soda suppresses immune function by 30 percent for three hours.
2. Stimulates yeast overgrowth. Yeast grows by fermenting sugar, and the yeast says thank you for eating sugar by making trillions of baby yeasties.
3. Amplifies symptoms of hypoglycemia, such as irritability when hungry . . . and the associated need for marriage counseling and divorce lawyers (seriously).

Want to Have Your Cake and Eat It, Too?

Start by cutting out the sugary drinks. Eat an apple or an orange (2 teaspoons of sugar) instead, and enjoy up to an ounce of dark chocolate each day. Though dark chocolate is not low calorie, I consider it to be a health food. That's why I tell people, "Avoid sugar—except for chocolate!"

I think pleasure is good for you. So here are some delicious yet healthy sweet things to enjoy:

- Sugar-free chocolate. Lily's and The Good Chocolate brands are my favorite these days. Russell Stover also has a good line available in most supermarkets and drugstores.
- Instead of sodas, Zevia (available at Safeway or health-food stores) has a whole line of sugar-free sodas that are sweetened with stevia.

Nutritional Support Made Easy

The modern diet is awful. It is appropriately abbreviated as SAD, for the standard American diet. In addition to 18 percent of calories coming from sugar, another 18 percent comes from white flour (which is a nutritional wasteland). Then enough fat is added so that half of what we eat consists of "empty calories," which are basically devoid of vitamins and minerals. Because of this, for the first time in human history, the obese are often malnourished.

With over half of the vitamins and minerals being lost in food processing, it is almost impossible to get the optimal levels you need from an American diet. Therefore I recommend a good multivitamin for pretty much everyone.

I will begin by discussing simple nutritional support to help supply the nutrients we should be getting from our diet. I will then finish the chapter with a discussion of special energy herbals and nutrients made by our bodies specifically to make energy.

If it seems overwhelming, let me give you the bottom line. You'll be able to get most of what you need with one simple drink and two capsules each morning.

WHICH NUTRIENTS DO I NEED?

People often ask me which vitamins or nutrients they need.

The answer? All of them.

Fortunately, this is a lot easier than it sounds.

Whether you have day-to-day fatigue or CFS/FMS, optimizing nutritional supplementation can dramatically improve how you feel. Here's how to make it easy.

Vitamin and Mineral Supplements
The argument that the average modern American does not need vitamin tablets is simply not valid. One study reported in the *American Journal of Clinical Nutrition* showed that fewer than 5 percent of the study participants consumed the recommended daily amounts (RDAs) of all

their needed vitamins and minerals. What is frightening is that this study was conducted on US Department of Agriculture (USDA) research center employees, people who should be especially aware of proper nutrition.

Meanwhile, the news media panders to their processed food and pharmaceutical advertisers by misreporting studies on the effectiveness of multivitamins. The headlines say they don't help. The research they are reporting often shows quite the opposite.

For those who say that you are "just making expensive urine" by taking a multivitamin (because it goes out in the urine), I recommend they consider what would happen if they stopped drinking water—which also "just goes out in their urine."

Making Nutrient Support Simple

In addition to a healthy diet, it is important to get good nutritional support with supplements. To keep it easy, I recommend the Energy Revitalization System vitamin powder made by Enzymatic Therapy. One simple low-cost drink a day replaces more than thirty-five supplement pills (it would take most people over fifty pills), supplying virtually all the vitamins and minerals you should be getting from your diet (the exceptions being iron, potassium, and essential fatty acids). This is much better than a handful of pills. Try it yourself. Prepare to be amazed at how much better you feel.

The best way to mix powders is to put the powder in a dry glass, add 2 to 3 ounces of water, and give it a few stirs *with a fork* till any lumps are gone. Then add another 3 to 5 ounces of water. It's the most worthwhile thirty seconds you'll spend each day!

For those who don't like powders, another excellent multivitamin is called Clinical Essentials by Terry Naturally. This is also geared for people with sensitive stomachs. Either of these will be excellent.

It is helpful to know that any supplement containing B vitamins will turn your urine bright yellow. This is normal and simply shows that you are absorbing the B vitamins well. They come out in the urine *after* they're finished doing their job.

The vitamin powder includes optimal levels of each of the fifty key vitamins, minerals, energy cofactors, and amino acids that you should be getting from your diet.

So, overall, aim to eat whole foods instead of junk, avoid excess sugar, drink plenty of water (or other sugar-free beverages), and take the Energy Revitalization System vitamin powder. I add a 5-gram scoop of SHINE D-Ribose or add the Smart Energy System (see page 72) to the vitamin powder each morning to turbocharge my energy.

See, I told you it would be easy.

Let's take a moment to look at a few other nutrients that can be very helpful in addition to what's in the vitamin powder and Smart Energy. We will begin by discussing deficiencies of nutrients that should be in our food. We will then finish with a discussion of herbals and special nutrients made by our body, which can be dramatically effective at increasing energy.

IRON

Iron is important because an iron level that is too low can cause fatigue, poor immune function, cold intolerance, restless leg syndrome, decreased thyroid function, and poor memory. I routinely recommend that anybody with fatigue or CFS/FMS have their iron level checked by doing a blood test called a ferritin level. Technically, this is normal if it is over 12, a level that, as previously discussed, misses over 90 percent of people with severe iron deficiency. So once again, ignore the normal range and aim to get your ferritin level up over 60 ng/mL.

If your ferritin is elevated, which can also cause FMS, your doctor should determine whether you have a genetic disease of excess iron called hemochromatosis. If caught early, it is easy to treat. If caught late, after causing diabetes and liver failure, it can kill you.

Although cosmetic issues may seem small relative to the debilitating nature of CFS/FMS, they are still important. This includes the severe hair thinning often seen in CFS/FMS. Iron deficiency contributes to hair loss and, according to Cleveland Clinic dermatologists, treatment of iron deficiency is important for restoring hair growth. In their opinion, "Treatment for hair loss is enhanced when iron deficiency, with or without anemia, is treated." They aim to keep the ferritin level over 70 ng/mL, but not higher than 150, as too much iron can also be toxic. Therefore, if you are taking iron, it's good to keep an eye on your ferritin blood levels every three to six months. Especially in men and non-menstruating women. Low thyroid and simply the stress of the CFS/FMS can also contribute to hair loss. When these are treated, most often hair growth resumes after nine months.

Take the iron at bedtime on an empty stomach. Do not take iron supplements within six hours of your thyroid dose, as it blocks thyroid absorption. It is normal for iron to cause constipation and a black stool.

Fortunately, if you take the iron every other day, you get almost as much benefit as taking it daily—with lower side effects. If the ferritin level is under 60 ng/mL, I give 25 to 50 milligrams of iron a day, making sure that the supplement also has at least 60 milligrams of vitamin C and other nutrients to enhance absorption.

The iron supplement that I recommend is called Iron Complex by Integrative Therapeutics (25 milligrams per soft gel). For those who cannot tolerate iron because of upset stomach or constipation, Floradix makes a liquid iron supplement that has 11 milligrams of iron per dose, is well absorbed, and does not upset the stomach.

A final note on iron: I am repeating myself because it is that important. Ferritin levels that are elevated, especially if the iron percent saturation test is over 45 percent, can be dangerous and may reflect a genetic disease called hemochromatosis, which can kill you if missed. So be sure your physician addresses this if your ferritin level is elevated.

New Help for Thinning Hair

Until now, all we could do was optimize nutritional support with the Energy Revitalization System vitamin powder, optimize thyroid function, and make sure that the ferritin blood test for iron was at least 100. Although these frequently help considerably, all too often it is not enough.

Most often, hair loss is caused by a condition called telogen effluvium. This is where a severe stress or infection (such as FMS, any of a number of infections, adverse changes in thyroid hormone levels, or even the stress of modern life) cause many of your hair follicles to all go into the resting (telogen) phase. Then two to three months into this resting phase, the hair falls out, making you want to cry when you look at your hairbrush.

Most often, if one is healthy, the hair will then grow back. But all too often, the hair stays thin.

The good news? Now there is something you can take to help, and people are loving it. It is called Hair Renew by Terry Naturally and contains a number of unique and key nutrients. But what makes it especially powerful is millet seed oil and the herb horsetail, combined with 5,000 µg of biotin and key amino acids.

Horsetail is a unique plant that has immune-supporting, remineralizing, and regenerating effects. It is a rich source of flavonoids, potassium, and silica. Put simply, large amounts of these three are needed for rapidly growing tissue, such as healthy hair and skin. The level of silica in the body decreases with age, which also results in nail and hair brittleness, along with decreased resistance to fungal and bacterial infections.

But especially powerful for hair growth are the components found in millet seed oil. In two studies, this was found to be very effective after three months of use—not just in getting hair out of the telogen phase, but even in people with the most severe health problems.

Eighteen studies have also found biotin to be helpful, especially when illness is contributing to poor hair growth. All these together markedly decrease hair loss over three months, while improving hair thickness and shine.

Got hair thinning? Combine the Energy Revitalization System and Hair Renew for three months. And watch your hair start coming back.

Coenzyme Q10

Coenzyme Q10 is a key energy nutrient. Take 200 milligrams each morning with a meal containing some fat or oil, so you absorb it. A special note: Most cholesterol-lowering drugs deplete coenzyme Q10 and in my experience can cause and worsen fatigue and pain. Anyone taking cholesterol-lowering medications (called statins) should also take 200 milligrams a day of coenzyme Q10.

Fish Oils for Everyone

The two key omega-3 essential fatty acids in fish oil are eicosapentaenoic acid (EPA) and docosahexaenoic acid (DHA), the latter being a major component of brain tissue. Perhaps the old wives' tales were right in calling fish "brain food."

Fish oil essential fatty acid levels are often low in most people, and even worse in those with CFS/FMS. Research shows that supplementation has many benefits. Even in healthy people, fish oil supplements decrease depression and inflammation.

The best way to get these essential fatty acids is by eating three to four servings of a fatty fish each week such as salmon, tuna, or sardines (fried fish does not count). It is also reasonable to supplement with essential fatty acids, and this is part of my daily regimen.

Most brands require taking eight to sixteen fish oil capsules a day to see the results observed in research studies. This is not only irritating and high cost but also causes fish oil burps. I like cats as much as the next guy, but having them follow me around all day waiting for me to burp got annoying.

The good news? Research has shown that a new way to extract and vectorize the fish oil essential fatty acids dramatically increases absorption. So all you need is one tablet a day of Vectomega by EuroPharma instead of eight a day of most fish oils. Out of thousands of natural products added each year, Vectomega won an award as one of the three best new products of the year by New Hope Network.

Special Nutrients and Herbals

DOUBLE YOUR ENERGY IN ONE MINUTE

What if you could double your energy in just one minute each day? Healthfully. At low cost.

You can. Here's my morning combo:

The Energy Revitalization System multinutrient powder supplies fifty key nutrients that should be in our diet and at optimal dosing. But there are six specialized nondiet nutrients and herbals that also powerfully boost energy production. These can easily be found in combination in a product called the Smart Energy System. Consuming these two products, one drink and two capsules, will keep your healthy energy turbocharged all day.

Let's look at the six powerhouses in Smart Energy.

D-RIBOSE: THE NATURAL BODY ENERGIZER

To understand energy production, it helps to look at critical "energy molecules" such as ATP (adenosine triphosphate). These represent the energy currency in your body and are like the paper that money is printed on. You can have all the fuel (calories) you want, but if it cannot be converted to these molecules, it is useless—and simply gets turned into fat.

B vitamins are a key component of many of these molecules. We find that these are helpful, but a key component is missing. In looking at the biochemistry of these energy molecules, we saw that they were also made of two other key components—adenine and ribose. Adenine (which is also called vitamin B4) is plentiful in the body. So we turned our attention to ribose, which is made in our bodies in a slow, laborious process. We found that ribose is low in energy-deficient states, making it hard to get your energy furnaces working again without it.

This was a eureka moment when things came together. Not having ribose would be like trying to build a fire without kindling—nothing would happen. We wondered if giving ribose to people with CFS/FMS, one of the worst energy deficiencies in the world, would jump-start their energy furnaces. The results amazed us.

I am the lead author on two published studies, which included almost three hundred people with CFS/FMS at fifty-four different clinics. Ribose was given at a dose of 5 grams three times a day for three weeks. People reported their energy increased an average of about 61 percent by three weeks. In addition, mental clarity, sleep, and overall well-being improved significantly, while pain levels dropped.

Ribose is available over the counter and is one of the few natural products that started with physicians and then moved into health-food stores.

Let's look at ribose in more detail to see what it does.

The Results of Our Study on Ribose in FMS

In our study, 203 patients completed the three-week treatment trial. D-ribose treatment led to both statistically ($p < .0001$) and clinically highly important *average* improvements in all categories:

- 61.3 percent increase in energy
- 37 percent increase in overall well-being
- 29.3 percent improvement in sleep
- 30 percent improvement in mental clarity
- 15.6 percent decrease in pain

Improvement began in the first week of treatment and continued to increase at the end of the three weeks of treatment. The D-ribose was well tolerated.

Source: Jacob Teitelbaum, Janelle Jandrain, and Ryan McGrew, "Treatment of Chronic Fatigue Syndrome and Fibromyalgia with D-Ribose: An Open-Label, Multicenter Study," *The Open Pain Journal* 5 (2012): 32–37.

D-Ribose Accelerates Energy Recovery

D-ribose (which is what I am referring to when I say ribose) is a simple five-carbon sugar that is found naturally in our bodies. But ribose is not like other toxic sugars, such as table sugar (sucrose), corn sugar (glucose), and fructose (fruit sugar). When we consume ribose, the body recognizes that it is different from other sugars and preserves it for the vital work of actually making the energy molecules that power the heart, muscles, brain, and every other tissue in the body—making it healthy and helpful even for people who can't tolerate sugar.

The amount of ATP we have in our tissues determines whether we will be fatigued or will have the energy we need to live vital, active lives. Ribose provides the key building block of ATP, and the presence of ribose in the cell stimulates the metabolic pathway our bodies use to make this vital compound. If the cell does not have enough ribose, it cannot make ATP. So, when cells and tissues become energy-starved, the availability of ribose is critical to energy recovery.

The Link Between Ribose, Energy, and Fatigue

Two very interesting studies in animals showed how dramatic the effect of ribose could be on energy recovery in fatigued muscle. These studies were conducted by Dr. Ron Terjung, one of the top muscle physiologists in the United States. In their research, Dr. Terjung and his coinvestigators found that ribose administration in fatigued muscle increased the rate of energy recovery by 340 to 430 percent.

Although this groundbreaking research was done in animals, it was instrumental in defining the biochemistry and physiology associated with the use of ribose in overcoming heart and muscle fatigue in humans. But most of us with CFS and FMS are neither top athletes nor research animals, so the question most of us wanted explained remained unanswered: "How will ribose affect me?"

Research in ribose and CFS/FMS began with a case study that was published in the prestigious journal *Pharmacotherapy* in 2004. This case study told the story of a veterinary surgeon diagnosed with fibromyalgia. For months, this dedicated doctor found herself becoming more and more fatigued, with pain becoming so profound that she was finally unable to stand during surgery. As a result, she was forced to all but give up the practice she loved.

Upon hearing that a clinical study on ribose in congestive heart failure was underway at the university where she worked, she asked if she could try the ribose to see if it might help her overcome the mind-numbing fatigue she experienced from her disease. After three weeks of ribose therapy, she was back in the operating room, practicing normally, with no muscle pain or stiffness, and without the fatigue that had kept her bedridden for many months.

Being a doctor, she was skeptical, not believing that a simple sugar could have such a dramatic effect on her condition. Within two weeks of stopping the ribose therapy, however, she was out of the operating room and back in bed. So, to again test the theory, she began ribose therapy a second time. The result was similar to her first experience, and she was back doing surgery in days. After yet a third round of stopping (with the return of symptoms) and starting the ribose therapy (with the reduction of symptoms), she was convinced, and she has been on ribose therapy since that time. This was the start of countless numbers of people around the world getting their life back with ribose.

Interestingly, one of our study patients had an abnormal heart rhythm called atrial fibrillation. Ribose is outstanding in the treatment of heart disease as well because it restores energy production in the heart muscle. Because of this, it was not surprising that this man's atrial fibrillation also went away with the ribose treatment, and he was able to stop his heart medications as well. It is common that people with even crippling heart disease feel dramatically better after six weeks on ribose. If you know anybody with heart disease (including heart failure, angina, and abnormal rhythms), have them use the recipe below. It can markedly improve heart function efficiency. After six weeks, they will often have their lives back.

A Recipe for Optimizing Heart Function

Heart disease is a common cause of fatigue. Whether the problem is heart failure, angina, or abnormal heart rhythms, increasing heart muscle efficiency can result in remarkable and measurable improvement. It can also be lifesaving. I recommend the following for heart health:

- **Ribose:** Take 5 grams three times a day for six weeks, then twice a day.

- **Coenzyme Q10**: Take 200 milligrams a day. Take it with a meal that has oil in it.
- **Energy Revitalization System vitamin powder:** Drink one-half to one scoop a day.
- **Acetyl-L-carnitine:** Take 500 milligrams three times a day for six weeks, then once a day.
- **Hawthorn Phytosome by Enzymatic Therapy:** For severe cases, take two capsules three times a day plus magnesium orotate 3,000 milligrams a day.

Use the above with the okay of your holistic physician. Two cautions: People taking the blood thinner Coumadin (warfarin) *must* get their physician's okay before adding any supplement or medication, and magnesium must be used under a doctor's supervision in those with kidney failure.

I recommend using SHINE D-Ribose to optimize energy. This contains the Bioenergy form used in the study, as I have heard back from people that they sometimes don't get the same results with generic forms. But the Bioenergy form was quite expensive, so I decided to bottle it, cut out the middleman, and cut the price in half. Each scoop contains 5 grams. For most people, a scoop each morning, or even twice a day, will give a dramatic energy boost within a month. For very severe fatigue, I begin with a 5-gram scoop three times a day for three to six weeks. To make things easier, the new Smart Energy System includes 5 grams of the Bioenergy ribose per scoop, along with five other key energy boosters.

But first a bit of background: I have a special interest in medical anthropology, feeling that there is so much we can learn from history. In fact, in medical school my nickname was "The Ghost." Why? I could often be found at two in the morning going through old journals from the medical school library.

My routine was to select four issues of the same journal—one from one hundred years ago, one from fifty years ago, one from twenty years ago, and a current one. Then I would scan through them to give me a perspective of what was happening in medicine over time. As a medical student, I was amazed to read studies written by the professors my textbooks were named after.

Doing this also showed me very clearly when the pharmaceutical industry had its rise and appeared to suppress pretty much all other research except for surgery. This was quite an eye-opener for a young med student. Of course, now you may be starting to see how I got my college nickname of "Rambling Jack." So here's where I am going with all of this: There are herbals that have been incredibly popular for literally millennia that have gone by the wayside.

Why?

Largely because mass farming and harvesting have bred plants that have lost most of their potency and effectiveness. So the products no longer work. But here's a secret: There are a few forms of these herbs that do. And they can rock your world.

Ashwagandha (KSM-66)

Ashwagandha is the most popular herb in Ayurvedic medicine, the healing art that stems from India. But again, the way the herbs are farmed and processed often destroys their potency.

My friend Chris Kilham (see www.medicinehunter.com) is one of the world's most respected herbalists. He travels all around the world hunting new herbs and making sure old ones are managed properly. He turned me onto the KSM-66 form of ashwagandha, and I am very thankful to him for this. This is the main form being used in research now, because they have taken measures to restore its old potency.

Here's what the (mostly placebo-controlled) research using specifically the KSM-66 ashwagandha shows. This ashwagandha is remarkable when it comes to:

- **Mood and stress relief.** In a placebo-controlled study, depression, anxiety, and stress were reduced significantly ($p<0.001$) by 77 percent, 76 percent, and 64 percent respectively after two months.
- **Memory and cognition.** Short-term memory and brain processing speed were improved.
- **Thyroid function.** Free T3 levels went up 47 percent and free T4 level increased 23 percent, which may account for the weight loss.
- **Muscle mass and endurance.** Exercise ability and endurance measured by the maximum oxygen consumption (VO2 max) in healthy athletic adults increased 12 percent and 14 percent respectively at Day 56 and Day 84. It also resulted in a 139 percent increase in muscle strength for the bench press, and a muscle size increase of 8 percent, 17 percent, and 3 percent for thigh, arm, and chest respectively.

- **Sleep.** It helped people fall asleep more quickly and stay asleep more efficiently.
- **Female sexual health.** Scores for arousal, lubrication, orgasm, and satisfaction improved significantly, by 62 percent, 59 percent, 82 percent, and 62 percent respectively.
- **Male libido.** Testosterone levels increased 17 percent; sexual fantasy/functions, arousal, orgasm, and sexual drive improved significantly, by 4 percent, 18 percent, 6 percent, and 11 percent respectively. I guess it's best for the man and woman to use it together, so they can keep up with each other. But careful if you're not looking to have children yet, because . . .
- **Male sperm count.** Sperm count increased 167 percent; sperm motility increased 57 percent.
- **Weight management.** KSM-66 ashwagandha supplementation resulted in a 3 percent reduction in body weight. That translates to losing 4.5 pounds in someone who weighs 150 pounds. It decreased body fat an average of 16 percent—a nice side benefit.

I think you're starting to see why ashwagandha is the most popular Ayurvedic herb for the 1.3 billion people living in India.

RHODIOLA

Rhodiola rosea, also called golden root, grows in arctic and mountain regions throughout Europe, Asia, and America. It has been an accepted medicine in Russia since 1969 for the treatment of fatigue and infectious, psychiatric, and neurologic conditions, and as a psychostimulant to increase memory, attention span, and productivity in healthy individuals.

Research shows pronounced anti-stress effects, enhanced physical work and exercise performance, increased muscle strength, and reduction in mental fatigue. It seems to work by supporting hypothalamic function as well as the brain transmitters serotonin, dopamine, norepinephrine, and endorphin. All of these tend to be low in fibromyalgia, and many in the population in general.

I first became aware of the research when I stumbled across studies being done by the Russian space program. They found that Rhodiola markedly improved stamina in the cosmonauts. Many with day-to-day down-to-earth fatigue and even fibromyalgia have found the same thing.

SCHISANDRA

Numerous studies, although many still in the animal study phase, show widespread benefits of the Schisandra plant. Especially important are its mitochondrial protection and insulin function.

GREEN TEA EXTRACT (*CAMELLIA SINENSIS*)

We've all heard about the health benefits of green tea. Many if not most of the benefits come from a component called epigallocatechin gallate (EGCg), which has very potent antioxidant properties. Use supplements that have at least 35 percent EGCg. Here are just a few of the studies:

- **Exercise endurance.** Fourteen men who consumed green tea extract for four weeks increased their running distance by 11 percent. It is especially potent at protecting against the free radicals caused by exercise.
- **Insulin sensitivity.** Reduced total cholesterol by 4 percent and LDL cholesterol by 4 percent; lowered blood pressure (only in people with high blood pressure).
- **May lower weight.** Thermogenesis is the process by which your body burns calories to digest food and produce heat. Green tea has been shown to boost this process by making your body more effective at burning calories, which can lead to weight loss. Healthy men burned 4 percent more calories during the twenty-four hours after consuming a green tea extract.
- **Younger skin.** Taken by mouth or even topically, green tea extract seems to help prevent skin conditions like loss of skin elasticity, inflammation, and premature aging. Therefore, it is often added to cosmetics.

GLYCYRRHIZIN (LICORICE EXTRACT)

Glycyrrhizin slows down the elimination of your body's stress hormone, called cortisol. This can make it dramatically effective for helping adrenal fatigue.

My goal is to make optimal supplementation easy and very affordable. To help with this, optimal levels and forms of ribose, ashwagandha, Rhodiola, Schisandra, green tea extract, and glycyrrhizin (licorice) can all be found combined in a simple but very powerful mix called Dr. Teitelbaum's Smart Energy System (available at www.endfatigue.com). Taking one scoop and two capsules in the morning, with an optional second dose at lunch, can change your life.

Though it doesn't contain everything in the Smart Energy and Energy Revitalization System, the Clinical Essentials Multivitamin plus Adaptra (a mix of Rhodiola and ashwagandha) are also superb for those who don't like supplement drinks.

For most of you, simply taking the morning drink and two capsules (combining the Energy Revitalization System and Smart Energy System) will leave your healthy energy feeling turbocharged all day. In many people, it will more than double their energy after one month—in under one minute a day.

Here's What I Take Each Morning

1. The Energy Revitalization System and the Smart Energy System: I add one scoop of each to 6 to 8 ounces of water and stir it with a fork.

2. Vectomega: I take one each morning for omega-3 support.

3. Coenzyme Q10: I take 200 milligrams with my breakfast.

4. CuraMed: I take 750 milligrams each morning, not for any problem I'm having but simply because the research shows its health benefits to be totally incredible. These include decreasing inflammation and cancer risk, helping mood, and more.

5. HRG80 Red Ginseng: I take one daily.

So one drink and a few pills, and my energy is flying high all day. This is with a work, travel, and writing schedule that would leave most people's head spinning.

Two More Amazing Herbals

Ginseng: The Asian Miracle Recovers

For over a millennium, ginseng has been the most popular herb in China and much of Asia. Unfortunately, the overharvesting of wild ginseng led to it becoming insanely expensive. The newer farmed ginsengs just didn't work as well, so its popularity started to wane.

Old wild ginseng produces over fifty different ginsenosides as a protective response to insect attacks and difficult weather, but these are usually not found in farmed ginseng. And the ginsenosides they produce are poorly absorbed by humans unless converted into "rare" ginsenosides.

But now, a unique new farming technique that reproduces the plant's challenges faced in the wild has allowed grown ginseng to have the same active component profile as the old wild plants—without the high pesticide levels found in most ginsengs—creating powerful new health possibilities.

Key Effects of Rare Ginsenosides

There are over fifty active ginsenosides. The key ones are found in red ginseng, which is made from the whole root and is then steamed. But these then need to be converted to what are called rare (or noble) ginsenosides to be able to be absorbed and active. Unfortunately, the levels of these in current farmed ginseng is very low. So, they can be helpful, but nowhere near as much as the old wild ginseng.

Here are ten of the key actions of ginseng:

1. Markedly improves energy production and decreases pain. This was shown in several studies using both healthy people as well as those with CFS and fibromyalgia as a model.
2. Markedly improves the ability to handle stress. Ginseng acts as an adaptogen, like Rhodiola, to balance the body, moving things in the direction needed instead of only increasing or decreasing a process. So for adrenal issues, for example, adaptogens can help whether cortisol is high or low.
3. Is anticancer.
4. Decreases inflammation.
5. Addresses a key component of pain called microglial activation (the cause of central sensitization pain); also acts as an NMDA receptor antagonist.
6. Helps memory in general and may even help in Alzheimer's.
7. Increases insulin sensitivity, which also increases energy levels.
8. Increases erectile function and sexual pleasure (part of what made it so popular in China).
9. Decreases lung inflammation.
10. Even helps hangover.

Unfortunately, the old potent ginseng is hard to come by. Farmed ginseng root goes for $50 a pound; wild ginseng often sells for over $700 a pound.

HRG80 to the Rescue

The potency of wild ginseng can now be affordably found in HRG80 Red Ginseng by Terry Naturally. They have one form for energy, and another one that also has been shown to help male sexual function. I am so impressed with the research on it that it is the topic of my tenth book. Read *The Healing Power of Red Ginseng* for more information.

CURCUMIN

In India, this isn't even used so much as an herb; rather, it is simply a staple of the diet, coming from turmeric. When I went to India to learn more about curcumin, it was fun to look in the supermarkets. They would have over thirty large barrels of different kinds of turmeric powder.

One of the biggest frustrations in my forty years of being a doctor has been curcumin. There have been over a thousand tantalizing studies showing an incredible array of health benefits, including prevention and treatment of cancer, lower risk of Alzheimer's, marked anti-inflammatory properties, dramatic pain relief, being more effective than sertraline (Zoloft) for depression, and even helping diabetes.

Unfortunately, the amount that you needed to take to see these effects was so high that basically you had to be eating an Indian curry diet for three meals a day, which I did while I was in India—and I must admit I was a very regular guy.

Before you run out and get some, it is sobering to look at a few numbers:

- Only about 2 percent of turmeric is curcumin, so it takes fifty capsules of turmeric to get one capsule of curcumin.
- Curcumin is poorly absorbed. To get the effective amount used in the studies takes seven to fourteen capsules a day.

Then research showed that by adding in the turmeric's essential oil, called turmerone, absorption of the curcumin was increased 693 percent.

So suddenly one capsule replaced seven. This new form, available as CuraMed (and for pain as Curamin), changed everything. Now one capsule was as or more effective than 350 capsules of turmeric.

Suddenly, over a thousand studies could now actually help people. I was so elated that I was going to write a book on it, but my friend and cancer researcher Ajay Goel, PhD, beat me to it, saving me a lot of time. I happily recommend his book, *Curcumin: Nature's Answer to Cancer and Other Chronic Diseases.*

For Athletes

Forget steroids. Here is an amazing (and legal) mix to dramatically increase endurance and performance:

1. The Energy Revitalization System multinutrient powder

2. The Smart Energy System

3. Recovery Factors

Recovery Factors is a unique porcine peptide support formula. It is discussed in detail in Chapter 17, "Nutrition Intensive Care." I recently completed a study on this and the results, which can be seen at www.recoveryfactors.com, are very powerful. In the study, we used four tablets twice a day for maintenance.

Here is information from Emile Kok, who has had over a decade's experience helping thousands of people with the Recovery Factors supplement:

> The most we have given anyone was forty tablets in one day, given to an ultra-marathon runner before and during a 110-kilometer ultra-marathon in Vietnam. He improved his time from the previous year by one and a half hours and had no pain the next day. Had he had six or eight tablets, I'm pretty sure he would not have experienced that level of benefit—it gets used up under severe stress, duress, or energy expenditure and in those cases higher dosages are required.
>
> We have what we call a sports protocol, which is to take half the dosage twenty minutes to half an hour before exercise and half immediately after . . . which then increases both performance and recovery. If there is a lot of endurance required, typically an additional half dosage would be taken halfway through the event

(especially in the case of a marathon or cycle race), which gives the athletes "a fresh pair of legs."

A top cyclist who won't cycle without the product anymore says that the lactate threshold changed for him and he is able to push harder than before.

For the athletes out there, I invite you to give this trio of supplements six weeks—and prepare to be amazed! Please email me at fatiguedoc@gmail.com if you would like to share your experience.

Important Points

1. Eat whole foods instead of processed foods whenever it's convenient.
2. Remove sugar and other sweeteners from your diet. Stevia, a sweet-tasting herb, is a healthy substitute.
3. Take one scoop of the Energy Revitalization System multivitamin powder plus the Smart Energy System daily. Put both in a glass, add 8 ounces of water, and stir with a fork. This will supply more than fifty key nutrients and herbals in one drink and two capsules, and replaces more than forty-five capsules of supplements. Prepare to be amazed!
4. Take HRG80 Red Ginseng.
5. Treat a too-low iron level with an iron supplement.
6. If you have dry eyes, dry mouth, depression, or inflammation, take fish oil (Vectomega supplies all you need in one tablet a day).
7. If you are on cholesterol medications (called statins) or have severe fatigue, add coenzyme Q10. Take 200 milligrams a day with a meal containing oil.

Exercise: Does Sex Count?

5

BFF Summary

1. Find a way to exercise that feels good. Do it with a friend on a regular schedule.
2. "No pain, no gain" is stupid.
3. Start slowly. A little bit can go a long way. See how many steps you are taking each day, and add about fifty steps every few days as is comfortable.
4. Get an exercise app like Fitbit, and slowly increase the lengths of your walks as feels best, aiming for six thousand to ten thousand steps a day. Take your time reaching this goal—there is no hurry.
5. Have a regularly scheduled exercise routine—with a friend.
6. For those with CFS and fibromyalgia, however, the rules are different and will be discussed in Chapter 18, "Exercise Intensive Care."

If exercise was a pill, everyone would take it.
That's because exercise can effectively help prevent or treat just about *every* health problem out there and is critical for optimizing vitality. Because our body has a "use it or lose it" approach to efficiency, the more exercise you do, the better conditioned your body will

be—and more energy you will have. (For those with CFS/FMS, however, the rules are different and will be discussed in Chapter 18, "Exercise Intensive Care.")

The need for exercise is obvious, so mostly I'm going to focus on some simple tips to make exercising easier. Let's start with the basic rules:

- **Rule #1: "No pain, no gain" is stupid.** "No pain, no gain." You've heard that slogan, of course. It reflects the belief that unless exercise *hurts*, it's not doing its job. I have another slogan I want you to say to yourself instead: "Pain is insane." "No pain, no gain" is stupid. Pain is your body's way of telling you, "Don't do that." Unless you're conditioning for highly competitive sports, exercise should be virtually pain-free.
- **Rule #2: Start slowly: A little bit can go a long way.** A common exercise error: You start a new exercise program by doing way too much, way too soon. People who do this usually *stop* exercising quickly as well—because they hurt. The body likes *gradual* change, so it can easily and comfortably adapt to new situations. So remember: A little movement is better than no movement at all. Even twenty to forty minutes of walking a day can make a massive difference.
- **Rule #3: Find an exercise you enjoy, or you won't stay with it.** Find an activity *you* love to do, look forward to, and that fits into your routine. Whether you're doing a dance class, going for a walk in the park, doing yoga, or even shopping, doing something you love makes it more likely that you'll stick with it.
- **Rule #4: Have a regularly scheduled exercise routine—with a friend.** Meet with a friend to do the exercise. The obligation of meeting somebody means that you're also more likely to show up.

Your Low-Cost Fitness Coach

It's funny. In the last edition we were talking about pedometers. The technology has changed so much that it feels like we were talking about rotary phones. Now we have fitness apps that can act like your exercise coach. Here are a few of the best:

- **Fitbit.** This is a device you wear like a watch that not only counts steps but monitors calories burned, duration, heart rate, sleep, and many other helpful measures. Likely the most popular app on the market.
- **Fitness Buddy.** This workout app will count steps and offer exercise routines and even meal plans.
- **Body Space.** Can't find a friend to work out with? No problem. This app is like an exercise Facebook, connecting you with an online exercise community.
- **Charity Miles.** Feeling generous? This app will donate money to charity when you run, bike, or even walk. So far, they have given over $2.5 million!

It is not necessary to push for high intensity. It's better to simply aim to walk six thousand to ten thousand steps a day (this is around three to five miles). Walking is a great exercise, especially if done outdoors in the sunshine.

It also is enlightening to see where you're starting from. When I first put on a pedometer and then excitedly checked it at the end of the day, it showed I had taken a whopping 687 steps for the whole day! This got me off the couch and out on the walking trail. By taking a half hour and doing a quick two- to three-mile walk, I added four thousand to six thousand steps a day—leaving me a whole lot less embarrassed.

Bottom line: Fitness apps show you exactly how much you're walking, so you get instant feedback and can set a goal to walk more.

And yes, sex is one of many good exercises. It also stimulates growth hormone, appropriately called the "fountain of youth" hormone.

6 Emotional and Spiritual Optimization: A Critical Foundation for Overall Health

BFF Summary

1. Our minds have no idea what is authentic to us—who we are and what we really want. Our minds simply know what we were taught to do to get approval.
2. But our feelings are tied directly to our authenticity. If something feels good, it is generally what our soul/psyche really want. If something feels bad, it is not authentic to us and generally reflects a false belief that we have about something.
3. Let what feels good (not what you *think* feels good) be how you set your life's GPS. Once you program in the "address" that feels good, then your mind, like the GPS, is brilliant at getting you there.
4. A simple three-step program will get you there.
   A. Fully feel whatever you are feeling. When it no longer feels good, then it's time to let the feeling go. It is not critical to understand why you feel that way. Simply feel the feelings.
   B. Make life a no-fault system. As long as we are blaming somebody else, we are giving up our power to fix the problem. In addition, most of the time we are projecting our own self-blame onto others.
   C. Choose to only keep your attention on things that feel good.
5. For those of you interested in exploring this further, I invite you to read my e-book *Three Steps to Happiness: Healing Through Joy.*

6. Learn to forgive yourself and others. I am happy to recommend an excellent book *The Magic Words: Your Pathway to Peace, Joy, and Happiness* by my friend Jon Lovgren.

In my forty-two years as a physician, I have learned something very important, something we were never taught in medical school. Part of healing from any illness sometimes includes a key piece of information. It is important to understand how an illness may actually help an individual. This seems an odd concept, but it really makes good sense once we look at it.

I have routinely found that if I help somebody get well just so they can go back to what made them sick in the first place, they will usually get a new illness. For example, their illness took them out of a very toxic job situation; then they got well while at home with their kids as they'd always wanted. Then when they reentered the workforce and found themselves back in a job they hated, their pain and symptoms returned.

Put simply, an important part of both recovering from illnesses and staying healthy is being authentic to yourself.

Claiming Your Authenticity

A simple insight is key to this: Our minds have no idea who we are. Although an amazing part of ourselves, our minds are simply the product of how they were programmed by society, news media, parents, government, friends, and so on. But the simple truth is that our minds have no idea what is authentic to us—who we are and what we really want. They simply know what we were taught to do to get approval.

But our feelings are tied directly to our authenticity. If something feels good, it is generally what our soul and psyche really want. If something feels bad, it is not authentic to us and generally reflects a false belief that we have about something.

Think of it using the analogy of a GPS. If you tell the GPS to take you where you want to go, it has no idea. Keep asking, and an advanced GPS may look up what is most popular for everybody else or what their advertisers recommend.

The GPS is like your mind. It has no idea where you want to go.

Instead, see how things feel. Let what feels good (not what you *think* feels good) be how you set your life's GPS. Once you program in the "address" that feels good, then your mind, like the GPS, is brilliant at getting you there.

It is critical, as Socrates said, to "know thyself."

As you get to know yourself, I will add in two other qualifiers in following your feelings:

- Don't do anything to hurt anybody else. In the short term, you may confuse the feeling of wanting to hit somebody over the head with a two-by-four with actually doing it. There are many times this *idea* feels good. But as you get to know yourself, you'll find that doing so never does.
- See how it works out for you. For example, running up your credit cards or bingeing on high-sugar foods may feel good in the short term but not so much in the long term.

You may be shocked as you discover who you really are. Still not convinced? If I'm right, you'll find yourself healthy and happy. If not, the worst-case scenario is you'll have lived a life that feels good.

Three Steps to Happiness

A simple three-step program will get you there. A little bit before the new millennium, I wrote a simple book to help guide the people I treat called *Three Steps to Happiness: Healing Through Joy.* I did a small print run of six thousand copies. This quickly sold out and I moved on to other books. About ten years ago, I found used copies of the book selling on Amazon for about $300. So, I put it out again as a simple $10 e-book, but here's the gist of it.

FULLY FEEL WHATEVER YOU ARE FEELING

When it no longer feels good, then it's time to let the feeling go. How about feelings that feel bad? Like anger or grief?

You'll be surprised at how good these can feel. Just ask my wife. She can vouch for how much fun I have during a good self-righteous hissy fit! Even grieving can be a healing process. But when the emotion stops feeling good, that means it's done and it's now time to let go of it.

It is important to realize that all feelings are valid. But what we think is causing the feeling usually has very little to do with what's really going on. The event we're tagging as the *cause* for our feeling was usually just the trigger. The depth of the feelings often relates to things that happened decades ago and often from a mix of numerous events.

Feelings don't necessarily need to be understood and certainly not solved or fixed. They simply need to be felt. Simply feel them and then let go of them.

We do not see things as they are; we see things as we are.

—Talmud

MAKE LIFE A NO-FAULT SYSTEM

As long as we are blaming somebody else, we are giving up our power to fix the problem. In addition, most of the time we are projecting our own self-blame onto others.

Want a trick so you can tell when you are doing this? Next time you get really ticked off at somebody or something and find yourself angrily pointing your finger, saying, "You [fill in the blank]," take note of this old Chinese expression: "When you are pointing at someone with one finger, you are pointing at yourself with three fingers." Notice where the bottom three fingers of your hand are pointing.

Then take a time-out and consider if what you are saying about the other person is really the truth about yourself. That you may be selfish, inconsiderate, arrogant, or any of the other things we project out onto other people. Then I invite you to find the part of yourself that is that way and love it unconditionally.

Why? Because I guarantee you it serves you to have that part of yourself. It may not be best for that part to always be active, but there are times that you really need it. For example, another description for selfish would be "personally responsible." You'll find that most people who call you selfish simply want your stuff for themselves, which is . . . selfish. Give it when it feels good to do so. Say no when it doesn't. And be okay with asking and having others say no as well.

After years of claiming and then unconditionally loving every part of yourself that arises, you will find that a remarkable thing happens. You will find that you totally and completely unconditionally love yourself. And others. Then you finally let love in from everywhere, and never have to fear losing love again.

There are six parts to the no-fault system:

- No blame
- No fault
- No guilt
- No judgment
- No comparisons
- No expectations

All these apply to yourself as well as others. So, don't feel guilty when you find yourself blaming somebody.

These six parts will not only result in reclaiming your power and becoming whole but also put you in the moment of *now*, where everything is really happening.

When you are pointing at someone with one finger, you are pointing at yourself with three fingers.

—Old Chinese Proverb

CHOOSE TO ONLY FOCUS ON THE THINGS THAT FEEL GOOD
You may say that you are ignoring reality when you are doing so. But let me offer a thought: Although the earth is one big stage, there are over seven billion movies going on simultaneously, with everyone being the star of their own movie. And the scriptwriter.

Ignoring the things that don't feel good is like going to a buffet and simply not picking those foods you don't like. Instead of constantly putting the food in your mouth and screaming at the management, "How dare you have this horrible food there!"

It also doesn't mean being uninvolved. It will feel good to be involved in righting injustices that matter to you, but only when you are doing so in a way that actually helps (although sometimes it does feel good to simply have a good hissy fit).

As you choose to only focus on the things in life, or in other people, that feel good, you will find an amazing thing happens. Over time, only those things start to show up in your "movie."

For those of you interested in exploring this further, I invite you to read my e-book *Three Steps to Happiness: Healing Through Joy.*

Forgiveness: A Key Part of Healing

There is an old quote that says, "Resentment is like swallowing poison and waiting for the other person to die."

God knows that people with CFS/FMS have a lot to be angry about. And it is healthy to feel the anger, but then, when it no longer feels good, it's time to let it go.

Meanwhile, it's not only people with CFS/FMS who have a lot to be angry about. Here is something interesting that I've observed: Humanity is going through a major period of awakening.

As we wake, we are getting glimmers of how broken some of our institutions are, including medicine, politics, education, and economics. Many of us are frustrated over our seeming inability to effect the changes we know are needed to truly change these institutions, and even changing our individual lives requires changing ourselves.

Doing so easily and quickly is the gift of an old Hawaiian technique called Ho'oponopono. As you do it, you will find yourself, and then the world around you, changing ever more deeply.

How can this be?

As I mentioned, each of us is the star of life's vast movie. By our choices and our actions (or all too often simply our reactions), we are both writing and producing the script in each moment. When we feel powerless, we are doing this by reacting unconsciously.

It is by becoming conscious that we reclaim wholeness and thus our individual power. We do this in several ways. One is by learning to unconditionally love and accept all the parts of ourselves. This requires self-forgiveness and forgiveness of others.

But here is the shocking truth: Forgiving others is mostly about forgiving ourselves. Self-forgiveness for feeling weak and powerless to say no, as has so often has been the story of our lives in fibromyalgia. For being afraid of intimacy. For feeling sexual. For wanting more. Even for beating ourselves up for being in pain.

All our perceived injuries, and the associated hurts that we carry, in truth come from how these things leave us feeling about ourselves. And it is in forgiving ourselves that we come to be able to love every part of ourselves. Then we realize that there is nothing left about the other person for us to forgive.

Then, when we have forgiven and lovingly owned all parts of ourselves, we truly step into the power that is wholeness. What others think about us is no longer important. Instead of guiding our lives by trying to please everybody else, we learn to tune into what feels good to us. Rather than doing what everyone else has told us that we should do to make them happy. In a word, we become authentic.

People with CFS/FMS have found that when they do this, the pain starts to dissipate. The physical and other cures start to flow naturally and easily into your life.

But how can we learn to forgive ourselves? In fact, how can we even become aware of the deep unconscious forces within us that shape our personal reality? We can try decades of psychotherapy, but this only takes people so far, and usually nowhere near far enough.

Now, ancient Hawaiian tradition offers us a simple and remarkably powerful tool. Simply repeat the four lines below in your mind when anger or other uncomfortable feelings seem to have hold over you.

These four lines make up Ho'oponopono (called "doing Pono"). As you repeat them in your mind, you'll find that what underlies your uncomfortable feelings will start coming to the surface in layers. Then, as if by magic, they start resolving and disappearing. It may seem unlikely that this is possible, but it is. You will see as you do it. You'll also start to understand how the sweet and beautiful Hawaiian aloha spirit came to be.

As you learn and practice Ho'oponopono, you will find yourself moving into self-awareness, self-acceptance, and self-love. Your life will change—dramatically, including your relationships, institutions, and, eventually, the world itself.

How to Do Pono

I am happy to recommend an excellent book called *The Magic Words: Your Pathway to Peace, Joy, and Happiness* by my friend Jon Lovgren. Using this simple technique cured his daughter's FMS, so helping those with this illness is near and dear to his heart.

Ho'oponopono simply consists of repeating these four lines in your mind when you have uncomfortable feelings. You are saying these to your-self, not the other person. Because at the end of the day all forgiveness is, in truth, self-forgiveness.

Simply repeat in your mind:

I love you.
I am sorry.
Please forgive me.
Thank you.

Repeat until the uncomfortable feelings resolve. It will leave you with a new understanding and vision of things.

LEARNING AUTHENTICITY, HOW TO BE HAPPY, AND FORGIVE-ness will change your life.

7 Making This All Simple: The Tune-Up Docs Program

BFF Summary

-A simple, free ten-minute quiz at www.tuneupdocs.com will analyze your symptoms and even pertinent lab tests, if available. It will then apply the key principles discussed in the previous chapters to let you know exactly what is triggering your fatigue and how to optimize *your* energy and overall vitality.

---

*T*he last few years may as well have written the obituary for the yearly medical checkup, though this has been largely ignored by the news and medical media. These annual evaluations were geared to seeing if you had "it" yet—"it" being some illness that is scary and expensive to evaluate and treat.

The message that yearly physicals should RIP has been resisted by many physician organizations who are finding that a big part of their revenue stream is disappearing, but it is what the research is showing. For example:

1. **Screening mammography.** An excellent study in *The New England Journal of Medicine* found that this test does not decrease mortality

from breast cancer. Rather it simply results in dramatic overdiagnosis, which results in women undergoing additional testing, increasing expenses, discomfort, and anxiety.

2. **Prostate-specific antigen (PSA) testing.** The test's developer, pathologist Richard J. Ablin, has called routine PSA screening a "public health disaster." The US Preventive Services Task Force (USPSTF) "recommends against prostate-specific antigen (PSA)–based screening for prostate cancer." It gives this test a grade of D. Looking at the actual statistics is sobering.

It is estimated that for every 1,000 men who undergo PSA testing, 240 will have a positive result and 100 will have a positive biopsy. Of those with positive biopsy results, 20.7 to 50.4 percent will actually have indolent disease that never advances or metastasizes. But 80 will opt for definitive treatment with surgery or radiotherapy. Following treatment, 50 of these men will experience long-term erectile dysfunction and 15, long-term urinary incontinence. While 1.3 deaths from prostate cancer will be prevented, 5 will still die from the disease despite having undergone treatment, plus any deaths from treatment, which are not tallied.

3. **Thyroid nodule screening.** And the list goes on and on . . .

What screening has withstood the benefits of scientific testing and time?

- Blood pressure and diabetes screening
- Glaucoma screening
- Colonoscopy (get one every ten years after age fifty)

4. **Pap testing.** Every three years from age 21 to 65.

Almost nobody comes away from their yearly physical actually feeling better, except perhaps some relief knowing they don't have cancer. But a phoenix is rising from the ashes of the yearly checkup. People are starting to realize that they can *feel* better. That the American myth of "aging isn't for sissies" is simply that. A false myth.

The new reality, which holistic physicians have known for decades, is that our job is not only to help people recover from illness but, perhaps more important, to help people prevent the illnesses in the first place, while creating optimal vitality. Most doctors know pieces of this puzzle, but they haven't yet organized them into a quick and highly effective form.

The good news? It's easy. Here's how.

Tune-Up Docs: A Ten-Point Program

There is a quick, free, and simple online questionnaire that you can do, where you check off what symptoms you have. This will quickly assess each of the categories below.

Then it will outline a simple approach, most of it nonprescription that will optimize the ten areas below. It's really that simple. The free quiz can be found at www.tuneupdocs.com.

These are the areas that are assessed:

1. Sleep
    A. Insomnia
    B. Sleep apnea
    C. Restless legs

2. Hormones
    A. Thyroid
    B. Adrenal
    C. Estrogen, progesterone, and testosterone (libido)
    D. Bladder and prostate

3. Microbial imbalance
    A. Sinus
    B. Candida

4. Energy
5. Overall nutritional support
6. Digestion
7. Mood
8. Cognitive function
9. Pain
10. Heart function

It's as easy as can be!

PART TWO

Getting
Pain-Free—Now!

BFF Summary

1. Pain is not an outside invader. Rather, it is like the oil light on your body's dashboard, telling you something needs attention. If you put oil in the car, the oil light goes out. If you give the body what it needs, the pain goes away.
2. There are ten main kinds of pain, both in the general population and in fibromyalgia. We will discuss each one and how to make it go away.
3. I would note that opioids are less toxic than chronic pain. Fortunately, by treating the root cause of pain, most people can get pain-free without opiates. But for those in need of them, they can be a godsend when used properly.

*I*n my experience having treated thousands of people with severe chronic pain, virtually all pain can be effectively eliminated or controlled. The problem is not lack of effective treatments, but rather a lack of physician education.

Unless there is something that can be operated on, most physicians' entire pain management training consists of:

1. Give arthritis medications (like ibuprofen), antidepressants or tranquilizers (especially in women), or simple pain relievers like acetaminophen.

If their training is "advanced," this may include epilepsy drugs (like gabapentin).

2. If the patient doesn't have cancer, don't use narcotics.

In real life, that's basically it. Most physicians do not know how to do much of a pain exam. Even fewer know how to do a muscle exam (despite most pain being muscular). And they are not aware of the research that shows that, for most pain, what is seen on the X-rays usually has little nothing to do with what is causing the pain. But since they don't know how to do a pain exam, they rely on the X-rays anyway.

For example, studies show that radiologists cannot distinguish who has back pain from who doesn't based on X-rays, although they almost always read out the report making it sound like your back is a disaster zone. This is because, being an upright species, virtually everybody has wear and tear in their spine by the time they are thirty years old. This is normal. Usually, though, this is not the cause of your pain. Your physician may blame the pain on the X-ray findings anyway. Research showed the same thing with CT scans of the jaw joint for TMJ.

So, most doctors truly have no idea how to diagnose or effectively treat pain. The result? One-third of Americans suffer *needlessly* with chronic pain. But once you understand what pain is, you will be able to make it go away.

Pain: The Oil Light on Your Body's Dashboard

Unlike infections, pain is not an outside invader. Rather, it is like the red warning light on your body's dashboard saying that something needs attention. But without having an owner's manual to explain what your body needs, it just gets very annoying.

Once you look at the owner's manual, it becomes clear what's going on and how to proceed. Same for your pain. It can be that simple.

There are ten key common types of pain. We will briefly discuss each type of pain, and then how to make it go away. This will include a less common but horrific type of pain called complex regional pain syndrome (CRPS/RSD). Fortunately, we now even have effective treatments for this. For those who want more detail on each kind of pain, I recommend my book *Pain Free 1-2-3*.

It is also important to realize that there is more to pain relief than simply taking pills.

Here are the four key domains for pain management:

1. **Biochemical.** For example, addressing inflammation and muscle pain caused by inadequate energy production in that muscle. This includes nutritional, herbal, and pharmaceutical treatments.
2. **Structural.** This means stretching the muscles, restoring range of motion, releasing the fascia, and even surgery to release trapped nerves when needed (most often it's not).
3. **Biophysics.** This includes things like acupuncture, vagal nerve stimulation, and an especially effective technique called frequency-specific microcurrent therapy.
4. **Mind-body-spirit.** What is going on in your body is often a metaphor for what is going on in your psyche. There's a good reason why some people are called a "pain in the neck" (or even lower). Meanwhile, old emotional traumas are often stored in our muscle and fascia memory. Part Four of this book will discuss how to address these.

8 The Ten Key Types of Pain

*T*hese are the ten most common kinds of pain. I would note that all of these can also be seen in fibromyalgia.

1. **Myofascial (muscle) pain.** A muscle is like a spring, in that it takes more energy for a muscle to relax than to contract. When muscles don't have enough energy, as results when you have fibromyalgia, they can become locked in shortened position, forming tender knots.

    Almost any kind of pain will throw the surrounding muscles into shortening as well. So muscle pain is critical to treat in all of the other kind of pain conditions below.

    Myofascial pain is the primary initial source of pain in most people, including those with fibromyalgia. Adding insult to injury, the presence of this chronic pain often leads to developing two other pains: central sensitization and small fiber neuropathic pain.

2. **Pain from inflammation.** This is the second most common cause of pain, and most often reflects as arthritis and tendinitis. Along with muscle pain, it is the main cause of pain in autoimmune illness as well. Often, tendinitis simply occurs because of the chronic muscle

shortening pulling on the tendons. For this, the solution is to also treat muscle shortening.

3. **Neuropathic (nerve) pain.** This feels like a burning, electric-like pain. Most often in the extremities like your hands or feet. In fibromyalgia, a condition called small fiber neuropathy is common.

4. **Migraines and other headaches.** Headaches lasting over twenty-four hours, with nausea and light and sound sensitivity.

5. **Abdominal pain.** This pain can result from indigestion, small intestinal bacterial overgrowth (SIBO), and irritable bowel syndrome. Improving digestion and treating the underlying infections are usually very effective for these.

6. **Nerve compression.** Pain such as carpal tunnel syndrome.

7. **Central sensitization.** Sometimes called brain pain, central sensitization is a form of pain that results in fibromyalgia, or any chronic pain condition, when sensitivity to pain increases in the brain itself. Think of it this way: The body starts with a simple pain signal to say what it needs. When it doesn't get it, it amplifies the pain to get your attention. This amplification occurs in the brain itself.

8. **Allodynia.** A type of skin pain where it hurts to be lightly touched, this tends to be a later stage of fibromyalgia and small fiber neuropathy. The medications memantine (Namenda), gabapentin (Neurontin), and/or pregabalin (Lyrica) can be very helpful for this kind of pain. Topical ketamine can be helpful in severe cases.

9. **Pelvic pain syndromes.** Pelvic pain syndromes usually come from muscle pain in the pelvic floor (the muscles, ligaments, and tissue that support your pelvic organs and pelvic joints) and include pain during intercourse. But the condition can also be neuropathic or come from localized tissue inflammation or dryness. Pelvic floor physical therapy combined with a prescription of the medications gabapentin (Neurontin) and amitriptyline (Elavil) usually help this.

10. **Sympathetically mediated pain.** Fortunately, this is much less common, but it is quite horrific. The most common form is called complex regional pain syndrome or reflex sympathetic dystrophy (CRPS/RSD). Fortunately, even this awful pain is becoming treatable.

We will look at each of these kinds of pain in Chapter 11. My goal is to keep the discussion very simple, focusing on a basic but highly effective overview of pain management, followed by the key treatments specific to each type of pain. A much more detailed discussion of pain can be found in my book *Pain Free 1-2-3*.

Let's start by looking at natural and prescription treatments that can address pain in general.

9   *Natural Pain Relief*

BFF Summary

1. Almost all pain can be effectively eliminated using the best of natural and prescription therapies.
2. Natural alternatives are often far more effective and generally much safer than prescriptions.
3. My favorite four natural options for pain relief in general (and these can all be combined with each other and with pain medications) are:
   A. **Curamin:** Take one to two capsules three times a day both to rebalance key inflammation pathways and to increase endorphins while melting inflammatory proteins. This is often a pain relief miracle for people.
   B. **End Pain:** Take one to two capsules three times a day to balance inflammation.
   C. **Topical comfrey cream:** I use only the Traumaplant form, rubbed over the painful areas three times a day to speed tissue healing and decrease pain.
   D. **Hemp oil:** I use 50 milligrams of only the Hemp Select brand by Terry Naturally, or hemp oil from licensed dispensaries, as otherwise quality control is a major problem. Any good hemp oil is a bit pricey, but the optimal dosing is three 50-milligram capsules twice a day and five at bedtime. CBD is only one of over a dozen active components of hemp oil, so I prefer using the whole hemp oil.
4. Even though benefits can begin in under an hour, it takes six weeks to see the full benefit of most natural and/or prescription pain treatments. Some prefer to begin each

treatment individually for the six weeks, adding the next treatments one at a time. This way, they can tell what is helping. If pain is severe, my preference is to start all of these at once, and then when the pain is controlled, to start weaning things down to see what is still needed.

5. Once you are pain-free for three months, many people find they can dramatically lower the dose of pain treatments. Pain is like putting out a fire. Once turned off for a while, it often stays off.

6. Although we are focusing on four natural pain options in this section, we will be discussing numerous others as we discuss each kind of pain.

7. There are many forms of bodywork that can eliminate pain by stretching your tightened muscles and fascia while restoring the full range of motion to your joints. Some excellent ones include Trager, Rolfing, myofascial release, chiropractic treatments, and acupuncture.

8. Biophysics offers many helpful options. Especially important? Frequency-specific microcurrent therapy.

9. Listening to calming music that distracts the mind from the pain has been shown to lower discomfort by 40 percent. I recommend piano music by Grammy Award winner Peter Kater.

Whether you have day-to-day pain from arthritis, muscle pains, headaches, or other causes, or the widespread and often very severe pain of fibromyalgia, relief is available. Naturally.

Many of you will have found that your pain is already less or even gone simply by doing those parts of the SHINE protocol that apply to you. But this takes time, and during that period it is not acceptable to leave people in pain. So even while going after the pain's root causes, I like to give treatments to help get people relief ASAP.

I prefer to start naturally. I would note that all the natural and prescription treatments we will be discussing can also be combined as needed to get pain-free. Some people do best with a mix of treatments.

A Simple Truth

It is simply not acceptable for you to be in chronic pain. You can become pain-free!

I want to repeat this, because so many doctors simply don't get it. Some seem to think that all pain is tolerable, as long as it is somebody else's.

It is simply not acceptable to be left in chronic pain!

I have found in treating thousands of chronic pain patients that almost everybody can get good solid pain relief. However, most physicians are simply not trained in pain management, resulting in one out of three adult Americans having often inadequately treated pain.

Unfortunately, the one pain treatment that most physicians are taught about is to give arthritis medications like ibuprofen (Motrin or Advil) or celecoxib (Celebrex). These are called nonsteroidal anti-inflammatory drugs (NSAIDs). In addition to not helping fibromyalgia or muscle pain, research shows that these medications cause about fifty thousand US deaths per year. Despite this, these medications are safer than being in chronic pain. But why not use safer options that work as well or better first?

Put simply, besides being cruel, leaving a person in chronic pain causes more physical toxicity than any medication, including narcotics.

Fortunately, there are much better ways to get pain relief. If your physician doesn't know how to safely and effectively get you pain-free, it doesn't mean you need to live with the pain. It just means that you need to find a pain or fibromyalgia specialist who knows how to *effectively* treat your pain. Fortunately, many if not most of you can even get pain-free simply by using the information in this book.

Let's start with some very safe and powerfully effective natural therapies.

Natural Pain Treatments

Many natural treatments can dramatically relieve pain. They can be used in combination with pain medications as well. In this section, I will focus on four key herbal treatments that are good for most kinds of pain. There are dozens of others, and many of these will be discussed under each specific kind of pain as well.

HERBAL TREATMENTS

There are two herbal mixes that are outstanding for pain in general. The first is an herbal mix called Curamin by Terry Naturally. This rather miraculous pain-relief product is a mix of a special, highly absorbed curcumin (called CurcuGreen), Boswellia, DLPA (DL phenylalanine), and nattokinase.

Although Curamin can start to work in minutes, it can take up to six weeks to see the full effect. I begin with one to two capsules three times a day. When the pain settles down, I lower the dose accordingly. It can be used every day or intermittently as needed. Let's look at its four components:

- **Curcumin**, which comes from turmeric, is the yellow spice in Indian food such as curry. There have been over one thousand studies done on this spice showing dramatic benefits for pain relief, inflammation, and even the treatment and prevention of cancer and Alzheimer's. The problem has been that it is so poorly absorbed that one had to essentially be living on Indian food to get enough to be meaningful. This changed dramatically when it was discovered that adding the essential oils back in, as is done in a special form of curcumin called CurcuGreen, increased absorption by almost 700 percent. This meant that one capsule could now do what seven of the next best used to do. This is the form present in Curamin.
- **Boswellia** is another name for the old biblical herb frankincense. It seems that the Three Wise Men knew what they were doing, as studies have shown that Boswellia can drop arthritis pain as much as 90 percent. Boswellia also helps with many kinds of inflammation beyond arthritis, including colitis and asthma.
- **DL phenylalanine (DLPA)** is an amino acid that increases levels of your body's own natural painkillers, called endorphins, and dopamine.
- **Nattokinase** helps break down inflammation, allowing the herbs and your body's healing mechanisms to get to the areas they need to in order to speed healing.

For most kinds of pain, I begin with the Curamin, and then I add a second herbal mix called End Pain by Nature's Way, if needed. Although they both have Boswellia, they can be combined, using one capsule three times a day of the Curamin if taking both together. The End Pain also contains cherry and willow bark.

Willow bark is the original source of aspirin but is much more effective than aspirin and less toxic. In head-to-head studies, willow bark was twice as effective as ibuprofen for chronic lower-back pain. Stomach endoscopy done after treatment trials with these medications showed that ibuprofen was associated with gastritis while willow bark caused no stomach inflammation.

These two herbal mixes have been outstanding for pain in general. In a number of head-to-head studies, both of these have been found to be as or more effective than celecoxib and ibuprofen.

TOPICAL COMFREY

Comfrey cream has been a mainstay of most healers' tool kits for many centuries. It has long been known to speed wound healing and in the old days used to be called bone knit, as it was used to speed the healing of broken bones. I find it useful for a wide array of pain.

Unfortunately, most comfrey also contains a component that can be toxic to the liver, called pyrrolizidine alkaloids. Fortunately, a strain is available that only contains the good components and none of the harmful ones. This is contained in a cream called Traumaplant.

I use it for most kinds of muscle or joint pains or injuries. Several studies show that it relieves pain, reduces inflammation and swelling, and speeds healing. In a head-to-head study against celecoxib (Celebrex), it was as effective for arthritis after six weeks.

Other helpful over-the-counter pain creams include doTERRA Deep Blue Rub and the Australian Dream Cream, both of which can be found online.

HEMP OIL AND MEDICAL MARIJUANA

Both hemp oil and medical marijuana can be remarkable for many kinds of pain. If cannabis were a pharmaceutical, every doctor would know about it and be using it every day in their practice, and it would likely be expensive. In fact, this is the current push, with the FDA recently approving the CBD "medication" Epidiolex ($30,000 per year) for treatment of a special form of refractory seizures.

CBD, hemp oil, and even cannabinoids are now legally available without prescription in many states and are reasonably priced. Most physicians are not yet familiar, however, with the research on how to use these.

THE RIGHT STUFF

It is important to note that not all hemp oil or CBD products are created equal. Although the products available through medical marijuana dispensaries tend to be of good quality, many if not most of those otherwise available over the counter are not.

This is important. Without experience, it is hard to tell how much of the active components are present in many products. *Many of them have labels that dramatically misrepresent their contents.* For example, it may say "CBD 100 mg" in bold type on the label and have less than 3 milligrams per dose.

A good form comes from concentrated European hemp (*Cannabis sativa*) stalk and seed oil. These can be found in 50-milligram capsules containing 20 percent CBD (i.e., 10 milligrams of CBD per capsule).

Because of this I'm very picky about what brand I use. I find a hemp oil called Hemp Select by Terry Naturally to be quite effective. The optimal dosing is three capsules twice a day and five at bedtime. Because the price of these capsules is about a dollar each, I start at this higher dose to determine optimal effectiveness and then drop to the lowest dose that maintains the desired effect. This is often as little as one capsule twice a day.

I find it more cost-effective to use a straight hemp oil product without added curcumin or other components. These are more cost-effective for body-wide pain when purchased separately. But if you just have a local area of pain, I would suggest the Hemp Select liquid and simply rub it over the area three times a day.

It may require six weeks of use to determine the full effects of hemp oil, but improvement in pain is often noted much sooner. It can be combined with any other pain medications or herbals as well. There is no upper safe limit; what limits the dose is the cost.

A BIT OF BACKGROUND

Cannabinoid receptors are critical for pain relief, sleep, immunity (including addressing cancers), and mood. There are over sixty active cannabinoids in the whole hemp oil. Although THC and CBD have been the most researched, the synergy of combining all ten different cannabinoids can be rather remarkable.

Let's take a closer look at this, beginning with pain.

Pain Relief and Cannabinoids

Although I hesitate to jump into the marijuana political quagmire, we have had such incredible feedback from people getting relief from hemp oil and marijuana that I am feeling the need to add my opinion.

The bottom line? These are powerful and very helpful tools. Fortunately, with hemp oil now being available and legal in all fifty states, people don't have to get high, or take the risk of getting arrested, to use it.

Key Biochemical Components of Pain Helped by Hemp Oil

It is important to hit pain from multiple directions. Most medications, and even most natural options, only address one or two pain types. Remarkably, different cannabinoids in hemp oil improve all ten of the below domains:

1. Muscle pain and shortening
2. Neuropathic pain
3. Inflammation
4. Nerve pain from other causes
5. Central sensitization or "brain pain"
6. Neurotransmitters (e.g., serotonin, dopamine, and NMDA and allodynia)

Contributing Pain Comorbidities

7. Insomnia
8. Anxiety and depression
9. Adverse response conditioning (fear of pain)
10. Tightening of fascia

The THC component of hemp can be helpful, but it comes with *significant* side effects and risks, for example:

- Poor functioning if you smoke marijuana (not a problem with hemp oil)
- Cost
- Jail (also not a problem with hemp oil)

SIDE BENEFITS OF HEMP OIL: SLEEP AND ANXIETY

Studies and clinical experience find hemp oil to be highly effective at improving sleep. Sleep is critical for pain relief, triggering growth hormone release and tissue healing. Hemp oil is one of the only sleep treatments that may actually help sleep apnea as well.

And it is remarkably helpful for anxiety.

The bottom line? Ignore the politics and go with the science.

OTHER NATURAL THERAPIES

We could fill a book talking about all of these (in fact, I did in my book *Pain Free 1-2-3* as well as in the *Cures A–Z* phone app). Here are a few of my favorites.

The (Piano) Keys to Fibromyalgia Pain Relief

Research on music and pain presents a novel therapy approach to easing pain.

The physiology of pain has two key components. The first is that a signal gets generated and sent to the brain. This electrical signal is no different than the signal the brain receives for heat, softness, cold, or countless other sensations. For pain, though, it is what the brain does with the signal after it is received that makes all the difference. This is the component that is called suffering.

The brain is receiving far more information every second than it can possibly process. *And* it naturally has the ability to tune out most of it. So, instead of the sensations being unpleasant, research has shown that the brain can easily be distracted to simply ignore many of the signals—including pain. Numerous studies have shown that the volume of pain signals go *way* down if the right kinds of music are used as a distraction.

A recent controlled research study looked at fibromyalgia pain and the effect of simply listening to the right kinds of music. For most new pain medications, if they can get the pain level to drop by 30 percent in just a third of the study population, this is hailed as a great breakthrough.

On the other hand, this study, simply using music, showed that for $12 you can get more effective pain relief then you can with $7,500 a year of medications. And instead of dizziness and weight gain, the only side effect is, perhaps, finding a big smile on your face.

This research group simply had people with fibromyalgia listen to music each day. They found that after fourteen days, pain levels went down an average of 40 percent. If the pharmaceutical industry had a drug that could do that, they would be ecstatic. Interestingly, pain levels continued to drop further day after day, and it is likely that beyond the fourteen days in the study, pain relief increased beyond the 40 percent drop. Remarkably, the music simply distracts your brain, so it starts to ignore the pain signal. Multiple studies show that this works for many kinds of pain, including cancer pain.

This doesn't mean that listening to just any music will work. You want something that will carry your mind off, away from the pain. My recommendation? Grammy Award–winning pianist Peter Kater's CDs. In addition to being brilliant, Peter Kater has an innate knack for understanding the role of sound in healing, and you will feel this as his music vibrates through your body. Listen to his music once a day, and let it carry you away to a comfortable place of peace, ease, and bliss.

STRUCTURAL THERAPIES/BODYWORK

There are many forms of bodywork that can eliminate pain by stretching your tightened muscles and fascia, while restoring full range of motion to your joints. Some excellent ones include Trager, Rolfing, myofascial release, chiropractic treatments, and acupuncture.

Some physical therapists are superb for pain. Others, well, aren't. If any bodywork therapist hurts you, let them know so they can ease back and work more gently. Remember, "no pain, no gain" is a good recipe for hurting yourself. As you research which techniques and practitioners are right for you, keep these guidelines in mind:

- Rolfing should be done only by a certified Rolfer with a lot of experience, as some people with minimal training claim that they do Rolfing and can work too aggressively.
- When talking with a physical therapist, ask if he or she is familiar with Dr. Janet Travell's work. If so, that is a very good sign. For those treating pain, I strongly recommend her two-part book series called *Myofascial Pain and Dysfunction: The Trigger Point Manual*.

A very large amount of discomfort caused by almost all the different types of pain comes from tight muscles. The center of the muscle where it bunches up into a tender marble is called a trigger point. Although SHINE gives the muscles the energy they need to release, structural problems can cause persistent localized muscle pain. These can often be helped by simple things that you can do at home to release these muscles. For more information on this, I recommend the book *The Art of Body Maintenance: Winners' Guide to Pain Relief* written by one of my favorite pain specialists, Hal Blatman, MD.

ADDRESS THE BIOPHYSICS

A biophysics approach is being taken by many different energy medicine disciplines. Whether doctors are using infrared or lasers to add energy to muscles, or using the Meridian or Chakra systems, these can all be classified under biophysics.

Many are highly effective, but there is one that I feel merits particular attention: frequency-specific microcurrent therapy. For persistent pain, especially if medications are not helpful or well tolerated, I highly recommend frequency-specific microcurrent therapy. The frequencies can be set to the specific tissue types, and offer a totally different and highly effective way of getting pain relief. For more information and to find a practitioner, go to www.frequencyspecific.com.

DON'T FORGET THE MIND-BODY CONNECTION

For this, see the many techniques in Part Four. Especially helpful? The trembling technique discussed by Dr. Peter Levine in his book *Waking the Tiger*. The treatment can be done on your own for the $10 it costs to buy the book. It can help release a lot of the muscle memory from old trauma that contributes to pain.

10 *Prescription Pain Relief*

BFF Summary

1. People get the most effective pain relief by using the entire healthcare tool kit. This includes treating the pain's root causes, while also using natural and structural therapies and, when needed, medications.
2. Because medications carry more risks, it is important that you have accurate information. Sadly, you will rarely get this information from physicians (who are not taught about it) or the media. For example:
   A. Arthritis medications such as ibuprofen, as previously mentioned, cause over fifty thousand deaths per year in the United States. It does this by increasing heart attack and stroke death risk by over 35 percent (shown in two large studies) as well as causing bleeding ulcer deaths. But these meds are still safer than chronic pain. I prefer to start with safe natural options that have been shown to be as or more effective, though.
   B. Including overdoses, acetaminophen kills a few hundred Americans a year.
   C. The pain herbals I discuss in the previous chapter kill zero Americans a year—and are frequently as or more effective than the medications.
   D. These numbers are taken directly from the scientific literature. If you had a different impression of safety from your physician or the media, you may want to start questioning why. I will give you a hint: Many physicians get most of their continuing medical education via the pharmaceutical industry, and the media is generally also

unwilling to upset their major advertisers. So we have a bunch of really good people, in a bunch of really broken systems.

3. Have a localized area of pain? Using compounded pain creams containing six to seven medications can be very effective after two to six weeks with minimal side effects. No need to soak 150 pounds of you with seven medications, when you can simply put them right into the muscles and tendons through the skin without side effects.

4. If you have fibromyalgia or any chronic pain, and you are not on narcotics, you should consider a compounded medication called low-dose naltrexone (3 to 4.5 milligrams at night). Give this at least two months to work. It can change your life.

5. Although some people are sensitive to any treatments no matter what, I have found the following treatments to be very helpful for many people with fibromyalgia pain and are often well tolerated: gabapentin, tramadol, tizanidine, and cyclobenzaprine.

6. I find the three FDA-approved medications pregabalin, duloxetine, and milnacipran to have more side effects, although they can be helpful in some people.

7. There are numerous other treatments that can help pain. I know you think you've tried them all, but you haven't. You can get pain-free.

---

*M*y preference is to use natural therapies for pain, but I will prescribe prescription medications when needed. They can be *very* helpful. All of the natural therapies I discuss can be combined with the prescriptions below. Doing so can decrease the amount of medication needed, while increasing their effectiveness and decreasing side effects.

I do *not* recommend using the ibuprofen (e.g., Advil or Motrin) family of medications (NSAIDs) for FMS, as they are minimally effective and can be dangerous. NSAIDs likely contribute to more than fifty thousand United States deaths a year. How? Two *British Medical Journal* meta-analyses of over 800,000 people show that NSAIDs are associated with a 35 percent or more increased risk of heart attack and stroke. Other research shows an additional four to sixteen thousand yearly deaths from bleeding ulcers. For those who would like the study references and calculations, they can be found in the *FFTF* notes at www.endfatigue.com.

Fortunately, there are safe and far more effective natural and prescription alternatives. Having said this, if you find that these medications are what work best for you, they are much less toxic than being in chronic pain.

Acetaminophen (Tylenol)

For occasional use, acetaminophen (Tylenol) is one of the safest medications available. The main problems are in people with underlying liver disease or in those taking over 3,000 milligrams daily. Acetaminophen can destroy the liver, and overdosing this drug is the most common reason for acute liver failure in the United States. This most often occurs because people are taking several different medications that contain acetaminophen without knowing it.

The main problem with long-term use of acetaminophen is that it depletes your body's glutathione—an amino acid compound that is a critical antioxidant. It is especially important for people with CFS/FMS.

For chronic pain, I therefore use other medications. But if acetaminophen is especially effective for you, you can simply take the supplement NAC (N-acetyl cysteine) along with it to help your body make more glutathione. I recommend taking 500 to 1,000 milligrams of NAC a day, making the acetaminophen much safer.

Pain Creams

These can be especially helpful, with virtually no side effects, for small localized areas of severe pain. Examples would be tendinitis or localized neuropathy. I recommend a topical prescription pain cream, which your physician can call into a compounding pharmacy such as ITC Pharmacy (www.itcpharmacy.com). These topicals typically include a mix of many pain medications. Simply rub a thin layer of the cream onto the skin over the painful areas two to three times a day for two to six weeks and then as needed.

This can often eliminate your worst pain spots—with virtually no side effects. You can use these products on up to three or four palm-sized areas at a time. Although usually not covered by prescription insurance, they are often moderately priced, and a 60-gram tube can last a long time.

Most compounding pharmacies can make this cream and can guide your physician on how to prescribe them. Unfortunately, instead of the usual approximately $90 per tube, a few compounding pharmacies were starting to play the pharmaceutical industry game and charging thousands of dollars. So if you find yourself at one of those pharmacies, even if they are simply charging this to your insurance company, I recommend you go elsewhere.

Although clinical experience and most studies show these creams to be effective, one study did not see efficacy. For many, however, it works very well after two to six weeks of use.

Low-Dose Naltrexone

This remarkable compounded medication can be very helpful for anybody with fibromyalgia, autoimmune illness, or chronic pain. See page 150 for more information on central sensitization.

Put simply, virtually anybody with severe chronic pain should be put on low-dose naltrexone (LDN) if they are not already taking narcotics. Interestingly, narcotics block the effect of the LDN, whereas high-dose naltrexone blocks the effect of the narcotics.

There is a very large body of both research and clinical experience showing this low-cost medication to be profoundly beneficial for chronic pain and autoimmune illness. Several studies have shown this for fibromyalgia alone.

The problem? The medication is off patent and relatively inexpensive, so it is nearly impossible to put through our regulatory process, regardless of the available research. But your physician can prescribe it through any compounding pharmacy. I like to use Skip's Pharmacy (www.skips pharmacy.com), and Skip is very knowledgeable about LDN.

If this was a patentable medication (and God knows they are trying to patent it despite it being generic), it would have sailed through the FDA process, the treatment would cost a good $25,000 per person per year (instead of the current $250 a year), and every physician would be convinced by the pharmaceutical industry's PR department that everyone should be on it.

Bottom line? Your physician has likely never heard about it except for its blocking the effect of narcotics. But you might be able to talk them into writing you a prescription for 50-milligram pills (see below) so that you don't ask for narcotics.

A couple of key things to know about this treatment:

1. It won't work if you are taking narcotics.
2. Doses over 4.5 milligrams at nighttime usually lose effectiveness (although we do see exceptions). A recent study of veterans with chronic pain found the 3-milligram dose to be more effective than 4.5 milligrams. The standard dose used by most physicians (to block the effect of narcotics in drug addicts) is 200 milligrams a day, and they come in 50-milligram pills from the standard pharmacy.
3. Some people find that it disrupts sleep in the beginning of treatment and may even trigger vivid dreams. It only does this in a modest percent of people and this side effect does go away with time for most. Because of this concern, many compounding pharmacies offer a "starting pack" of low-dose naltrexone, which starts you at an even lower dose and slowly moves your dose up to avoid this problem. Overall, that's a good idea.
4. It takes two full months to start working. When I first started using the treatment about twenty-five years ago, I only gave it three to four weeks to work, so I didn't see the effectiveness. Give it time.
5. In people under 150 pounds I usually go with 3 milligrams at bedtime. In those who weigh over 150 pounds, I am more likely to go with 4.5 milligrams.
6. After two months on the full dose, I give people the option of getting naltrexone 50-milligram tablets from their regular pharmacy so it will be covered by insurance. I have them grind the tablet up very finely with a mortar and pestle, then mix it with about 3 ounces of water (83 milliliters, if you want to be exact) and shake it well. Taking 1 teaspoon (5 milliliters) a night will supply the 3-milligram dose. For the 4.5-milligram dose, mix the ground 50-milligram tablet in with 55 milliliters (just under 2 ounces) of water and take 1 teaspoon a night. This will give eleven doses.

This treatment after two months not only can dramatically decrease pain, but can also improve energy, cognition, and numerous other processes.

Oral Medications

There are dozens of medications and other treatments that can be helpful for pain in general, including fibromyalgia pain. Interestingly, the cost of a medication has *absolutely nothing* to do with its effectiveness, and everything to do with whether your physician hears about it. Here are a few that I find most effective.

Tramadol (Ultram)

This medication affects both serotonin and endorphin (narcotic) receptors. Like fluoxetine (Prozac), though, you can see withdrawal symptoms if it is stopped suddenly. In my experience, even this is much rarer than what I see with antidepressants. Nonetheless, because tramadol does have a component that's about 1/1000 the effect of codeine, it is currently being attacked in the current drug war.

But in real life, it is quite safe and often very effective. I've also seen no problem with dose escalation as with narcotics. The recommended regimen is one to two 50-milligram tablets up to four times a day as needed for pain. The most common side effects are nausea and vomiting (when people use more than six tablets a day) and sedation. These effects generally wear off with continued use and can often be avoided altogether by starting with a low dose and slowly working up to the level that most effectively treats your pain.

Gabapentin (Neurontin)

This medication helps nerve pain, central sensitization, pelvic pain, and overall fibromyalgia pain while also helping both muscle and nerve pain along with sleep and restless leg syndrome. It is also generic and low cost, so you can see why I hold it in such high regard for fibromyalgia. It is not addictive, although, like any medication, if high doses are used for long periods, it should be tapered off over time instead of being stopped suddenly. The main side effect is sedation, so I start with a low bedtime dose and then increase as tolerated. Unintentional overdoses are quite uncommon.

The main problem? If somebody is taking high-dose narcotics along with anything that can be sedating, they are more likely to overdose on the narcotics. But if you're not also taking narcotics with them, it is not an issue.

Nonetheless, the current government war on people in pain is attacking pretty much anything that helps pain, even if it is much safer than standard over-the-counter medications. I find that gabapentin is an excellent medication if your body tolerates it comfortably. As with any medication, don't use it if it doesn't. Dosing can range anywhere from just 100 milligrams at bedtime to over 3,000 milligrams a day.

TIZANIDINE (ZANAFLEX)

This acts as a muscle relaxant and can be very helpful for pain. The dose is 2 to 4 milligrams up to three times a day. Most people simply take 2 to 4 milligrams at bedtime to help sleep. Caution: Do not take it along with the antifungal medications fluconazole or itraconazole.

CYCLOBENZAPRINE (FLEXERIL)

This is a cousin to the medication amitriptyline (Elavil) that seems to keep most of its benefits and very little of the side effects. It acts as a muscle relaxant and can also be helpful for sleep. The trick is to keep the dose low enough to get the muscle relaxant benefits without the sedating side effects. Interestingly, although the standard dose used to be 10 milligrams three times a day, simply taking 2.5 to 5 milligrams at bedtime, and even up to 5 milligrams three times a day, can often be very helpful with minimal side effects. Some people find that other medications in the same family such as amitriptyline (Elavil) can be very helpful, often at very low doses.

All four of the above medications can be taken together, and I may give two or three at the first visit for patients to try individually, and then in combination if needed. The key problem is that of serotonin levels going too high by combining several serotonin-raising medications (e.g., antidepressants or tramadol). This can trigger something called serotonergic syndrome. If you start getting anxiety from these medications, check with your physician, who should consider lowering the dose.

Because all of these medications are available in low-cost generics (i.e., they are off patent), they cannot be put through the expensive FDA-approval process to get an additional recommendation for fibromyalgia.

An Important Note About Pain Medications

Many people find that they are not able to tolerate any pain medications because of the side effects. When this occurs, it is usually because too high a dose was used initially. Some people tolerate the higher doses without difficulty, so it is not unreasonable to start at the high dose to see if one can get quick pain relief. But if you get side effects that are uncomfortable, instead of abandoning the medication, simply drop to a very low dose and then slowly work the dose up to the recommended dose as is comfortable.

This works because, unlike narcotic medications, which work best in the beginning and then may lose effect, it takes a while for your body to adapt to the side effects of the medications we are discussing, but the pain-relieving effects tend to increase over time.

In addition, as with many other medications we discuss in this book, most of the benefits occur at lower doses and most of the toxicities occur at higher doses. So, it often works best to use a low dose of several medications instead of a very high dose of one. Sometimes, even a tiny dose can be very helpful for pain.

Three FDA-Approved Medications for Fibromyalgia

PREGABALIN (LYRICA)

This is my favorite of the three. It has the benefit of improving sleep, but at doses over 450 milligrams, it can increase weight gain and ankle swelling. Although when this drug is taken by itself, higher doses are necessary to see the optimal effect, when it is combined with the other treatments we discuss, many people find that simply taking 250 to 300 milligrams at bedtime can help pain and sleep without the side effects. I use either this or gabapentin, but generally not both together. Pregabalin was quite expensive at about $8 per capsule, but has now gone generic and costs 30 cents.

Duloxetine (Cymbalta)

This antidepressant medication raises both serotonin and norepinephrine. It can be especially helpful for nerve pain and tends to be energizing instead of sedating. But it can cause *severe* withdrawal symptoms when stopped. I find that if 60 milligrams a day is not helping, increasing the dose is unlikely to add anything besides side effects. This is one of the few medications where it is dangerous to break the pill. So if you want to try a lower dose, have your doctor prescribe a lower-dose tablet.

Unfortunately, the company did not make a low enough dose tablet to allow people to wean themselves off the drug safely. And the pills cannot be broken. This has resulted in some horrific withdrawal issues. There is a trick to weaning off safely by gently cutting open the pills and using the small beads inside to lower the dose very slowly. But this is best done with a knowledgeable physician's or pharmacist's supervision (although most physicians are not familiar with this trick).

Milnacipran (Savella)

I consider this an expensive form of the medication amitriptyline (Elavil) and have not been especially impressed with its usefulness.

Other Helpful Medications

The natural and pharmacologic treatment options we've discussed will provide excellent pain relief for most people. In some cases, however, more aggressive treatment is needed. For more detailed information on pain relief, I recommend my book *Pain Free 1-2-3*. I would note that there are well over thirty different treatments that we use for pain. We are giving just a few key ones to start with.

If other medications are needed, here are a few others that can be helpful for stubborn pain cases:

- **Baclofen (Lioresal).** This is a powerful muscle relaxant that can be increased to a dose as high as 20 milligrams four times a day. The main limiting side effect is sedation.

- **Oxcarbazepine (Trileptal).** Take 150 milligrams twice a day, or as high as 600 milligrams twice a day.
- **Lamotrigine (Lamictal).** Take 25 milligrams at bedtime for one week. I then increase to 25 milligrams three times a day for one week. It can slowly be increased to the maximum dose of 100 milligrams four times a day as is needed and tolerated. Although rare, it can cause a rash that, if you stay on the medication, can be fatal. Most rashes would not be a cause for concern, but to be on the safe side: *Stop Lamictal at first sign of any rash.* Research has shown that this can be combined with the oxcarbazepine (Trileptal).
- **Topiramate (Topamax).** I begin with 25 to 50 milligrams daily, and increase it by 25 to 50 milligrams a week until the person gets the desired effect. This medication is usually given twice a day at a total daily dose of 50 to 100 milligrams for migraines and 200 to 300 milligrams a day for nerve pain, although lower doses can also be effective. This is a medication that I have seen work wonderfully in patients for whom numerous other treatments failed, and sometimes it starts working within a few days. If you get side effects, decrease the dose and perhaps later increase it more slowly until you get the desired effect. The most common side effects are diarrhea, loss of appetite, sedation, and nausea. The nausea will often go away after one has been on the topiramate for three months. It also has the benefit of causing weight loss as well as pain relief. Besides sedation, its most worrisome, albeit unusual, side effect is that it can make your body very acidic, to the point where it is dangerous. Because of this, it is reasonable to check a blood bicarbonate level every so often (especially if you start developing symptoms such as fatigue) to make sure that the test result is okay (over 17 mEq/L).

Feeling Guilty About Taking Pain Medications?

I suspect that you get no bonus points in heaven for having suffered through the pain instead of taking the medications needed to be comfortable.

I often tell people I treat the story about a pious man trapped by floodwaters. The National Guard came into the city and told everyone they had to evacuate, or they would drown. This man refused to leave, saying that he had faith in God and that God would protect him.

The floodwaters came and soon the Coast Guard boat arrived, floating by the man's second-story window. They beseeched him to climb in the boat and be saved, but he refused, once again saying that he had faith in God to protect him.

Pretty soon he was up on the top of his roof and a helicopter came by and yelled at him to get in. Once again, he refused—and the man drowned.

He went to heaven, and God came by. The man was very angry at God and said, "I had full faith in you and you let me drown!"

God said, "What are you talking about? I sent the National Guard, the Coast Guard, and a helicopter."

The medications are like the National Guard, the Coast Guard, and the helicopter. It's okay to use them!

11 Addressing Each of the Ten Most Common Pains

I am purposefully keeping each part of this chapter brief, simply addressing the key things you need to know to get relief for each of these kinds of pain. As most of these are short and to the point, we will not include a BFF Summary for these.

1. Myofascial (Muscle) Pain

A muscle is like a coiled spring. It takes more energy for a muscle to relax (stretch) than to contract. When muscles don't have enough energy, as results when you have fibromyalgia or even day-to-day muscle pain, they can become locked in shortened positions, forming tender knots.

Almost any kind of pain will throw the surrounding muscles into shortening as well. So addressing associated muscle pain is *critical* in all other pain conditions. Sadly, the muscle component is usually missed by physicians, despite the muscle pain routinely contributing to much if not most of the pain.

Myofascial pain is the primary initial source of pain in most people with fibromyalgia. Our published research and clinical experience have shown that using the SHINE protocol decreased pain more than 50 percent.

To further complicate this problem, the presence of untreated chronic muscle pain often leads to the development of two other pains: central sensitization and neuropathic pain.

TREATMENT

Treat with SHINE. When you have frequent muscle pain, or even a localized area where it just won't go away, treating the underlying factors that control energy production can help the muscles finally release.

The letters in SHINE stand for:

Sleep
Hormonal deficiencies
Infections and inflammation
Nutritional supplementation
Exercise as able

RECOMMENDED SUPPLEMENTS

CURAMIN
A special mix of BCM-95 curcumin, Boswellia, DLPA, and nattokinase has been a pain relief miracle—even for many whose pain has lasted decades. Take one to two capsules three times a day till the pain resolves.

WILLOW BARK AND BOSWELLIA
The End Pain herbal mix is especially helpful for back pain and combines both willow bark and Boswellia. For acute or chronic pain, you can take two tablets three times a day For acute pain, relief can be provided by Curamin or End Pain individually or you can even combine them.

The pain relief may begin quickly, sometimes in as little as 30 minutes. It builds over a week and maximizes at six weeks. The dose can often then be lowered to one or two a day as needed. It's like putting out a fire. Once the pain is gone for six weeks, you may no longer need the natural treatments or may only take them "as needed"—with a lower dose doing the job.

TOPICAL COMFREY
The only form of this I use is called Traumaplant. Other forms of comfrey cream can have a component that is toxic. This is not present in Trauma-

plant. This cream not only helps pain but speeds healing. Apply it three times a day as needed.

OTHER HELPFUL CREAMS
Try different ones to see what works best for you. Others that people find very helpful are Australian Dream Cream and doTERRA Deep Blue Rub.

OTHER THERAPIES AND ADVICE

RELEASING TIGHT MUSCLES
There are many ways to stretch your muscles, releasing them and the pain. These include chiropractic, osteopathic manipulation, and a host of excellent types of massage and bodywork. Unfortunately, most MDs have virtually no training in treating muscle pain, except for having been taught that chiropractors (who *do* know how to treat muscle pain) are quacks. Medical school training in this area is both pathetic and (I say this as an MD) embarrassing. I view chiropractic as an essential specialty in the healing arts. Some MDs who practice physical medicine and rehabilitation (PM&R or physiatrists) are finally learning about muscle pain.

For any health practitioner working with chronic muscle pain, treatment is blind if you're not familiar with myofascial trigger points and their referral zones. If you take nothing else from this book, I strongly recommend that you get the textbook *Myofascial Pain and Dysfunction: The Trigger Point Manual* by Dr. Janet Travell and Dr. David Simons. This will dramatically increase your effectiveness.

Acupuncture can also help. Some 70 percent of acupuncture points correspond to muscle trigger points (the belly of the muscle where it causes a painful knot). Put a needle in a trigger point and the muscle will release (though much more is also happening with acupuncture).

STRUCTURAL ISSUES
Other treatments can release the muscles, but if you don't treat the structural stresses (such as carrying a twenty-pound purse around, having uneven hip heights, or working in an "ergonomically incorrect" workplace), the muscles will get strained, lose energy, and go back to their shortened position.

Meanwhile, any bodywork that stretches the muscles will feel better. For a few days. But unless you treat the underlying cause of the energy crisis, the muscles will go right back to their shortened position and hurt again. So it may be best to treat the biochemistry with SHINE, and then do the massage, chiropractic, or other technique to stretch the muscles. This way they will stay released after the treatments.

ICE AND HEAT

Ice acts as an anti-inflammatory, and heat brings in healing blood flow. Either can be used for up to twenty minutes at a time (so you don't overheat or overcool the muscle). And if using both together, start with ice followed by heat. Ice is best used in the first thirty-six hours after an injury. Heat can be used anytime.

One especially helpful technique is to add 2 cups of Epsom salts to a tub of hot water and soak away. Epsom salts are made of magnesium, which will soak into your tissues with the heat, relaxing your muscles and loosening any tight joints. Often, you can feel the pain flow right out as your muscles relax.

RELEASING TIGHT MUSCLES ON YOUR OWN

I again happily recommend the book *The Art of Body Maintenance: Winners' Guide to Pain Management* by Dr. Hal Blatman, an outstanding pain specialist in Cincinnati, Ohio.

Ehlers-Danlos Syndromes

These represent a broad group of genetic connective tissue disorders, encompassing a wide range of severity and patterns. Symptoms may include hyper-flexible loose joints, overly stretchy skin, and other disorders of the connective tissue that vary based on the individual's genetics.

Consider this diagnosis if you have overly flexible joints or skin. More information can be found online (as usual, most places give the scariest information instead of noting mild forms). This can be one more trigger for fibromyalgia.

Physicians specializing in this area know the standard things to look for. But again, they may not be familiar with the natural treatment options. If you have this condition, look up the Cusack protocol. This natural approach can markedly strengthen the connective tissues over time, and you can do it on your own. Ask to join their Facebook page, which has over sixteen thousand members.

---

2. Pain from Inflammation

This is the second most common cause of pain, and most often reflects as arthritis and tendinitis. Along with muscle pain, it is the main cause of pain in autoimmune illness as well, usually accompanied by secondary (and usually missed) muscle pain.

For tendinitis, I like to use Curamin plus compounded pain creams containing ketoprofen and other medications. If your physician lets the local compounding pharmacist know it is for tendinitis, the pharmacist can guide them on what to prescribe. This combination tends to be highly effective for tendinitis after six weeks of use, along with avoiding overuse and straining of the tendon and muscle.

Now let's take a look at arthritis, and how to make it go away.

ARTHRITIS AND AUTOIMMUNE ILLNESS

BACKGROUND
Natural remedies can dramatically decrease most kinds of arthritis pain and improve function. This is especially important because some arthritis medications can be particularly dangerous (see page 110). Fortunately, arthritis pain is very treatable naturally—with many natural options being as, or more, effective than the medications. Instead of side effects, the herbals cause "side benefits," such as a lower risk of cancer, Alzheimer's, and premature death.

TREATMENT
Natural remedies can dramatically decrease most kinds of arthritis pain and improve function. Give them six weeks to see the full effect. You will be amazed at how much better you feel. You can often stop or lower the dose treatments (as able) after three months of being pain-free. To improve joint comfort and function, I recommend following these four steps.

Step 1: Feed Your Joints

I do this with:

- **Nutritional support.** Take the Energy Revitalization System vitamin powder.

- **Glucosamine sulfate plus chondroitin.** Take 750 milligrams of glucosamine sulfate two to three times a day. If severe, add 400 milligrams of chondroitin two times a day. Research shows that this combination is essentially equivalent to Celebrex. This was also found in the large National Institutes of Health (NIH) study comparing the two, but you would never know it from looking at the study abstract or media reporting.

  The headlines? "Glucosamine Plus Chondroitin Ineffective for Arthritis." What the data showed? They were statistically and clinically equivalent, with the glucosamine chondroitin combination often being more effective.

  Meanwhile, large studies have shown a 22 percent lower rate of death versus those not taking glucosamine. So switching to glucosamine would save even more lives.

Other nutrients have also been shown to help arthritis, including hyaluronic acid. The above three, plus three others, can be found in a combination herbal called Be Mobile. For arthritis, I combine this with the Curamin as my starting approach.

Step 2: Balance Inflammation

I do this with:

- **Herbals.** I combine the Curamin and End Pain. Two head-to-head studies of Curamin versus Celebrex showed Curamin to be equally effective for arthritis, and another study showed the same for rheumatoid arthritis.
- **Comfrey cream.** Head-to-head studies have shown that topical comfrey (Traumaplant) was as effective for arthritis as Celebrex after six weeks.
- **Fish oil.** If you have overtly inflammatory arthritis (red, swollen joints, as in rheumatoid arthritis), add 1 teaspoon of fish oil or three 800-milligram capsules two to three times a day of regular fish oil or just one or two tablets a day of Vectomega.

Step 3: Exercise and Stretching

Walking (in a warm-water pool, if it is too painful on the ground) is good exercise for arthritis below your waist. If you have decreased flexibility, put heat on the affected joints (herbal beanbags that can be heated in the microwave are very good for this). After five to ten minutes in the heat, slowly and gently move the joints (as able) to reclaim your full range of motion. Do this two to three times a day until your joints are limber.

Step 4: For Stubborn Cases

If symptoms persist despite these treatments, look for and treat food allergies with a special form of acupressure called NAET. An elimination diet can help you tell if food allergies are a problem.

ADDRESSING AUTOIMMUNE ARTHRITIS

For inflammatory arthritis associated with autoimmune disease, such as lupus or rheumatoid arthritis, I add low-dose naltrexone (3 to 4.5 milligrams a night; see page 121). This can have dramatic benefits after two months.

If you have rheumatoid arthritis, large studies have shown that long-term antibiotic treatment with 100 milligrams of minocycline twice a day was highly effective. If you are using this, it is important to prevent candida overgrowth with once a week Diflucan (see Chapter 3). But as minocycline was five cents a dose instead of $24,000 a year, the research has been largely ignored. It is not clear whether the antibiotic works by fighting an infection or by directly settling down microglial activation (which this antibiotic uniquely does; see the section on central sensitization on page 150).

I do agree with using the expensive immune-modulating medications along with the natural therapies and LDN for rheumatoid arthritis. I suspect that this combination best protects your joints and improves long-term function. My concern is that because these disease-modifying anti-rheumatic drugs (biologic DMARDs) are highly profitable, this is pretty much all that your physicians will hear about; therefore, I recommend the comprehensive arthritis protocol above.

3. Neuropathic (Nerve) Pain

BACKGROUND

Nerve pain (neuropathy) is characterized by pain that is burning, shooting (often to distant areas), or stabbing. It also has an "electric" quality about it. Tingling or numbness (paresthesias) and increased sensitivity with normal touch being painful (allodynia) are also commonly seen.

Nerve pain can be triggered by malfunction of nerves associated with illness (e.g., diabetes or low thyroid), infections (e.g., shingles), pinched nerves (e.g., from muscles or disc disease), nutritional deficiencies (e.g., vitamins B6 and B12), injury (e.g., stroke, tumors, spinal cord injury, and multiple sclerosis), fibromyalgia, and medication/treatment side effects.

TREATMENT

NUTRITIONAL SUPPORT

Nutritional support is critical. Use the Energy Revitalization System vitamin powder. Be careful not to take more than 45 milligrams total of vitamin B6 (the amount in the powder specifically for this reason), unless it is in the form of pyridoxal 5 phosphate, because high-dose vitamin B6 can aggravate nerve pain.

In addition to the B vitamins, magnesium, biotin, and 1,000 units of vitamin D already in the powder, add the following supplements to support nerve health:

- **Coenzyme Q10:** Take 200 to 400 milligrams a day with food that has fat in it.
- **Lipoic acid:** Take 300 milligrams two times a day.
- **Acetyl-L-carnitine:** Take 1,000 milligrams three times a day.
- **Vitamin D:** Take another 2,000 units a day or more (in addition to the 1,000 units in the vitamin powder). In one study, this decreased diabetes nerve pain by 47 percent. The vitamin D can be obtained from many sources, including sunshine and the vitamin powder.

Give these six to twelve months to work (it takes time for nerves to heal), though you'll likely feel better much sooner. These, especially acetyl-L-carnitine, may also prevent nerve pain from developing (as it might during chemotherapy).

MEDICATIONS
Lidocaine (Lidoderm) Patches and Topical Creams

Many medications can be very helpful for nerve pain. For small areas, begin with the Lidoderm patch (very expensive) and compounded topical creams. Your physician can call in a prescription for Nerve Pain Cream to ITC Pharmacy (www.itcpharmacy.com or 888-349-5453) and they will mail it to you. Apply the cream to the painful area(s) two to three times a day and give it two weeks to start working. The lidocaine patch can be put over the compounded pain creams, leaving an area without the cream at the periphery, so the patch will stick.

Oral Medications

For large areas, or if the patches are not effective, I prescribe the oral medications gabapentin (Neurontin), amitriptyline (Elavil), tramadol (Ultram), duloxetine (Cymbalta), and pregabalin (Lyrica), often giving these in combinations, followed if needed by over a dozen other medications that can help nerve pain. A fair treatment trial is six weeks. Read the nerve pain chapter in my book *Pain Free 1-2-3* for more detailed information on over a dozen medications that can be helpful. Ibuprofen and other NSAIDs and even codeine/narcotic medications are *not* very helpful for nerve pain.

If side effects occur, this does not mean you can't use the medication; it means it may be necessary to start with a lower and more comfortable dose. The body adapts to the medication, which will allow the dose to be increased over time without side effects, while the medication's benefits persist.

OTHER THERAPIES AND ADVICE

- **Blood tests.** Do blood testing to check for diabetes, low thyroid, or vitamin B12 deficiency. I give B12 injections if the B12 level is under 540 mg/mL in a patient with nerve pain.
- **IV gamma globulin.** For a type of nerve pain called small fiber neuropathy, IV gamma globulin can be very helpful after four months of use.

4. Migraines and Other Headaches

Headaches are a major source of chronic pain. Although most people get an occasional headache, as many as forty-five million Americans get them on a regular basis.

If you are having a new very severe headache of a type that you have not had before, see your physician ASAP to be sure there is not something dangerous causing it.

MIGRAINE HEADACHES

BACKGROUND

Migraine headaches can be very severe and usually last for several days. Migraines are often preceded by an "aura," which may consist of visual disturbances such as flashing lights. The headaches are often associated with nausea, sweats, dizziness, and light and sound sensitivity. The cause is still controversial, with muscle contraction, low serotonin, and the relaxation (dilation) of blood vessels all playing a role.

TREATMENT

After three months of being on the supplement regimen below, continue to use the Energy Revitalization System, as even on its own this may be enough to help. Natural approaches can commonly eliminate even frequent and horribly severe migraine problems, but remember that it usually takes two to three months to see the effect, so give them time to work.

Recommended Supplements to Stay Headache-Free

- **Multivitamin powder.** Take the Energy Revitalization System vitamin powder. This has a good maintenance level of magnesium and vitamin B2.
- **Vitamin B2.** Take 300 milligrams of vitamin B2 (riboflavin) in the morning. This decreased migraine frequency 69 percent after six weeks in two placebo-controlled studies.
- **Magnesium.** Take 200 milligrams of magnesium at night. Although magnesium is already in the vitamin powder, adding this amount for three to four months can be helpful. An excellent product called Neuro

Comfort by Douglas Labs contains the riboflavin, magnesium, and a number of other things helpful for migraine headaches in two capsules a day.

- **Butterbur.** Butterbur (Petadolex) can both prevent and eliminate migraines. Take 50 milligrams three times a day for one month and then 50 milligrams twice a day to prevent migraines. You can take 100 milligrams every three hours (for a maximum of 300 milligrams in a twenty-four-hour period) to eliminate an acute migraine.
- **Magnesium IV.** In the hospital emergency room or holistic doctor's office, placebo-controlled research shows that 1 gram of intravenous magnesium over fifteen minutes can effectively eliminate an acute migraine within minutes (to find a holistic physician, see page 317). This makes intravenous magnesium more effective than narcotics. Because this medication costs approximately ten cents per dose, few emergency room doctors have heard about this research. Most of the cost is starting the IV.
- **Melatonin.** Take 3 milligrams at bedtime. Do *not* use a time-release form.

MEDICATIONS

During a migraine, medications are also reasonable (and can be taken with the natural therapies). Though your tendency with regard to many medications may be to wait to see if you really need them, the earlier the migraine is treated, the more successful the treatment is—and spending two days with a migraine is a lot less healthy than taking the medication.

Aspirin, Acetaminophen, and Caffeine

In the United States, medications in the triptan family (Imitrex) remain the first choice of physicians use for the treatment of acute migraines. No one is paying to give the physicians the research showing that the old combination of aspirin, acetaminophen (Tylenol), and caffeine (cost approximately 20 cents versus $10 to $25 per dose) is equally effective. So don't forget that you can use these if needed (e.g., one to three Excedrin Migraine or Excedrin Extra Strength; the dose recommendations on the bottle are fairly low).

Midrin

Midrin, which is a prescription mix of three medications, can also be effective. Two capsules are taken immediately, followed by one capsule every hour until the headache is relieved (to a maximum of five capsules within a twelve-hour period).

Triptans (Imitrex)

The triptans have proven to be effective for migraines—but, unfortunately, they can be a bit expensive. A fascinating study can guide you on when to use triptans versus when to go with other therapies: 75 percent of migraine patients get painful sensitivity to normal touch around their eyes (e.g., wearing eyeglasses). If you use a triptan before you get the pain and tenderness around the eyes, it will knock out the migraine 93 percent of the time. If the pain and tenderness around the eyes has already set in, a triptan only eliminates the migraine 13 percent of the time (although it still helped the throbbing). In other words, if you are one of the lucky ones who does not get pain around the eyes, a triptan can knock out your migraine at any time. If you are one of those who do get pain and tenderness around the eyes, it is a race against the clock to take the medication before that pain starts. This means that you should take a triptan early in the attack (within the first five to twenty minutes) before the skin hypersensitivity gets established.

OTHER THERAPIES AND ADVICE
Food Allergies

Avoiding hidden food allergies can reduce or eliminate migraines in 30 to 85 percent of patients. In one study, the most common reactive foods were wheat in 78 percent of patients, oranges in 65 percent, eggs in 45 percent, tea and coffee in 40 percent, chocolate and milk in 37 percent, beef in 35 percent, and corn, cane sugar, and yeast in 33 percent. Clinical experience also suggests that the artificial sweetener aspartame (NutraSweet) can trigger migraines and other headaches (although this is controversial). You may find that instead of avoiding foods that trigger your migraines for the rest of your life, you may be able to eliminate the sensitivities/allergies using a simple yet powerfully effective acupressure technique called NAET (visit www.naet.com).

Estrogen Patches

In women, if the migraines are predominately around the time of menstruation or ovulation, or they are associated with taking oral contraceptives (where you wake up with a headache), the key is to prevent the *fluctuating* estrogen level. One way to do this is to use an estradiol estrogen patch for one week beginning a few days before your period is expected (e.g., a Climara .1 patch).

These migraine headaches around ovulation and menses require the hormonal treatments, as they often respond very poorly to the other medications. In fact, this is the main cause of treatment-resistant migraine headaches.

If your migraines are usually in pretty much the same area of the head each time, this suggests that muscle trigger points related to that referral pain pattern are contributing. See a massage therapist, chiropractor, or osteopath familiar with myofascial release; show them the pattern of your headache; and ask them to release the muscles that may be the source of that pattern.

TENSION HEADACHES

Tension headaches account for about three-quarters of all headaches. They cause moderate pain on both sides of, and across, the forehead, tend to both start and fade away gradually, and are the result of muscle tightness coming from the (sternocleidomastoid) muscles in the neck. These are the muscles that turn your head from side to side. With tension headaches, you can often find a tender knot right in the middle of the muscle, three fingers widths below your earlobe. This knot, called a trigger point, refers pain and tenderness to the sides of your forehead (the temple area), and then sends the pain across your forehead. Although putting a hot compress or a pain cream on the temples and across the forehead may help temporarily, they are more effective when placed over the tender knots in the muscles on both sides of the neck.

Occasionally, tension headaches are felt at the base of the skull, on the top of the head, and/or behind the eyes. For these headaches, the pain is often coming from the muscles where they attach to the base of the skull at the top of the back of your neck. If you push on those muscles (called the suboccipital muscles) where they attach at the base of the skull during a headache, they will be very tender and can make the headache better or worse. When the pain is reproduced by pushing on the area, you know that these muscles are part of the source of that headache. If this is the case, use heat (and menthol pain creams, like Tiger Balm or Icy Hot) over those tender areas.

If your headaches are severe and last over twenty-four hours, are associated with nausea or light and sound sensitivity (you hunt for a dark quiet room to lie down in), or you see flashing/shimmering lights before the headache, see the section on migraine headaches (page 138) and consult your physician.

TREATMENT

Because tension headaches are muscular, the same treatments discussed in muscle pain or in the SHINE protocol will often decrease or even eliminate their recurrence.

Recommended Herbal Mixes

- Curamin Headache Relief
- End Pain
- Tiger Balm or Icy Hot cream rubbed over the painful muscles

Medications

- **Acetaminophen.** Take 325 to 500 milligrams, which is safe if used occasionally. Ibuprofen and other aspirin family medications can be used if acetaminophen is not effective, but these carry much greater risk, so use the herbals or acetaminophen first. Do not exceed 4,000 milligrams a day of acetaminophen. Check all medications (prescription and OTC) to see how much acetaminophen you are getting total, as several medications you are taking may include it. If using acetaminophen regularly, take 500 to 650 milligrams a day of NAC (N-acetyl cysteine) to protect the liver. For most people using acetaminophen only occasionally, the 250 milligrams of NAC in the vitamin powder gives good protection.

Other Therapies and Advice

- **Soak your muscles.** For tension headaches and other muscle pains, add 1 to 2 cups of Epsom salts to a tub of hot water and take a nice leisurely soak. Use a bathtub pillow for added comfort.
- **Myofascial release.** Stretching the muscles that are triggering the headache can prevent and eliminate the pain. A chiropractor is much more likely to be able to help than most physicians. They will release

the muscle causing the headache, but be sure to use the SHINE protocol or your muscles will tighten again in a few days.

5. Abdominal Pain

New abdominal pains need to be evaluated by a physician, but most often they turn out to be either indigestion (felt in the solar plexus) or gastroesophageal reflux disease (GERD), felt under the chest bone. If the pain goes away quickly when you take a liquid or chewable antacid, this is very suggestive of an acid-related problem.

HEARTBURN AND REFLUX

BACKGROUND

Do you think your problem is too much stomach acid? If you think so, keep this in mind: The older people get, the more likely they are to use antacids. This is interesting since stomach acid production decreases dramatically as people get older.

We seem to forget that having stomach acid is both necessary and normal. In fact, the body has gone to great lengths to be able to produce stomach acid without digesting the stomach itself. Your body needs to have proper nutrition, however, to make the mucous lining that protects the stomach. Instead of giving the stomach what it needs to heal, we sometimes make the mistake of turning off our stomach acid to solve the problem.

What goes on in real life is that most of the enzymes we need to digest the food we eat are naturally present in the food. This occurs because enzymes are what a fruit or vegetable uses to ripen.

Many decades ago, food processors realized that they could prolong the shelf life of food from days to years by destroying the enzymes present in the food. Because of this, most of the enzymes present in processed foods, which we need in order to digest our food, have been eliminated over the last thirty-plus years. This corresponds to the period of time in which we have seen a dramatic increase in degenerative diseases, autoimmune conditions, food allergies (with wheat going from being the "staff of life" to the stuff of allergies), and indigestion.

When you can't digest your food properly, the acid starts to reflux up into your chest and you get burning in your solar plexus (just below the bottom of your ribs) and mid-chest (called indigestion or acid reflux). As a simple hint: food should be past the stomach less than an hour after you eat it. If you're still tasting what you ate over an hour ago when you burp or have acid reflux, you're not digesting properly and should take digestive enzymes.

An additional cause of indigestion and ulcers is a stomach infection with bacteria called *H. pylori*. But the presence of *H. pylori* is not necessarily unhealthy. Most physicians are not aware that half of healthy adults will have this bacteria in their stomach, causing no problems at all.

The Problem with Acid Blockers

Though turning off stomach acid helps you feel better in the short term, acid blockers used for over two months can be both dangerous and addictive. In rare cases, such as precancerous changes in the esophagus, they may be needed long term (so discuss with your physician who prescribed them). But even in those cases, research suggests that the chronic use of acid blockers is more likely to cause harm than to prevent esophageal cancer.

Overall, acid blockers are being grossly overused, resulting in osteoporosis and nutritional deficiencies (again, we make stomach acid for a reason). The proton-pump inhibitors (PPIs), like prescription or over-the-counter omeprazole (Prilosec), have also been associated with a 44 percent higher risk of developing Alzheimer's disease and a 25 percent higher risk of early death. In addition, acid blockers have been shown to be addictive, causing a rebound of massive acid secretion when you stop them. So, wean off them using the treatments we discuss instead of stopping them suddenly.

I would note that the histamine-2 blocker medications (H2 acid blockers) cimetidine (Tagamet) or famotidine (Pepcid) are much safer and preferred, but improving your digestion and then weaning yourself off these medications is the best route to take.

Treatment
General Diet Advice

- **Drink warm liquids with meals.** Cold temperatures inactivate your digestive enzymes. Save ice drinks for between meals.
- **Drink refrigerator-cold diet colas.** Cola has the same acidity as stomach acid, so drinking some diet cola with large meals (e.g., Zevia cola) can actually improve digestion. Drink these at only refrigerator

temperature as opposed to ice cold. Vinegar-based salad dressings can also help.

Recommended Supplements

- **Plant-based enzymes.** Take 100 percent plant-based enzymes (not animal sourced, which don't work for digestion) to help digest your food. CompleteGest by Enzymatic Therapy is excellent. Take two capsules with each meal (or with larger meals) to help digest your food properly. If the enzymes are irritating to the stomach, wait till your stomach feels better on the licorice and mastic gum (see below) before resuming the enzymes.
- **Licorice.** The herb licorice is as effective as cimetidine (Tagamet) in head-to-head studies, but instead of turning off stomach acid, it actually helps heal your stomach's protective lining, which is a good thing. I like the brand Advanced DGL, which does not need to be chewed and so avoids the heavy licorice taste. Take one twice a day to help heal your stomach, and give it six weeks to work. Licorice tea can also help, but there is no licorice in licorice candy.

Advanced Herbal Remedies for Heartburn Relief

Add one capsule a day of Advanced Heartburn Rescue by Terry Naturally, a special mix of limonene (which can kill the indigestion-causing *H. pylori* infection in your stomach) and sea buckthorn oil, which may help heal your stomach's natural protective lining. This can give you long-term relief. Another option for killing these bacteria is 1,000 milligrams of mastic gum twice a day for one to two months (and thereafter as needed). Either can treat the *H. pylori* infection in your stomach, and both work well together. I usually give these before antibiotics for an *H. pylori* infection.

Medications

- **Cimetidine (Tagamet).** After a month on this regimen (using the plant-based enzyme plus the licorice treatment recommendation together), your doctor will often be able to stop your acid-blocker medicine if you've been on them. Instead of stopping them suddenly, I recommend you switch to cimetidine (Tagamet), an over-the-counter medicine that decreases stomach acid without turning it off, for a month. By the second month, you'll usually be able to stop all treatments, though you may prefer to continue the digestive enzymes and something to supply more stomach acid. The treatments above can be used intermittently if you have a recurrence of indigestion.

- **Antibiotics.** Your physician may prescribe a mix of antibiotics and acid blockers to kill the *H. pylori* ulcer-causing bacteria. Often, the natural treatments above can take care of the problem. If you do take the antibiotics, take 500 to 1,000 milligrams a day of vitamin C with the antibiotics to increase their effectiveness, along with the Advanced Heartburn Rescue or mastic gum.

For Night-Time Reflux

The treatments above will help with daytime acid reflux or GERD, but it is often nighttime reflux that leaves your esophagus chronically irritated. Though it's a bad idea to keep your stomach acid "turned off" during the day (you need it to digest food), you don't need stomach acid at bedtime while sleeping. So addressing the nighttime reflux as well for three months can allow the esophageal irritation to resolve. Here are a few tips:

- **Bicarbonate of soda.** Take ½ teaspoon of bicarbonate of soda (e.g., Arm & Hammer) in 4 ounces of water at bedtime to neutralize the acid in your stomach (not for children under sixteen years old). If you have high blood pressure, substitute food-grade potassium bicarbonate (available on Amazon). Don't eat for two hours before bedtime and take two capsules of a plant-based digestive enzyme such as CompleteGest sixty to ninety minutes before sleep. This will complete digestion and ensure your stomach is empty when you sleep, so there is nothing to reflux for a few hours.
- **Sleep with your upper body elevated.** Raise your upper body at least six to eight inches when in bed (just raising your head with pillows won't work). One way to do this is to place a six- to eight-inch brick or book under the legs of the bed (just the two legs under the end of the bed where your head is). Another wonderful solution is to use a sleep wedge pillow. You can find one called the Sleep Improving Pillow Wedge online at www.hammacher.com.
- **Melatonin.** Take 5 to 6 milligrams of immediate-release melatonin at bedtime. This decreases reflux.

- **Acid blockers.** If other remedies don't work, try 200 milligrams of a mild acid blocker like cimetidine (Tagamet) at bedtime, which is less addictive than other acid blockers.

IRRITABLE BOWEL SYNDROME AND SIBO

If the pain is lower than your solar plexus (around your belly button) and associated with increased gas or bloating, most often it will turn out to be intestinal. It is important that you see your physician to rule out other causes, but if they don't find anything, it will usually be called spastic colon or irritable bowel syndrome. This is just a medical way of saying you have gas, bloating, diarrhea, and/or constipation and they don't know why. Here's why you have it . . .

BACKGROUND

When doctors do not know what is causing your symptoms, we give it the label "spastic colon" or "irritable bowel syndrome" (I use the terms synonymously), instead of more effectively searching for the source of your symptoms.

The most effective way to eliminate spastic colon is to treat the underlying causes. This condition is sometimes caused by food sensitivity, such as to lactose in milk or fructose in sodas. More often, however, it is caused by an infection, and most patients' spastic colon resolves when the underlying bacterial, fungal, and parasitic bowel infections are treated. Unfortunately, there is no reliable test for fungal overgrowth, which is why this is missed. Suspect yeast overgrowth if you also have chronic sinusitis or nasal congestion. These also often go away when the fungal infection is treated—along with the spastic colon. In addition, when you pass gas from candida, it usually doesn't have much odor to it.

Small intestinal bacterial overgrowth (called SIBO) can mimic spastic colon and responds to many of the same treatments, but may require treating for bacterial infection and low thyroid issues (even if blood testing is normal). SIBO, as well as lactose and fructose intolerance, can be diagnosed by hydrogen breath testing (HBT), though this is usually not needed. Instead, if your gas has a nasty sulfur smell (remember the "silent but deadlies" from grade school?), this suggests SIBO or parasites.

TREATMENT
General Diet Advice

- **Stop milk and fructose.** Don't consume milk and fructose (i.e., so-das) for ten days. If symptoms resolve, stop sodas (diet sodas are okay) and try lactose-free milk products. With lactose intolerance, most people can have some milk. They just don't have the enzymes to digest more than a certain amount, and then it causes gas (not dangerous—just a nuisance). Taking the missing enzyme called lactase by mouth (found in products such as Lactaid) may allow you to tolerate more dairy products. I also recommend avoiding excess sweets.

Recommended Supplements

- **Magnesium.** If constipation is a predominant symptom, increase fiber and water, and take 200 to 300 milligrams of magnesium a day.

Other Therapies and Advice

- **Check for candida.** See Chapter 3 for fungal/yeast treatment.
- **Check for and treat parasites.** Do stool testing for parasites only at a lab that specializes in this (e.g., Genova Diagnostics by mail, see www.genovadiagnostics.com).
- **Take an enteric-coated probiotic.** Probiotics support healthy bowel function. If it's not enteric-coated, your stomach acid will simply kill the healthy bacteria. I recommend taking one capsule of Pearls Elite a day. Make sure you buy the type with five billion bacteria.
- **Check for SIBO.** If you have the distinctive sulfur smell to your gas, begin with an excellent herbal mix called Ultra MFP Forte. Two twice a day for one month (one bottle) will usually take care of it. If not, I will often prescribe a safe antibiotic called rifaximin (Xifaxan), 550 milligrams a day for ten days. But this antibiotic costs about $650, so be sure it is covered by insurance before you get it. If symptoms recur, I also treat for an underactive thyroid (see page 29), a main cause of recurrent SIBO.

  Wonderful work by Dr. Mark Pimentel has shown that very severe chronic constipation is often associated with overgrowth of methane-producing bacteria, which put your intestines to sleep. When treating for this, I often add 500 milligrams of the medication neo-mycin four times a day for ten days to increase effectiveness.

If symptoms persist, ask your doctor to do a hydrogen breath test (HBT) to look for SIBO and lactose or fructose intolerance.

- **Look for and treat food allergies.** If the SIBO tests are negative, treat for food allergies using an acupressure technique by NAET (see www.naet.com).
- **Take peppermint oil capsules.** For gas pains, begin with enteric-coated peppermint oil capules (e.g., Peppermint Plus by Enzymatic Therapy), which eases the cramps.

6. Nerve Compression Pain

CARPAL TUNNEL SYNDROME

BACKGROUND

Carpal tunnel syndrome is characterized by pain, numbness, and tingling that occurs in one or both hands. It often wakes people from their sleep, leaving them feeling like they have to "shake their hands out" to make the pain and symptoms go away.

This syndrome is caused by the compression of a nerve (the median nerve) as it goes through a narrow tunnel in the wrist formed by the carpal bone, hence the name carpal tunnel syndrome. According to the American Academy of Neurology, 10 percent of the population suffers from the syndrome. It also affects up to 50 percent of industrial workers. All too often the syndrome is treated by surgery. Although this can be effective, it is also expensive and, though rare, can leave people with residual problems due to the formation of scar tissue that can occur after surgery.

TREATMENT

Fortunately, unless people are continuing to stress the wrist with repetitive stress injuries (e.g., handling heavy equipment or doing very large amounts of typing), carpal tunnel syndrome can often be relieved without surgery. In almost all of my patients, their carpal tunnel syndrome has resolved by simply using the advice here.

Unfortunately, your doctor may be totally unfamiliar with these conservative therapies—in today's medicine only expensive treatments tend to get attention. If surgery is recommended, ask your physician if you can try these conservative measures instead for six to twelve weeks.

Recommended Supplements

- **Vitamin B6.** Take 50 to 250 milligrams of vitamin B6 daily. Only use the P5P (pyridoxal 5 phosphate) form as this is safer for nerve problems.
- **Desiccated thyroid hormone.** Use Armour Thyroid even if your blood tests are normal.

Other Therapies and Advice

- **Use a "cock-up" wrist splint.** When your hand gets into funny positions while you are sleeping, it stretches and strains the nerve as it goes through your wrist. This is why you wake up in the night with numbness or tingling. Use a "cock-up" wrist splint to keep your hand in the neutral position (i.e., the position your hand is in while holding a glass of water), which takes the stress off the nerve. Be sure to wear the splint while sleeping, and take the vitamin B6 and thyroid for at least six weeks to give the treatment time to work. During that period, also wear the wrist splint during the day whenever you conveniently can.
- **Other conservative measures.** Other conservative measures can also be effective, including acupuncture, osteopathic manipulation, chiropractic manipulation, and myofascial release.

7. Central Sensitization Pain

A Beginner's Guide

Background

Central sensitization syndrome and microglial activation are very extensive topics that would take writing a book to fully discuss, but here's a very simple overview.

Pain is the body's way of saying that something needs attention, like the oil light on a car's dashboard. When that need is not being addressed (chronic pain, I suspect from almost any cause), the body can then amplify the alert (pain). It does this in the form of amplifying the pain both through signals in the spine and in the brain. Basically, the pain is trying to get your attention—just as if the oil light got brighter and more annoying as a car's oil level dropped.

In the brain, this occurs when brain cells called microglial cells become activated. Think of these cells as the usually mild-mannered gardeners in the brain that tend to and nourish the brain cells. There are many things that can then make these mellow gardeners become very aggressive. For example, if the gardeners see bugs in the garden (think infections), something injuring their plants (think traumatic brain injury), or perceive another threat or need (think chronic pain). Then the now manic gardeners start weeding frantically, overstimulating the brain and the pain.

Although this is a gross oversimplification, I hope you get the point. So how do you get these gardeners to become mellow again and settle the microglial activation?

TREATMENT

- Address any infections (viral or antibiotic sensitive).
- Get rid of the pain triggers in the periphery. In fibromyalgia, this is mostly muscle pain from chronic shortening initially, followed by secondary nerve pain (including small fiber neuropathy).
- Use any in a number of medications or supplements to settle down central sensitization as well. Here are just a few of them:

Supplements

- **Low-dose naltrexone.** This is by prescription from compounding pharmacies. I like to use Skip's Compounding Pharmacy (www.skips pharmacy.com) as Skip Lenz is especially knowledgeable, and they have great prices and quality. Take 3 to 4.5 milligrams at bedtime. It takes two months to see the effect. Sometimes LDN will disrupt sleep quality at first, in which case I have people start with a very low dose (the pharmacy will actually make a starter pack to allow you to raise the dose up slowly), or even begin by taking it in the morning. See more information about this on page 121.

- **Hemp oil.** I recommend Hemp Select to help numerous components of the pain cycle, including central sensitization. Although hemp oil is expensive, three capsules three times a day can be a godsend.

- **Palmitoylethanolamide (PEA).** Take 350 milligrams four times daily for two to four weeks, then twice a day (or three times a day if more helpful). Higher doses may be more effective. I recommend the brand Mirica, one to two capsules two to three times a day. Start slowly and work up.

- **SHINE.** Treating the entire process with the SHINE protocol generally settles down central sensitization as well.

Medications

- **Doxycycline or minocycline.** I will prescribe 100 milligrams twice a day if the person cannot take the low-dose naltrexone. These specific antibiotics have been shown to decrease central sensitization, but they can cause candida overgrowth over time unless a person is also using the natural antifungals such as Lufenuron and/or 400 milligrams of fluconazole (Diflucan) once each week.

- **Metformin (Glucophage).** 500 to 1,000 milligrams twice daily.

- **The big three.** Pregabalin (Lyrica), duloxetine (Cymbalta), and milnacipran (Savella) can all help central sensitization. You may have noticed that most of what you've heard about fibromyalgia pain is central sensitization, although this is just one of ten key types of fibromyalgia pain. And what you have heard about for treating it are likely Lyrica, Cymbalta, and Savella. Why? Because the companies making these three medications spent about $210 million per year on advertising, compared to just a few million dollars a year that the NIH has for fibromyalgia. This does not mean these medications are not helpful. It just means that they are a very small part of the healthcare tool kit for treating fibromyalgia.

8. Allodynia

WHEN EVEN SOFT TOUCH HURTS

BACKGROUND
Allodynia may occur in more severe cases of fibromyalgia pain. In these cases, even a light touch across the skin may hurt.

TREATMENT
Although medications for nerve pain may help, in a small subset even these do not. In these cases, I use a medication called memantine (Namenda), which inhibits special pain sensors called NMDA pain receptors. The antiviral amantadine (Symmetrel) also blocks NMDA receptors.

In addition, if the pain persists for over three months on the SHINE protocol, it is worth considering a trial of intravenous or subcutaneous infusions of gamma globulin. Giving the infusions at a dose of 1 gram of gamma globulin per pound of body weight three days in a row and then repeating every three to four weeks is one reasonable regimen. It is very expensive, so make sure it is covered by insurance. Allow the infusions six months to work.

The medications gabapentin (Neurontin) and/or pregabalin (Lyrica) can also be very helpful for this kind of pain.

Topical, or even intravenous or intranasal, ketamine can be helpful in severe cases. Because this is psychoactive, it can only be used by physicians trained in its use and is a controlled drug. It is now available as the intranasal spray for treatment of severe depression. The drug companies are charging about $800 a dose. Compounding pharmacies can make it for about $5 per dose.

9. Pelvic Pain Syndromes

INCLUDES PAIN DURING INTERCOURSE

BACKGROUND
Pelvic pain syndrome usually comes from muscle pain in the pelvic floor (the muscles, ligaments, and tissue that support your pelvic organs and

pelvic joints). But the condition can also be neuropathic or come from localized tissue inflammation or dryness. Pelvic floor physical therapy is highly recommended. There are many physical therapists specializing in pelvic floor pain who are superb. These are usually familiar with myofascial pain and trigger points. Combining this with a prescription of the medications gabapentin (Neurontin) and amitriptyline (Elavil) usually is very effective, although most people will have the pain go away simply with the medications and the SHINE protocol

In many people, especially women over forty-five years old, pain during intercourse is simply caused by vaginal dryness from inadequate estrogen production. For them, I recommend a compounded bioidentical estrogen and progesterone cream. After six weeks, this usually takes care of the problem and also decreases urinary incontinence and bladder infections. An excellent lubricant for intercourse is a liquid coconut oil. Nature's Way makes Always Liquid Coconut Premium Oil, which is excellent for this. Some of the synthetic lubricants can be irritating.

Pelvic Pain Syndromes in Fibromyalgia

These are very common and include:

- **Interstitial cystitis (IC).** This is a bladder problem characterized by *severe* urinary urgency, frequency, burning, and pain. I am not talking about the mild urinary urgency seen in fibromyalgia, but rather when it is so severe that people want their bladder surgically removed. Once bacterial infections have been ruled out, I prescribe 10 to 25 milligrams of amitriptyline (Elavil) at bedtime plus 300 to 900 milligrams of gabapentin (Neurontin) at bedtime and perhaps during the day as well. I then also treat the patient for presumptive candida with oral fluconazole (Diflucan) for three months. Many supplements including B vitamins and vitamin C may aggravate the bladder symptoms in a subset of people with IC.
- **Vulvodynia.** Defined as chronic vulvar itching, burning, and/or pain that is significantly uncomfortable, this condition causes vulvar/vaginal pain either only during intercourse or constantly present. In my experience, vulvodynia seems to occur as three main types: neuropathic, inflammatory, and muscle pain. I also add bedtime amitriptyline (Elavil) and gabapentin (Neurontin) for vulvodynia.

- **Prostate pain.** Prostate pain is fairly common in men. When no infection is found, it is called prostadynia. I suspect that prostadynia often occurs because of subtle infections and usually improves when these are treated. Taking 500 milligrams of the bioflavonoid quercetin twice a day decreases prostate symptoms in both prostadynia and prostatitis. I treat with fluconazole (Diflucan) for candida first, followed by an extended trial of ciprofloxacin (Cipro) or doxycycline if needed.
- **Endometriosis.** Endometriosis is characterized by abdominal and pelvic pain that is usually worse around the menstrual cycle. It is often associated with other symptoms suggestive of chronic fatigue syndrome and fibromyalgia, such as fatigue, achiness, cognitive dysfunction, and insomnia. For more information, read the book *Endometriosis: The Complete Reference for Taking Charge of Your Health* by Mary Lou Ballweg and the Endometriosis Association.

I discuss pelvic pain in more detail in my book *Pain Free 1-2-3*.

10. Sympathetically Mediated Pain

CRPS/RSD

BACKGROUND

Fortunately, this horrible pain from complex regional pain syndrome and reflex sympathetic dystrophy (CRPS/RSD) is relatively uncommon. I remember the first person I saw with this pain. This unfortunate woman had seen her rheumatologist and had her knee aspirated. It got infected and triggered CRPS. At that time, early in my medical career, I had never even heard of the condition. I had no way to treat her.

The pain was so severe that she wanted to get an amputation. I told her that would not help the pain, but she did it anyway. And it did not help. Since then, I have spent thirty years asking at every pain conference I went to if anybody had found anything to help CRPS.

Although it can spread throughout the body, most often it is in just one hand or foot. If I walk into the exam room and see the person hiding an extremity behind them to avoid anybody brushing against it, I look for this illness. Fortunately, even this awful pain is becoming treatable.

But few physicians are familiar with even diagnosis, let alone treatment.

The pain is so severe, and this area so important, please forgive my making this discussion lengthier than the others.

TREATMENT

It is important to recognize that multiple kinds of pain are involved in CRPS. In addition to the pain caused by sympathetic reflex issues and neuropathic pain, there is a very large component of secondary muscle pain that may also be a severe cause of discomfort, so looking for and treating all of the components is important.

How to Begin

- Look for a pain medicine specialist (someone who specializes in physical medicine and rehabilitation–a physiatrist). Most of these specialists come from either an anesthesia background (focusing on surgical and injection techniques) or more of an internal medicine background, which includes treating myofascial/muscle/nerve pain. In the beginning of the illness, the former is most helpful as the nerve blocks can be most beneficial in the first twelve to eighteen months. After that, somebody who knows how to do trigger point therapy and other muscle techniques may be more effective.
- Watch the excellent video by Dr. Pradeep Chopra called "CRPS/ RSD: Update on Treatments," at www.youtube.com/watch?v=6_Nzh nAXX2c. He is my favorite CRPS/RSD specialist, and his video has a wealth of helpful information and is a good place to begin. If you can see him for CRPS medical care, this would be highly recommended as well.

There are many other steps as well, but these offer a very good beginning and can be extremely helpful for what has been a very challenging condition in the past.

Next Steps

For treating the root causes of CRPS, try the following:

- **IV Bisphosphonates.** Use whatever is available locally. Use 90 milligrams of pamidronate administered once over three to four hours (give in 500 cc normal saline). Per Dr. Pradeep Chopra, use 300 milligrams of clodronate IV daily for ten days, or 7.5 milligrams of alendronate (Fosamax) IV once. Both can cause initial flaring of symptoms in acute CRPS, so this is better for chronic cases. He also uses 60 milligrams of pamidronate IV. Neridronate was the bisphosphonate used in a 2013 Italian study by Dr. Massimo Varenna, which showed significant and sustained benefit in CRPS. Long-term treatment is often necessary to maintain benefits.

- **Low-dose naltrexone (LDN).** I give 3 to 4.5 milligrams at night. This is very helpful and simple, and it can settle down what is called central sensitization, a key component of the pain. Higher doses will not work. LDN is available from compounding pharmacies. It usually costs about a dollar a day and may initially disrupt sleep a bit. If this happens, take it in the morning and begin with lower dosing and work up instead. The benefits can be marked over time and usually begin after about two to three months, with side effects disappearing. LDN cannot be taken if one is on narcotics. In that situation, taking 100 milligrams of doxycycline twice a day can help with the central sensitization, but it can cause candida/yeast overgrowth. The next two treatments also help with central sensitization, though I find the LDN to be the most effective and safe of these, and usually just use LDN for central sensitization unless I am not able to. See page 150 on central sensitization.
- **Quinapril (Accupril).** I give 10 milligrams of this blood pressure–lowering medicine that also blocks microglial activation and central sensitization.
- **Pentoxifylline or metformin.** These can also help central sensitization.
- **IV ketamine protocols.** These can be *very* helpful. Physicians who use these protocols will usually know the dosing, but it should be at least 1 milligram per kilogram of body weight. Some physicians who give IV ketamine will also give intravenous lidocaine. Both of these increase in effectiveness over time.
- **Dimethyl sulfoxide (DMSO).** Topical 50 percent DMSO (available from compounding pharmacies) applied three times a day has been shown to significantly diminish CRPS symptoms over several months. This is low cost with the only real side effect being a garlic smell.

For Pain

- **Gabapentin (Neurontin).** I give 100 to 900 milligrams three to four times a day as needed for pain. Other medications in this family used along with nortriptyline can also be quite helpful.
- **Baclofen (Lioresal).** I give 10 milligrams (one or two tablets) three to four times a day for muscle pain. Start low, as it can be very sedating.
- **Compounded cream.** Use a topical nerve pain cream including at least ketamine, gabapentin, baclofen, and lidocaine. This is available from ITC Compounding Pharmacy (888-349-5453) by prescription. Your physician can call the pharmacist there who will guide them. Apply topically one to three times a day to the painful areas and give it six weeks to start working.
- **SHINE.** It is common for a secondary fibromyalgia to be present in CRPS. This also needs to be treated using our SHINE protocol. If fatigue, widespread pain, and poor sleep are present, then you likely have a secondary fibromyalgia.

GENERAL CRPS/RSD SUPPORT

Use the following over-the-counter supplements:

- **Vitamin C.** This reduces free radicals and decreases the risk of recurrent CRPS. The suggested dose is 500 milligrams by mouth once daily.
- **Fish oil.** This reduces inflammation and enhances the immune system. Take two tablets of Vectomega a day. This markedly decreases the number of pills needed.
- **Energy Revitalization System vitamin powder or Clinical Essentials multivitamin.** These have B vitamins, magnesium, vitamin C, and vitamin D along with numerous other critical nutrients needed to help settle pain from a number of causes. If using the Clinical Essentials, add 1,000 units of vitamin D daily.
- **Acetyl-L-carnitine.** This reduces free radicals and blocks T-type calcium channel. The suggested dose is 500 to 1,000 milligrams by mouth three times a day. This and the two below take three to six months to start working.
- **Lipoic acid.** Take 300 to 600 milligrams twice a day to markedly help nerve discomfort. It can be combined with IV lipoic acid.

- **NAC (N-acetyl cysteine).** Take 500 to 1,000 milligrams daily to increase glutathione.

Holistic physicians may also give 1 to 2 grams of magnesium over one to two hours plus 1,000 milligrams of lipoic acid IV as often as two to three times a week for a few months until pain settles down, and then it can be given less often. Lipoic acid is especially helpful and has been widely studied for neuropathic pain, but not yet for CRPS—it is reasonable to give, however. The main side effect of lipoic acid at intravenous doses over 600 milligrams is a drop in blood sugar, so the doctor should have a glucose IV on hand to administer as needed. (This is easy to address and not a big deal.)

My Favorite CRPS Specialist in the Whole World

Dr. Pradeep Chopra is a pain management specialist in Pawtucket, Rhode Island, and a Brown University School of Medicine professor. He has a ketamine IV clinic as part of his office. He is frequently the keynote speaker for the Reflex Sympathetic Dystrophy Syndrome Association (RSDSA), and you can view his conference videos on YouTube or at www.rsds.org. He is one of the most compassionate and knowledgeable CRPS doctors there is.

One of his patients says:

> He does not take insurance. He and his team literally spent five hours one-on-one with me. He sets up a basic treatment protocol that you can share with your primary physician. After the appointment, if you email him, he answers your questions and may even give you treatment options or new referrals.

Contact Dr. Chopra at 401-729-4985 or www.painri.com.

FOR ACUTE FLARES OF RSD/CRPS

From "Tips for Managing Complex Regional Pain Syndrome" by Jim Ducharme, MD (https://rsds.org/wp-content/uploads/2014/12/Tips-for-Managing-Complex-Regional-Pain-Syndrome.pdf):

Given the cause of the pain flare-up, the treatment needs to be directed at stopping the NMDA activity. This is best accomplished with ketamine, an NMDA antagonist. A patient can only receive intravenous ketamine in a hospital environment, so emergency physicians need to be able to recognize and treat these severe pain flare-ups.

Treatment is straightforward:

1. Initial bolus of 0.2–0.3 mg/kg of ketamine infused over 10 minutes. Giving this dose as an IV push will produce a high rate of dissociative side effects (up to 75 percent of patients) and should be avoided. Almost diagnostic is the patient's response: severe pain should be resolved by the end of the 10-minute bolus.

2. An infusion of ketamine (0.2 mg/kg/hr) for four to six hours. Although the medical literature for this is almost nonexistent, clinical experience has shown that an infusion of this duration resets the NMDA activity to baseline. Patients can return home on their usual medications, with the expectation that the flare-up, which can normally last weeks, will be over. Return rates for the same flare-up after ketamine treatment approach zero. For readers who feel four to six hours is too long, I encourage them to try shorter periods (two or three hours) and publish their results. No discharge prescription from the emergency department will be required.

Patients do not require admission, and they should not receive opioids. They do require the acute ketamine intervention, or they will suffer severe pain for weeks as a result of the flare-up. To date, there is no other effective treatment for a CRPS pain flare-up. Some researchers have studied an infusion of 5 mg/kg of lidocaine over a 60-minute period* as an alternative treatment plan, but results are variable. Referral of newly diagnosed patients to physiotherapy and a comprehensive pain program is critical.

---

* I consider 3 milligrams per kilogram over twenty to thirty minutes, and then 2 to 3 milligrams per minute of intravenous lidocaine over three hours to be safer and more effective.

To Avoid Recurrence/Spread with Surgery

Take 1,000 milligrams of vitamin C a day. In general, the 500 milligrams in the Energy Revitalization System vitamin powder should be taken daily to decrease recurrence risk.

I hope this is helpful for you. CRPS has been one of the hardest pain conditions to treat for decades, but it is finally giving way to effective treatment. The problem now is lack of physician education. The above will give you the tools you need. Please share them with your physician and others.

PART THREE

SHINE

Intensive Care

*Recovering from Chronic Fatigue Syndrome
and Fibromyalgia*

BFF Summary

Research shows that fibromyalgia is very treatable, with average improvements of over 90 percent using the SHINE protocol. A major part of the protocol can be done naturally without a physician's prescription.

To make things easy, there is a free brain fog–friendly fifteen-minute quiz at www .energyanalysisprogram.com, which can analyze your symptoms (and even key lab tests if available). It uses and organizes the principles discussed in this book. The quiz will quickly determine the key issues draining your energy, and tailor a protocol to optimize energy production in your case.

Introduction: CFS and Fibromyalgia Are Now Very Treatable

What if CFS and fibromyalgia were now *very* treatable? The good news? They are!

Our published randomized, double-blind, placebo-controlled study (the gold standard for research design) showed that 91 percent of people improved, with an average 90 percent improvement in quality of life using the SHINE protocol. This is far more effective than treatments for many other illnesses. We very much appreciate the researchers at the NIH who helped us design the study.

As a reminder, SHINE stands for addressing and optimizing:

Sleep
Hormones and hypotension
Infections and immunity
Nutrition
Exercise as able

In CFS/FMS, we add "hypotension" to the H. This includes conditions like postural orthostatic tachycardia syndrome (POTS) and neurally mediated hypotension (NMH).

The info in Part One lays the foundation to healing, even in CFS/FMS. We know comparing CFS/FMS to day-to-day fatigue is like comparing a lit match to a nuclear meltdown. But trying to recover from CFS/FMS without starting with the basics is like trying to build a house without a foundation. It just doesn't work. Once you've read and done the treatments in Part One, *then* the information here can rock your world.

Having read Part One, you've made a great start toward recovery. You've read the key parts of your body's "owner's manual" and learned what the different warning lights mean. But by the time CFS or fibromyalgia hit, your body was already pulled over to the side of the road, with no power, and out of the game. But though it may feel permanently damaged, or just this side of dead, it's not. You simply tripped a circuit breaker (or for those of you old enough to remember the expression, "blew a fuse") called the hypothalamus.

Ready for some good news? CFS/FMS doesn't happen to everyone who has an overwhelming energy crisis. Instead they get things like cancers that do kill them. Getting the illness instead may have saved your life.

If it saved your life so you can live like this, you may think, *Fat lot of good that did me*. But our research shows you *can* turn the circuit breaker back on and get your life back.

I'll show you how in this section.

More good news? Ever see a mutant-superhero movie? Where the character gets some superpower from their illness or spider bite? There is a superpower gift you may find you got from the illness (I did). I'll share it with you at the end of this book.

This dramatic improvement with the SHINE protocol has also been shown in the thousands of people that we have treated. It has been so incredibly personally gratifying to watch them get their lives back. Meanwhile, outcomes continue to improve even more, by adding the newer treatments in this book.

The Science Shows That CFS and Fibromyalgia Are Very Treatable

So why aren't physicians applying the research? This is occurring for several reasons. Fortunately, you can get well anyway.

This is why we have created tools such as the *free* Energy Analysis Program (www.energyanalysisprogram.com) to make this simpler, so everyone can get treatment. This patented free fifteen-minute quiz can analyze your symptoms, and even key lab tests if available, to determine what is causing your energy crisis. It will then tailor a protocol to optimize your energy using a mix of natural and prescription therapies.

Basically, it applies a large part of the information in this book, making things very simple. Much of this can actually be done on your own. This is part of our goal of making effective treatment available for everyone.

Here's how to proceed in getting well:

1. Read through this book. It is okay to simply look at the BFF Summaries so you can understand what is going on with your body. Even with brain fog, most of you will be able to do this fairly simply. This understanding will leave you feeling much more comfortable and help you learn what you need to do to get well.
2. Even if you begin with just the natural therapies by themselves, you can make a major difference.
3. Do the free Energy Analysis Program (www.energyanalysisprogram .com) to apply the principles in this book to easily figure out what problems you need to address to recover your health. This will give you a detailed protocol. It is okay to start with the Energy Revitalization System vitamin powder, Recovery Factors, and the Smart Energy System. After one month, most people see significant benefits with only these three supplements. Then go down the list and add in more of the recommendations as you're comfortable.

You will be amazed how much you can improve simply by using the natural options we discuss, and then, in Part Five, I will show you how to encourage your doctor to write for some key prescriptions.

Many people with CFS/FMS are financially devastated and can't afford very much at all. I was homeless when I had the disease, so know that I understand. See "Surviving Prescription Costs" on page 324. Fortunately, the cost of a treatment has absolutely nothing at all to do with its effectiveness.

Also, see my article on how to treat fibromyalgia at low cost at https://www.vitality101.com/health-a-z/low-cost-treatments-for-cfs-and-fibro myalgia.

If you have the option of getting a health insurance policy that includes a medical savings account (MSA), this is an excellent idea. Then you can use this for supplements and holistic practitioners.

Ready to move on to the next step of getting well by applying SHINE Intensive Care? Read on . . .

Staying Up-to-Date on the Newest Fibromyalgia Research

I invite you to sign up for my free email newsletter at www.endfatigue.com or www.vitality101.com. It comes out, well, whenever I feel like I have something to say. But this way you don't have to wait for the next edition of this book ten years from now to get current information.

I also highly recommend Cort Johnson's website, www.healthrising.org.

12 What Are Chronic Fatigue Syndrome and Fibromyalgia?

BFF Summary

1. Chronic fatigue syndrome (CFS) is characterized by the paradox of inability to sleep despite being exhausted, brain fog, and, if fibromyalgia (FMS) is also present, widespread pain. You may have a variety of other symptoms as well. Common symptoms include increased thirst, weight gain, low libido, nasal congestion/sinusitis, and frequent infections.
2. CFS and FMS occur when you expend more energy than you can make. This overloads your circuits, causing you to "blow a fuse" in the part of the brain called the hypothalamus.
3. There is no currently accepted test for making the diagnosis. It is not needed. Testing is needed to determine the *cause(s)* of your CFS/FMS, and how to treat it.
4. Research shows that effective therapy is available for 91 percent of people with CFS/FMS by simply treating with the SHINE protocol (increasing and addressing sleep, hormones, infections, nutrition, and exercise as able).

---

*A*re you exhausted? Are you having widespread pain, experiencing brain fog, and having trouble sleeping? If you answered yes, you're one of 6 to 18 million Americans, and one of over 250 million people worldwide, with a CFS- or FMS-related process. Meanwhile, one out of every three Americans suffers with inadequately treated chronic pain and 31 percent of adults are *chronically* fatigued.

People with CFS/FMS are like the tip of an iceberg that is rapidly coming to the surface. As the numbers of cases grow, these conditions will become increasingly hard to ignore.

So you are not alone, even if sometimes you feel that way.

Put simply, CFS/FMS represents a severe energy crisis in your body, where you essentially blow a fuse. Just like there are many ways to trip a circuit breaker in your home, there are many ways to do so in your body, causing CFS and FMS. In this book we will teach you how to get rid of these energy leaks while turbocharging your energy production. This way, the circuit breaker kicks back on will reset, and your body will feel like it is coming back to life.

Let's start with the basics.

Making the Diagnosis: The Standard Way

There are differing definitions that are used clinically and in research. Just to offer an idea of these, I have included three common ones. The first two are pretty irrelevant for your day-to-day care, so feel free to skip them:

1. The 1994 US Centers for Disease Control criteria for CFS (a definition with which I am wholly *un*impressed) require the presence of the following:

   A. Clinically evaluated, unexplained, persistent, or relapsing chronic fatigue that is of new or definite onset (has not been lifelong); is not the result of ongoing exertion; is not substantially alleviated by rest; and results in substantial reduction in previous levels of occupational, educational, social, or personal activities.

   B. Concurrent occurrence of four or more of the following symptoms, all of which must have persisted or recurred during six or more consecutive months of illness and must not have predated the fatigue:

- Self-reported impairment in short-term memory or concentration severe enough to cause substantial reduction in previous levels of occupational, educational, social, or personal activities
- Sore throat
- Tender cervical [neck] or axillary [underarm] lymph nodes
- Muscle pain
- Multi-joint pain without joint swelling or redness
- Headaches of a new type, pattern, or severity
- Unrefreshing sleep
- Post-exertional malaise lasting more than twenty-four hours

2. The old 1990 American College of Rheumatology (ACR) diagnostic criteria for fibromyalgia. This required a person to have persistent widespread pain, and eleven of eighteen tender points on the tender point exam, which most doctors have absolutely no clue how to do.

3. In 2011, the ACR modified the diagnostic criteria for fibromyalgia, which no longer uses the tender point exam and is a marked improvement. These have been updated in the 2016 ACR criteria, and I find either of these acceptable to use.

THE 2011 MODIFIED ACR FIBROMYALGIA DIAGNOSTIC CRITERIA

A patient satisfies the diagnostic criteria for fibromyalgia if the following conditions are met:

1. Widespread Pain Index (WPI) ≥7 and Symptom Severity (SS) scale score ≥5, or WPI 3 to 6 and SS scale score ≥9.
2. Symptoms have been present at a similar level for at least three months.
3. The patient does not have a disorder that would otherwise explain the pain.

Take this test and add:

1. Widespread Pain Index: Circle each area where you've had pain over the last week, then count how many you circled. (Your score will be between 0 and 19.)

Shoulder girdle, left	Hip (buttock, trochanter), left	Jaw, left	Upper back
Shoulder girdle, right	Hip (buttock, trochanter), right	Jaw, right	Lower back
Upper arm, left	Upper leg, left	Chest	Neck
Upper arm, right	Upper leg, right	Abdomen	
Lower arm, left	Lower leg, left		
Lower arm, right	Lower leg, right		

2. Symptom Severity scale score: For each of the three symptoms below, score its severity over the past week, using the following scale:

0 =	No problem
1 =	Slight or mild problems, generally mild or intermittent
2 =	Moderate, considerable problems, often present and/or at a moderate level
3 =	Severe, pervasive, continuous, life-disturbing problems

_____ Fatigue (score 0 to 3)
_____ Waking unrefreshed (score 0 to 3)
_____ Cognitive symptoms ("brain fog") (score 0 to 3)

Then add *JUST 1 point* for each of the following three symptoms that have occurred during the previous six months:

_____ Headaches (score 0 to 1)
_____ Pain or cramps in lower abdomen (score 0 to 1)
_____ Depression (score 0 to 1)
_____ Total SS scale score (adding the 6 items above). The final score is between 0 and 12.

Technically, the 2011 ACR modified diagnostic criteria are not supposed to be used by the patient, but only by doctors. I don't believe that this limitation is really necessary. Happily, though, in real life there is a much simpler way to tell if you have a CFS/FMS-related process and are likely to improve with SHINE treatments.

A really simple way to tell if you have the diagnosis? Go to www .vitality101.com and do the free quiz at Step 2. It will quickly tell you if you meet the diagnostic criteria for chronic fatigue syndrome or fibromyalgia.

Diagnosing CFS and/or FMS Made Easy

Simply answer these four questions:

1. Do you have severe fatigue, along with insomnia and perhaps brain fog?
2. Have you been checked by your doctor, and no other overt cause was found? (Being told you're depressed or crazy because the doctor was clueless doesn't count.)
3. Has it lasted over three months? If yes to these three, you likely have CFS until proven otherwise.
4. Do you also have widespread pain? If yes, then you also have fibromyalgia.

In most cases, it is that simple.

ANOTHER NAME FOR A CONDITION WITH RELATED SYMPtoms is myalgic encephalomyelitis (ME). This diagnosis tends to be used more in Canada and Europe. Although there are differences in how they are defined, and every case is different, I consider CFS, FMS, and ME to be related and overlapping conditions that all respond well to the treatments discussed in this book, so I use the term CFS/FMS to refer to all of these.

A Quick Tip

Though in most cases CFS and FMS are two names for the same condition, because of current politics and the social stigma attached to the diagnosis of CFS, you will generally do better to use the FMS label instead. Some good news from an unexpected quarter? The pharmaceutical industry spent nearly $210 million a year on advertising to make the diagnosis of FMS medically and socially acceptable, so it could create a larger market for its three FDA-approved FMS medications.

What CFS and FMS Feel Like

CFS and FMS occur in varying degrees of severity, ranging from moderately disruptive to leaving some people bedridden. And no, these are *not* happening because you are depressed or "you're getting older." They're happening because you have CFS/FMS.

There are dozens of symptoms that can be seen with CFS/FMS. Doctors not familiar with the illness, even excellent physicians, have difficulty making sense of this wide array of symptoms, so their reactions may have left you and your family confused and concerned. Some especially clueless physicians may have even implied that since *they* don't know what's wrong, *you* must be crazy.

So let's clear this up for you right now.

The most common complaints among chronic fatigue and fibromyalgia patients include:

- **Overwhelming fatigue.** Most people with CFS/FMS have significant or overwhelming fatigue. Occasionally, they experience short periods during which they feel better. However, after several hours or days of feeling energetic, they typically crash back down into severe fatigue.

    Often, CFS/FMS patients wake up feeling tired and spend the day that way. Oddly, they often have the most energy between 10:00 p.m. and 4:00 a.m. This is due, in part, to their day-night cycles being reversed. In addition, too much exercise often makes the fatigue worse.

When CFS/FMS patients try to exercise, they feel worse that day and as if they were hit by a truck the next. If you have CFS/FMS, this "post-exertional fatigue" occurs because you can't make enough energy to condition your body to exercise and simply deplete what little energy you had. This causes further deconditioning and discouragement. A better approach is to walk as much as you can, but only to the point where you feel "good tired" after the exercise and better the next day. After approximately ten weeks of gentle, slow walking to begin reconditioning, while doing the treatments discussed in this book, most people find that they can start to increase their walking by up to one minute a day as their energy levels increase. Once you can walk for about an hour a day, then you can start slowly increasing the intensity of exercise. See Chapter 18, "Exercise Intensive Care."

- **Severe insomnia.** People with CFS/FMS are lucky to be able to sleep five hours a night despite being exhausted. Meanwhile, it's like an alarm clock goes off every night between two and four in the morning. Restless leg syndrome and sleep apnea are also much more common in people with CFS/FMS.

- **Brain fog.** People with CFS/FMS often suffer from poor short-term memory and difficulty with word finding and word substitution. Sometimes you may even have to think for a moment to remember your children's names. About one-third of people will also have rare, brief episodes of disorientation, lasting thirty seconds to two minutes. These most often happen when taking an exit ramp while driving or making a turn in a store aisle. It can feel frightening, but it is not dangerous and passes quickly.

  Brain fog is one of the most frustrating symptoms for some people and is often the scariest. Many people are afraid that they are developing Alzheimer's disease. A simple way to differentiate between brain fog and dementia is that with brain fog, you may constantly forget where you left the keys. With Alzheimer's, however, you may forget how to *use* your keys. They are not the same, and the brain fog also routinely improves, and often resolves, by using the SHINE protocol.

- **Achiness and pain.** Achiness in both muscles and joints is also common and may progress to nerve pain as well. Initially, it feels like you have achy muscles in many different parts of your body. As you shift positions, the pain may move around to different areas over time. In the beginning, this pain is predominantly from tight muscles and is associated with tender knots in the muscles called trigger points (where the belly of the shortened muscle bunches up). These feel like tender marbles when someone gives you a massage.

As the condition progresses, some people develop numbness or tingling in their hands or feet (paresthesia and carpal tunnel syndrome), and sometimes burning/shooting pains (nerve pain or neuropathy). Sometimes the skin is even sensitive to touch (called allodynia). All of these pains can be effectively treated and are discussed in Chapters 9, 10, and 11.

- **Increased thirst.** Because of hormonal problems, people with chronic fatigue and fibromyalgia often have decreased ability to hold on to salt and water, which increases urine output and thirst. A classic description of CFS/FMS is that you "drink like a fish and pee like a racehorse." Drinking a lot of water and *increasing* salt intake becomes important and will help you feel better. As we discuss regarding low adrenal function in Chapter 14, "Hormone and Hypotension Intensive Care," trying to restrict salt when you have CFS/FMS is a quick way to crash and burn. When people ask me how many glasses of water to drink a day, I tell them a much better approach is simply to check your mouth and lips. If they are dry, you are thirsty and need to drink more water.

  It is important to note that dry eyes and dry mouth that do not improve when you drink more water (called sicca syndrome) are also common. These symptoms can often be resolved by taking fish oil (Vectomega) and sea buckthorn oil (Omega 7 by Terry Naturally) supplements, B vitamins, and magnesium.

- **Frequent infections.** Many CFS/FMS patients have:
  - Recurrent respiratory infections, sore throats, and swollen glands and seem to catch every cold that's going around. This tends to resolve with adrenal support (see Chapter 2).
  - Chronic sinusitis, nasal congestion, and postnasal drip. This is most often caused by candida/yeast.
  - Digestive disorders, including gas, cramps, and alternating diarrhea and constipation. These are usually attributed to irritable bowel syndrome (sometimes still called spastic colon). Irritable bowel syndrome simply means that you have these

symptoms and your doctor does not know why. In CFS/FMS, these are usually triggered by bowel infections, especially candida, and improve with treatment. If your gas smells like sulfur, you likely also have SIBO (small intestinal bacterial overgrowth).

- Continuing body-wide flu-like symptoms. These patients often have reactivation of an old virus.

- **Allergies and sensitivities.** CFS/FMS patients often have a history of being sensitive to many foods and medications. I find that food sensitivities and other sensitivities usually improve when the adrenal insufficiency and yeast or parasitic overgrowth are treated. Desensitization techniques such as NAET (Nambudripad's Allergy Elimination Technique) can also be very helpful in more severe cases (more about this in Chapter 19).

- **Anxiety and depression.** Approximately 12 percent of people with CFS have marked anxiety, sometimes with palpitations, sweating, and other signs of panic. Metabolically, CFS/FMS sometimes leaves people more prone to hyperventilation as well as a rapid resting pulse. These symptoms, too, often improve with treatment. Depression is also more common in any illness, including cancer, where severe pain or debility are present. This does not mean that the person doesn't have cancer. Unfortunately, some physicians will simply label a person as depressed if they can't figure out what is wrong with them, instead of honestly saying they don't know. This is simply unacceptable for any physician to do. Fortunately, this kind of nonsense is becoming less common as physicians are learning more about these illnesses.

So how can you tell if you are depressed? Well, for starters, ask yourself. Research shows that simply asking is as reliable as fancy depression scales. Another way to tell? Do you have many interests? If you have a lot of interests but are frustrated that you don't have the energy to do them, you are probably not clinically depressed.

As with any severe chronic illness, if you feel that working with a psychologist or mental health professional would be helpful, please do so. Find one familiar with CFS/FMS. Somebody with metastatic cancer would not dream of working with a psychologist who doesn't believe cancer is a real illness. The same applies to CFS/FMS. This can be one more helpful tool in your healing tool kit.

- **Weight gain.** Studies done in our research center show that people with CFS and fibromyalgia gain an average of thirty-two pounds with their illness. I suspect this occurs because of changes in metabolism caused by low thyroid function, yeast overgrowth, a deficiency of acetyl-L-carnitine, insulin resistance, immune dysfunction, and poor sleep. Many patients are thrilled not only to feel better and have their pain go away with treatment but also to find their weight dropping (see Chapter 20).
- **Decreased libido.** When asked how their libido is, most people with CFS/FMS (73 percent in one of our studies) answer, "What libido?" In addition to pain and a general yucky feeling, hormonal deficiencies also contribute to this symptom. However, libido often improves with treatment, though it may take six to nine months.
- **Other common symptoms.** These include occasional shortness of breath (not with exercise), non-exertional chest pain (usually benign chest wall muscle tenderness, but check with your doctor to be safe), occasional dizziness on standing, and even bladder and pelvic pain. We discuss these more elsewhere in the book.

You may have recognized yourself as you read through this list. If you did, please be assured that you are not alone. You are part of a large group of over one hundred million people worldwide.

What Causes CFS and Fibromyalgia?

Poor sleep, poor nutrition, an overwhelmed immune system, hormone system malfunctioning, and the increased speed of modern life are all contributing to people blowing a fuse. But why are there so many diverse symptoms?

THE ROLE OF THE HYPOTHALAMIC CIRCUIT BREAKER

As noted above, the energy crisis in CFS/FMS causes people to have a major control center, called the hypothalamus, go into hibernation mode. I call this blowing a fuse. I grew up with a fuse box in our home, and when I came down with CFS, it felt exactly like I blew a fuse, so this is the expression that I will use here. But I recognize that fuse boxes have largely disappeared. Nowadays, instead, what occurs is tripping a circuit breaker, so I will use the expressions "blowing a fuse" and "tripping a circuit breaker" interchangeably.

The hypothalamus, a critical control center in the brain, goes offline first during an energy crisis because it uses more energy for its size than any other area in your body. This is because it controls so many different functions, as I'll discuss below.

Fortunately, no damage is done to the hypothalamus during this process. When energy production is restored, so is hypothalamic function.

The Hypothalamus: A Major Control Center

Understanding the four key functions controlled by the hypothalamus explains most of the symptoms seen in CFS/FMS. These functions are:

1. **Sleep.** The hypothalamus is a major sleep control center. When it goes offline, people get horrible insomnia despite being exhausted. This is why the inability to sleep despite being exhausted is such a good marker distinguishing CFS/FMS from fatigue with other causes.

2. **Hormonal function.** The hypothalamus controls our body's entire hormonal system through the pituitary gland, which is located right below the hypothalamus. Because of this, people with CFS/FMS have symptoms of low thyroid (tired, achy, brain fog, and weight gain), low adrenal (irritability when hungry and crashing during stress), and low estrogen or testosterone.

3. **Autonomic nervous system regulation.** This is what controls blood pressure, pulse, sweating, and bowel function. This is why we often see low blood pressure, rapid pulse, unusual sweating patterns, and acid reflux.

4. **Temperature regulation.** Although you may sometimes feel feverish, you'll find that your temperature is usually below 98.6°F. In fact, in people with CFS and fibromyalgia, a temperature over 99 usually reflects a fever.

SO HOW CAN I TELL WHAT BLEW MY FUSE?

Often, the problem that caused the initial stress is long gone (e.g., a car crash), and the treatments in this book will simply turn the circuit breaker back on. In other cases, it will be important to avoid what caused you to blow your fuse in the first place. For example, if you get well so you can go back to a toxic job that made you sick in the first place, you will likely blow a fuse again. (We'll talk about how to avoid this in Chapter 6.).

Below are some of the most common triggers to consider.

If your illness began suddenly:

- Viral, parasitic, or antibiotic-sensitive infections
- Injury (even mild fender benders)
- Pregnancy (usually beginning soon after the baby is born)
- Toxic exposures (especially if others around you also got sick)

If your illness came on gradually, consider:

- Yeast (candida) overgrowth—especially if you have sinusitis or nasal congestion and/or spastic colon
- Hormonal deficiencies (even if your blood tests are normal)— especially low thyroid or low hormone levels due to perimenopause
- Chronic stress, including both at work and within relationships— these syndromes commonly affect hardworking "adrenaline junkies"
- Autoimmune disorders (e.g., lupus, rheumatoid arthritis, Sjögren's syndrome)
- Mold toxin illness
- Anything that disrupts sleep, including sleep apnea, restless leg syndrome, or a spouse who snores

If you think about tripping a circuit breaker in your home, it makes this concept a bit easier to understand. Although it is annoying, a tripped circuit breaker protects your home from burning down during a power surge. In the same way, I do not view CFS/FMS as the enemy. Rather, I see them as attempts on the body's part to protect itself from further harm and damage in the face of any number of overwhelming stresses.

I suspect that the root cause of the hypothalamic suppression can be found in the mitochondria, or the energy furnaces in the cells. The good news is that restoring adequate energy production using the SHINE protocol can jump-start your healing process by optimizing mitochondrial energy production and restoring function in your hypothalamic circuit breaker. There is no single magic bullet to get well, however. People who suffer from CFS/FMS usually have a combination of several different problems, and the exact combination varies considerably from individual to individual. It is important to look for and treat all of the factors simultaneously.

SO WHY DO I HAVE PAIN?

When muscles do not have enough energy, you might think that they would go loose and limp, but that is not the case. Think about writer's cramp. When this happens, the muscles in the hand or arm get so tired that they become tight—often stiff as a board—and they will hurt. The multiple little painful knots (called trigger points) are the belly of the muscles where they have bunched up. As people feel pain from these knots, they start shifting their weight to take the strain off the uncomfortable areas. Unfortunately, this puts more strain on other areas, and the pain starts moving around your body.

In addition, when you're not able to get deep sleep, your muscles do not heal from the day's activities, and this also contributes to pain. Many of you have probably noticed that the few nights you can get a good night's sleep, the pain decreases.

To compound the problem, once you develop chronic pain, the brain actually starts to amplify the pain, and the brain itself can then trigger the pain. This is called central sensitization. Central sensitization is what you hear about most in discussions of fibromyalgia pain. This is not because it is the main problem, but I suspect this is because the three FDA-approved medications for fibromyalgia target central sensitization. This is just one modest piece of the pain process, with the key source and root cause of the pain being from the tight muscles.

In addition, chronic pain of many types can also commonly trigger a secondary nerve pain, called chronic inflammatory demyelinating polyneuropathy (CIDP), and low thyroid (despite normal lab tests) also increases the tendency of getting carpal tunnel syndrome (found in 45 percent of people with fibromyalgia). This is where tissue swelling compresses a nerve going through the wrist, causing numbness, tingling, and pain in your hands. This generally also goes away with thyroid and vitamin B6 (see Chapter 9, "Natural Pain Relief").

Bottom line? You'll be amazed at how dramatically your pain can be decreased and usually eliminated as you get eight to nine hours of deep sleep a night, optimize thyroid function, restore energy production in your muscles (which is what this book is about), and stop sending excessive pain signals to your brain.

It never ceases to amaze me how quickly a case of FMS can resolve once the underlying problems are treated. In fact, the duration of the disease simply does not seem to affect how responsive it is to treatment. Two of the top authorities on muscle pain, the late and great Dr. Janet Travell and Dr. David Simons, devoted much of their life's work to studying muscle trigger points, and their research laid the foundation for much of what we discuss in this book.

THE GOOD NEWS

The good news is that everything I have discussed above is treatable. The trick is to sort out which problems are most active in each individual and to treat them all. We certainly have much more to learn, but we already know enough to help most people reclaim their lives.

Here Are the Tests I Order for My New Consult Visits

- Comprehensive metabolic panel including electrolytes, calcium, and magnesium
- CBC with platelet count,.ESR, ferritin, iron percent saturation, vitamin B12 level
- TSH, free T4, free T3, reverse T3, anti-TPO antibody
- Pregnenolone, DHEA-sulfate, total fasting morning cortisol, ACTH, HgbA1C
- Total IgE, urine analysis including microscopic exam to look for infections
- Free and total testosterone, fasting insulin, FSH, LH
- For females only: prolactin, estradiol, progesterone
- Draw fasting blood tests before 9:30 a.m.

13   *Sleep Intensive Care*

BFF Summary

1. Getting eight to nine hours of solid, deep sleep a night without premature waking or a medication hangover is critical to getting well.

2. Begin with natural sleep aids. I recommend the Revitalizing Sleep Formula by Enzymatic Therapy, Terrific Zzzz, and Nature's Bounty Dual Spectrum Melatonin 5 Mg.

3. Because of the severity of the sleep disorder in CFS and fibromyalgia, most patients will need to add prescription medications for at least six to eighteen months. A low dose of several medications is more likely to be effective without next-day sedation than a high dose of one medication. Zolpidem (Ambien), trazodone (Desyrel), gabapentin (Neurontin), and low dose cyclobenzaprine (Flexeril) are the four best prescription sleep medications. Most regular sleeping pills make you feel worse by keeping you in light sleep.

4. Take whatever combination of treatments you need to get your eight hours of solid sleep a night.

5. A weighted blanket (see Luna brand on Amazon) can be very helpful for pain and insomnia when medications aren't tolerated.

The Importance of Sleep in Fibromyalgia

The most effective way to eliminate fatigue and pain in CFS/FMS is to get eight to nine hours of solid, deep sleep each night on a regular basis. In fact, disordered sleep is, in my opinion, one of the key underlying processes that drive CFS/FMS. Usually, when I lecture, I ask, "How many of you who have CFS/FMS can get at least seven to nine hours of solid sleep a night without medications?" Generally, out of three hundred to four hundred people in the audience, only one or two people, if any, raise their hands. When I speak with these people later, I usually find that they have sleep apnea, narcolepsy, or another treatable cause for their fatigue in addition to or besides CFS/FMS.

Basically, if you can get a good night's sleep without taking anything, there's a good chance that you may not have CFS or FMS. This doesn't mean that the SHINE protocol won't help you; in fact, it helps many types of fatigue. I teach doctors that the first thing to ask when people complain about fatigue and widespread pain is, "Can you get a good night's sleep?"

Why? Because the hypothalamic circuit that goes offline in CFS and fibromyalgia controls sleep. That's why asking about insomnia separates out CFS/FMS from other conditions so well.

If you have addressed the suggestions in Chapter 1, you can be sure that poor sleep hygiene is not your problem. This is important because your doctor may want to blame your insomnia on this. It is important to let them know that your problem is not poor sleep hygiene; it is hypothalamic sleep-center malfunction.

The hypothalamic sleep disorder in CFS/FMS is usually too severe to be dealt with by any single prescription or natural remedy. What works best is to mix these until you find a combination that gives you eight to nine hours of solid restorative sleep a night, without a hangover.

Whatever treatments you use, though, it is important that they not only increase the duration of sleep but also maintain or improve the deep-sleep stages. Unfortunately, many sleeping pills in common use—for example, diazepam (Valium)—actually worsen deep sleep. You want to be certain that the treatments and medications you use leave you feeling better the next day, not worse. In addition, long-term use of these addictive benzodiazepine medications may be associated with risks that are not seen with the other sleep aids we discuss. I would note that alprazolam (Xanax) and clonazepam (Klonopin) are exceptions in the benzodiazepine family. These may actually improve deep sleep and have other benefits that could make their use worthwhile in fibromyalgia. Clonazepam (Klonopin) is the least addictive member in the benzodiazepines and the longest acting.

There are several approaches to using sleep treatments in CFS/FMS. Some doctors prefer to use a single medication or treatment and push it up to its maximum dose. If that works, great; if not, they stop that medication and switch to another. Other doctors prefer to use low doses of many different treatments together until the patient is getting good, solid sleep regularly.

I *strongly* prefer the latter approach in CFS/FMS, for two main reasons. First, my experience is that people with CFS and fibromyalgia can be *very* medication sensitive, especially if high doses are used. Most of a medication's benefits occur at low doses and most of the side effects occur at high doses.

Second, each medication is cleared out of the body on its own schedule, regardless of whether it is taken with other medications. If you take a low dose of a sleep medication, so that it is out of your body when it is time to wake up eight hours later, the blood level may not be high enough to keep you asleep all night. If you increase the dose to the level at which it does keep you asleep all night, it may not be cleared out of your body until 2:00 p.m. the next day, leaving you feeling very hungover.

If, however, you combine low doses of four or five different sleep aids, each of them will be cleared out of your body by morning. Meanwhile, the effective blood levels that you have during the middle of the night from each treatment are additive and will keep you asleep. Because of this, most people with CFS/FMS find that they do best taking low doses of anywhere from three to seven different treatments, combining them to get eight to nine hours of solid sleep each night.

Baby Yourself During Stress—So You Sleep Like a Baby

It is not uncommon to see your sleep worsen again during periods of increased stress— whether physical or emotional—and the flaring of your illness. During these times, I increase the treatments as needed to maintain at least seven to eight hours of solid sleep without waking prematurely or being hungover. I find that patients do not have a problem with continually having to escalate the dose, so I don't worry about increasing the treatments during periods of stress or flaring of your illness.

The best way to need less medication in the long run is to use as much as it takes to get eight hours of solid sleep each night for six months. When you are sleeping well and feeling better for six months, you can then start to reduce the treatments, as long as you continue to get eight hours of solid sleep each night.

Many people find that they can taper off most sleep treatments after about eighteen months. Other people need to take some of the sleep treatments for years. This is okay. Either way, I suggest staying on something for sleep long term to decrease the risk of your CFS/FMS coming back. This could simply be an herbal remedy or a small dose of a sleep medication.

Helpful Prescription Medications

There are dozens of medications that can help sleep in fibromyalgia. Below are my favorites. Do not drive or operate hazardous equipment if you are taking these medications. Also, as with almost any medication and most herbs, do not get pregnant during treatment.

As we've discussed earlier, CFS/FMS patients usually do better with combining low doses of several medications than with taking a high dose of just one.

With hypothalamic sleep-center dysfunction, it is inappropriate to stop taking your sleep medications prematurely. Just as with high blood pressure, it is reasonable to stay on your sleep medications for years, if needed. Fortunately, after people are feeling better for six months, they usually find that they can lower the dose of sleep medication as the sleep center (in the hypothalamus) recovers. Keep in mind that if you use adequate medication to get eight to nine hours of solid sleep a night for six to nine months, you will likely need less sleep medication in the long run.

Let's look at the prescription sleep medications that work best in CFS/FMS.

Zolpidem (Ambien)

This is my first choice of sleep medication for treatment in CFS/FMS because it is usually effective and well tolerated. It is also uniquely effective at helping people *fall* asleep, while the other medications help people *stay* asleep. Because zolpidem is short acting (that is, it is out of your body after six hours), it is less likely to cause side effects than many other medications, but it also may not keep you asleep all the way through the night. A dose of 5 to 10 milligrams will likely give you at least four to six hours of good, solid sleep as a foundation. Doses of 10 milligrams or less are also less likely to cause addictive issues than higher doses.

If my patients wake up in the middle of the night, I have them simply keep half of a 5-milligram tablet by their bedside. When they wake during the night (as long as they have at least four hours before they need to drive), they simply bite the half tablet between their front teeth to crush it, and put it under their tongue. Then they roll over and go back to sleep. It gets absorbed very quickly under their tongue, so it works in just a few minutes.

It is common to see severe rebound insomnia for about a week when you stop using this medication, so do not stop it suddenly. When tapering someone off this medication, I decrease the dosage by about 2.5 milligrams every two months, while giving them something else to assist sleep. In my experience, zolpidem can also be helpful for restless leg syndrome. I do prefer to keep the total dose under 10 milligrams a night to avoid both addiction and problems with memory.

Trazodone (Desyrel)

Desyrel is marketed as an antidepressant (at a dose of 300 to 450 milligrams a day), but its main use in CFS/FMS is to treat disordered sleep. A dose of 25 to 50 milligrams is usually optimal for sleep. A small percent of people will need higher dosing.

Gabapentin (Neurontin) or Pregabalin (Lyrica)

These medications are chemically related to gamma-aminobutyric acid (GABA), though their mode of action is more complex. Although they are related, one will often work and be well tolerated even if the others are not. They are all effective for pain and restless leg syndrome and can markedly improve sleep quality. The main side effects are sedation and dizziness. Pregabalin may also cause weight gain at doses of 450 milligrams or higher. These are also discussed in Chapter 10. I give 100 to

600 milligrams of gabapentin, or 50 to 300 milligrams of pregabalin at bedtime. I generally begin with the gabapentin first.

CYCLOBENZAPRINE (FLEXERIL)

This is a muscle relaxant and can be helpful for people who experience severe muscle pain with fibromyalgia. Interestingly, although the standard dose is 10 milligrams three times a day, studies show that just 2.5 milligrams at bedtime can be very effective in fibromyalgia for both sleep and lessening of next-day pain—with minimal side effects. I give 2.5 to 5 milligrams a night as feels best.

OTC ANTIHISTAMINES

I give 25 to 50 milligrams at night of doxylamine (Unisom), diphenhydramine (Benadryl), or dimenhydrinate (Dramamine). These antihistamines can be very effective and are usually well tolerated. Rarely, they can aggravate the brain fog.

Cuddle Yourself

Lying on the Cuddle Ewe mattress pad can help relieve pain when it interferes with sleep. This cushioning sheepskin pad is available at www.cuddleewe.com or 800-366-6056. In addition, getting wool sheets and pillowcases has been associated with a marked decrease in pain (especially when combined with wool long underwear during the day when it is cold outside) because the wool keeps your muscles warm, while wicking away any moisture from sweating.

Another medication-free tool that can be helpful is a heavy or weighted blanket. This has the same effect on calming your adrenal and nervous system as a swaddling blanket has with a baby. I've seen dramatic benefits for sleep and pain with these. Find a quality blanket where each pocket is filled with glass beads and is sealed and separate from the others. This keeps the weight from shifting around.

You can find weighted blankets on Amazon, and many people like the Luna brand. The blanket weight is based on your body weight, with the recommendation being 10 to 15 percent of your body weight. Check out the Amazon reviews that include "verified purchase" to get an idea of their popularity.

I adjust the mix of natural and prescription treatments to be sure people get at least seven to eight hours of sleep a night.

Getting Started

1. Be sure your sleep hygiene is okay (see Chapter 1).

2. Add natural remedies.
   A. Revitalizing Sleep Formula—two to four capsules at bedtime
   B. Terrific Zzzz
   C. Nature's Bounty Dual Spectrum Melatonin 5 Mg
   D. If you are wide awake at bedtime, try the Sleep Tonight herbal mix.

3. I add medications (usually in this order and with these starting doses):

   A. **Zolpidem (Ambien):** I give 5 to 10 milligrams a night. You can use part sublingually if you wake in the middle of the night.
   B. **Gabapentin (Neurontin):** I give 100 to 600 milligrams. If not well tolerated, consider 50 to 300 milligrams of Lyrica (pregabalin) at bedtime.
   C. **Doxylamine (Unisom) or diphenhydramine (Benadryl):** I give 25 milligrams at night. The antihistamines may also help pain.
   D. **Trazodone (Desyrel):** I give 25 to 50 milligrams at bedtime.
   E. **Cyclobenzaprine (Flexeril):** I give 5 milligrams, half to one tablet at bedtime.

OTHER MEDICATIONS FOR SLEEP

While this will get most people with CFS/FMS sleeping their eight hours, in some cases much more may be needed. Then I keep in the treatments that helped somewhat, and add in the following one at a time:

- Clonazepam (Klonopin): 0.5 to 1 milligram
- Tizanidine (Zanaflex): 4 milligrams, half to one tablet (Caution: Do not take while on the fluconazole [Diflucan] antifungal.)

- Tricyclic or other antidepressants: I will only use one of the below at a time:
  - Doxepin (Sinequan): 5 to 10 milligrams, one to three capsules at bedtime, or 10 mg/cc in liquid form. If a lower dose is needed, you can start with one to three drops at night. This is a powerful antihistamine. Some people get the greatest benefit with the least next-day sedation with a dose of less than 5 milligrams a night.
  - Amitriptyline (Elavil): 10 milligrams, half to five tablets at bedtime. This may cause weight gain or dry mouth, and is especially good for people with nerve pain or vulvadynia (pelvic pain).
  - Mirtazapine (Remeron): 15 milligrams, one to three tablets at bedtime. This can be very effective, but may cause heavy next-day sedation. But it's definitely worth a try when nothing else is working.
- Olanzapine (Zyprexa): 5 milligrams, half to two tablets at bedtime. Although used as an antipsychotic medication, in these very low doses it tends to be very well tolerated and can be very effective for sleep. Its main downsides are that it can cause weight gain, especially with higher dosing. But it is one of the very few medications that increases deep (stage 4) sleep, which is what is especially missing in fibromyalgia. A relative to this medication called quetiapine (Seroquel); taking 25 to 50 milligrams can often be effective.
- GHB (gamma-hydroxybutyrate, or Xyrem): This was an excellent natural sleep option in fibromyalgia. It used to cost about $20 a month and be available in health-food stores. It deepens sleep far better than any other treatment on the market. It was so effective that the government was concerned that it might be being used as a date rape drug, and now it has gone from being inexpensive and over-the-counter to being tightly regulated and costing over $200,000 per year. If all else fails, this often works very well; however, I've stopped prescribing it because government regulation has made it far too expensive and difficult to obtain.

Side Effects of Sleep Aids

For all of the medications listed in this section, any side effects that you may notice will usually occur the same day that you take the medication. I have not seen any "fly now, pay later" side effects from prolonged use of nonaddictive sleep meds. The exception is that less than 1 percent of people who take zolpidem (Ambien) for more than a year develop an unusual and severe depression, which dramatically resolves one to seven days after stopping the sleep medication. In these rare situations I simply take the person off Ambien. I have not seen zolpidem worsen symptoms in patients with preexisting depression. I've also seen sleepwalking and sleep eating in approximately one patient per thousand. These side effects mostly occurred when the individuals were taking over 10 milligrams a night.

An Important Sleep-Related Disorder in CFS/FMS

In Chapter 1, we discussed sleep apnea and restless leg syndrome. While frequently seen in CFS and FMS, these are also common in the general population. But there is one other important form of sleep-disordered breathing to be aware of in CFS/FMS.

UPPER AIRWAY RESISTANCE SYNDROME (UARS)

This is where the inability to breathe through your nose while sleeping disrupts sleep quality. This diagnosis is usually made with a sleep study, but I will rarely bother with it for this. People know if they have trouble breathing through the nose at night.

In addition, there is a simple nose test to see if you are suffering from nasal resistance. Looking in a mirror, press the side of one nostril to close it. With your mouth closed, breathe in through your other nostril. If the nostril tends to collapse, try holding it open with the flat side of a tooth-pick. Test both nostrils. If breathing is easier with one nostril held open, using nasal dilators or strips when sleeping (see below) may help.

TREATMENT FOR UARS

Although a mild decrease in airflow while sleeping may not seem like a big problem, it has been shown to disrupt sleep enough to cause and/or perpetuate CFS/FMS.

Most people find that their nasal congestion and UARS go away after treating their candida (see Chapter 3). If the nasal congestion persists, however, a simple nasal dilator called Nozovent (available online) can be helpful. Another easy option is Breathe Right nasal strips, which are available at most pharmacies and many supermarkets.

14 Hormones and Hypotension Intensive Care

BFF Summary

1. In those with irritability when hungry, especially if their illness began with a viral infection (adrenal fatigue), I usually recommend the supplement Adrenaplex plus the bioidentical prescription hormone hydrocortisone (Cortef). At doses of 25 milligrams or more daily (equivalent to 5 milligrams of prednisone), this hormone can suppress your adrenals and have significant toxicity. But at doses of 20 milligrams a day or less, overall I find it to be fairly safe. People know within a month if these are going to help.
2. Acne, severe weight gain, darkening of facial hair, and irregular periods? Consider PCOS (polycystic ovary syndrome) in women. I do this by looking at test results for a fasting insulin over 10, or a high or high normal DHEA-sulfate or testosterone. The medication metformin, a low-carbohydrate diet (e.g., ketogenic), and birth control pills can all be very helpful.
3. Have trouble standing for extended periods without aggravating exhaustion, brain fog, and even dizziness on standing? These suggest orthostatic intolerance (POTS/NMH), which means the blood is rushing to your legs when you stand up, and staying there. A simple two-minute quiz will tell you if you have it (see page 199). Treatment is also discussed.
4. Tired, achy, weight gain, and cold intolerant despite being on thyroid hormone? Some people have become "deaf" to regular thyroid hormone because of the fibromyalgia. A significant percent of these people will feel dramatically better using a special form of

active T3 hormone called liothyronine (Cytomel). For this, you will need a holistic physician familiar with the protocol. When people hit the correct dose, they feel like "somebody turned the lights back on in my body." Although rare, this treatment carries the risk of unmasking heart disease if present.

5. Optimizing testosterone is important in both men and women.

6. Don't worry about getting pregnant (don't do so while on treatment). People with fibromyalgia usually do great during pregnancy. It is after delivery that they usually need help. Those of you with infertility can also email me for a free infertility information sheet.

Adrenal Intensive Care

WHEN IS CORTISOL OKAY?

The adrenal fatigue we discussed in Chapter 2 is critical and applies for those with CFS and FMS. But other considerations are also important here, as those treatments may not be enough. This occurs because research shows that the hormonal "mission control" center in the brain, called the hypothalamus, is malfunctioning. Some of the earliest NIH research pointing to hypothalamic problems in fibromyalgia and CFS looked at hypothalamic-pituitary-adrenal axis problems.

So, intensive care is sometimes needed. This can easily be done by supplying the hormones that the adrenal gland normally makes. Begin with the recommendations in Chapter 2.

USING BIOIDENTICAL CORTISOL

Most directly, and especially helpful in CFS/FMS, is treating the underactive adrenal problem with ultralow doses of adrenal hormones. Most important would be hydrocortisone (Cortef), but fludrocortisone (Florinef), pregnenolone, and DHEA are also sometimes helpful. This usually quickly banishes the symptoms of low blood sugar and can markedly improve energy and immune function.

I like to begin with bioidentical hydrocortisone (Cortef), available by prescription at most pharmacies. I usually keep the dose at or under 15 milligrams per day. This immediately gives your body the support that your adrenal glands are unable to give and may help you feel much better quickly. The added cortisol also takes some of the strain off your adrenals so that they can heal.

POTENTIAL TOXICITY OF CORTISONE

Adrenal hormones are essential for life. Without them, a person dies. But, as with any hormone, too much can be dangerous, and any cortisol supplementation should be closely monitored by your CFS/FMS specialist.

In the early studies using adrenal hormones, the researchers had no idea what dose was normal and what was toxic. When they gave injections of the hormone to arthritis patients, the patients' arthritis went away and they felt better. However, they gave patients many times more than the normal amount, and many patients became toxic and died. Because of this, the researchers became frightened and avoided using adrenal hormones whenever possible. Medical students were taught to avoid adrenal hormones unless no other treatment choices existed.

The use of adrenal hormones needs to be put into perspective, however. Imagine if early thyroid researchers had given their patients fifty times the usual dose of thyroid hormone. Thyroid patients would have routinely died of heart attacks. The thyroid researchers, though, were fortunate enough to stumble upon the healthy dose early on and to skip these negative outcomes (likely because too high a dose of thyroid caused immediate side effects). If they had not, people today would not be treated for an underactive thyroid until they were in a coma.

Medical science is just beginning to learn that a person can feel horrible and function poorly even with a minimal to moderate hormone deficiency. Waiting for the person to go off the deep end of the test's normal scale is simply not healthy.

Fortunately, research has shown that the very low doses of cortisol we are recommending are safe. To put it in perspective, 5 milligrams of bioidentical hydrocortisone (Cortef) is approximately equal to 1 milligram of the synthetic prednisone, and I consider the bioidentical to be both safer and more effective, unless one is treating inflammation.

Unfortunately, most physicians are not familiar with the research on the safety of ultralow-dose hydrocortisone. In fact, I had been so indoctrinated about the dangers of prednisone (cortisone) in medical school that it took me three years of researching the scientific literature to get comfortable with this approach. But the research showed that using doses of 20 milligrams of hydrocortisone (equivalent to about 4 milligrams of prednisone) or less daily was quite safe overall. It was the higher doses that were toxic.

For those of you who would like to have more information on this, I highly recommend the book *Safe Uses of Cortisol* by the late Case Western Reserve University endocrinologist and professor William Jefferies. The book is out of print but available from online vendors for about $60. The book is well worth it, if needed for peace of mind. He routinely would give patients with CFS/FMS 20 milligrams of cortisol daily over the long term, and he did so safely.

Most often, I use 5 to 15 milligrams daily. Most people find that either taking it all in the morning, or about two-thirds in the morning and one-third at lunchtime works the best. Some will take 2.5 to 5 milligrams at 4:00 p.m., but taking it much later than this will tend to keep people up at night.

Doses over 20 milligrams a day will start to cause adrenal suppression, putting your adrenal glands to sleep. Doses over 37.5 milligrams a day (a routine dose for overt adrenal failure called Addison's disease) start to show the severe toxicities associated with prednisone use. The Cortef (hydrocortisone) is the bioidentical hormone, and I find it works much better than prednisone.

To summarize, if your CFS/FMS symptoms started suddenly after a viral infection, if you suffer from hypoglycemia (and irritability when hungry), or if you have recurrent infections that take a long time to resolve, you probably have underactive adrenal glands. About two-thirds of my severe CFS/FMS patients have underactive or marginally functioning adrenal glands or a decreased adrenal reserve. Although I go predominantly based on symptoms and response to treatment, a fasting morning cortisol under 14 mcg/dL, especially if the ACTH is under 25 pg/mL, or glycosylated hemoglobin of 5.2 or less suggests that treatment is warranted to see if it helps. I give the hydrocortisone (Cortef) along with the Adrenaplex supplement.

Although I prefer natural products to pharmaceuticals, in this situation I am comfortable adding ultralow-dose standardized bioidentical cortisol to the natural therapies in those with CFS/FMS. This can markedly improve function and help your body heal.

DHEA AND DHEA-S

Although what this hormone does is not yet clear, DHEA (dehydroepian-drosterone) is the most abundant hormone produced by the adrenal cortex. If it is low, you will feel poor. DHEA-S (dehydroepiandrosterone sulfate) levels normally decline with age but appear to drop prematurely in CFS/FMS patients. Patients often feel much better when their DHEA-S levels are brought to the mid-normal range for a twenty-nine-year-old. Most women need 5 to 10 milligrams a day (already present in the Adre-naplex) and men need 25 to 50 milligrams each morning.

In women, half of their body's testosterone is made from adrenal DHEA, so taking DHEA can also correct low testosterone levels. But more is not better. If you have side effects, such as acne or darkening of facial hair in women, this suggests the DHEA dose is too high.

Interestingly, for women with autoimmune illnesses such as lupus, 200 milligrams a day of DHEA significantly improved how they felt. We don't know if this would be the case in rheumatoid arthritis as well, but we do know that prednisone treatment (5 milligrams or more) for any illness will lower DHEA-S levels. My suspicion is that low DHEA levels increase the prednisone's toxicity, so I consider it reasonable to supplement DHEA at 10 to 25 milligrams a day for anybody on prednisone.

The only test I will do for DHEA is called the DHEA-S (DHEA-sulfate).

PREGNENOLONE

This is the "mother hormone" that all of the other adrenal steroid hormones are made from. Think of it like the bricks that make up a house you are building. You can have all the workers and other materials needed, but no way to build the house if you don't have bricks.

We very frequently find that people with fibromyalgia have pregneno-lone levels in the lowest 2 percent of the population. The cause is not clear, but things like viral infections, cholesterol-lowering statin medications, and immune changes can all block the pathway that makes pregnenolone. When this hormone is low, I will supplement. The Adrenaplex also has 15 milligrams of pregnenolone in two capsules. This is enough for most people and keeps it simple. I will sometimes add 25 to 100 milligrams each morning, though.

Polycystic Ovary Syndrome (PCOS)

We have also found that roughly 5 to 10 percent of women with CFS/FMS actually have elevated DHEA-S and testosterone levels. When I see this, I suspect and look for polycystic ovarian syndrome (PCOS) and insulin resistance. If a fasting morning insulin level is higher than 10 units/mL (suggestive of insulin resistance), especially if ovarian cysts or infertility are also present, these patients often improve significantly with a diabetes medication called metformin (Glucophage). I prescribe 500 to 1,000 milligrams one to two times a day to improve insulin sensitivity. This can also assist with restoring fertility, as well as helping the patient lose excess weight.

Interestingly, a recent study showed that in people with FMS and elevated insulin or glycosylated hemoglobin (hemoglobin A1C) levels, metformin significantly decreased pain. I do not find that this medication helps pain in the absence of these tests being elevated. This does make sense, though, as when insulin levels are high, this also likely starves the cells for energy, which will increase FMS pain.

As metformin can cause vitamin B12 deficiency, it is critical that a multivitamin containing vitamin B12, such as the Energy Revitalization System vitamin powder or Clinical Essentials, be taken with it. Polycystic ovarian syndrome may also improve with low-dose hydrocortisone and with chromium supplementation of 1,000 micrograms daily.

Neurally Mediated Hypotension and Postural Orthostatic Tachycardia Syndrome

If your blood pressure is low, you get dizzy upon standing, you crash after exercising, and you get a rapid pulse and a drop in blood pressure on standing, you might have neurally mediated hypotension (NMH) or postural orthostatic tachycardia syndrome (POTS). Often, NMH and POTS are simply labels given to some people with chronic fatigue syndrome. If so, adrenal support becomes especially important.

Association Between POTS/NMH and CFS
Unfortunately, when conventional doctors make a diagnosis of POTS or NMH, they typically don't recognize their association with CFS. Research shows that they need to.

Researchers at Vanderbilt University School of Medicine studied forty-seven patients with POTS. In POTS, when you stand up you have a fast heartbeat and low blood pressure, causing symptoms like dizziness, nausea, poor endurance, and fatigue. Of these, 93 percent had severe fatigue and 64 percent were diagnosed with CFS. The folks with CFS had far worse cases of POTS than the others. "Fatigue and CFS-defining symptoms are common in POTS patients," concluded the researchers in an article published in *Clinical Science.*

But weak adrenal function isn't the only cause of POTS in CFS patients.

The area in your brain called the hypothalamus, the "circuit breaker," that controls energy for many key functions within your body, such as sleep and hormone production, also controls blood pressure and heart rate through what is called the autonomic nervous system—a system that depends on healthy adrenal glands in order to function optimally. NMH and POTS are disorders of this autonomic function.

A diagnosis of POTS or NMH is likely to be a part of a larger CFS process if:

- Your fatigue is severe
- You have insomnia
- You're young (five to thirty years old)
- You tend to have a fast heart rate

One way to confirm this diagnosis is to undergo the tilt-table test. In this test, you are strapped to a table and held upright to see if you pass out. Though it's the best diagnostic test for POTS/NMH, in my opinion it doesn't add much (except for expense and making you feel sick).

I'm comfortable treating POTS/NMH in CFS patients on the basis of symptoms alone. The simple quiz below was shown to be about as reliable as the tilt-table test in a study in the peer-reviewed journal *Mayo Clinic Proceedings*. In addition, see the "poor man's tilt-table test" discussed on page 202.

The good news is that treating with the SHINE protocol can help not only CFS/FMS but POTS as well.

Orthostatic Intolerance Quiz
Below is a quick quiz that has been shown in the *Mayo Clinic Proceedings* to be a good screening test for orthostatic intolerance.

QUICK ORTHOSTATIC INTOLERANCE SCREENING QUIZ

Below is a quick screening test that gives a good idea about the presence of orthostatic intolerance, especially when it's combined with the ten-minute pulse test discussed below. It looks for the presence and severity of orthostatic symptoms. These symptoms include worsening dizziness, fatigue, racing heart, or brain fog when standing. Circle 0–4 below as best applies to your situation.

A. How often do you get orthostatic symptoms when standing?

0 *never or rarely*
1 *sometimes*
2 *often*
3 *usually*
4 *always*

B. Activities of daily living—orthostatic symptoms

0 *do not interfere* with the usual activities of daily living (e.g., work, fixing meals, dressing, bathing)
1 *mildly interfere* with the usual activities of daily living (e.g., work, fixing meals, dressing, bathing)
2 *moderately interfere* with the usual activities of daily living (e.g., work, fixing meals, dressing, bathing)
3 *severely interfere* with the usual activities of daily living (e.g., work, fixing meals, dressing, bathing)
4 *severely interfere* with the usual activities of daily living (e.g., work, fixing meals, dressing, bathing). My symptoms often leave me *bed- or wheelchair-bound*

C. How severe are your orthostatic symptoms when you stand up?

0 *none*
1 *mild*
2 *moderate.* I *sometimes* have to sit back down to relieve them
3 *severe.* I *frequently* have to sit back down to get relief
4 *severe.* I *sometimes faint* if I do not sit back down

D. **Conditions causing orthostatic symptoms**

0   *never* under any circumstances

1   *sometimes* have symptoms that occur during normal activity (e.g., walking, eating, or prolonged standing), or during exposure to heat (e.g., hot day, hot bath, hot shower)

2   *often* have symptoms that occur during normal activity (e.g., walking, eating, or prolonged standing), or during exposure to heat (e.g., hot day, hot bath, hot shower)

3   *usually* have symptoms that occur during activity (e.g., walking, eating, or prolonged standing), or during exposure to heat (e.g., hot day, hot bath, hot shower)

4   *always* experience orthostatic symptoms when I stand, regardless of the activity or conditions

E. **Standing time**

0   usually I can stand *as long as I need* without developing orthostatic symptoms

1   usually I can stand *more than 15 minutes* without developing orthostatic symptoms

2   usually I can stand *5 to 14 minutes* without developing orthostatic symptoms

3   usually I can stand *1 to 4 minutes* without developing orthostatic symptoms

4   usually I can stand *less than 1 minute* without developing orthostatic symptoms

Add up your scores from the five sections above for the total score.

_____ **Total Score**

Scores of 9 or higher strongly suggests orthostatic intolerance. In CFS/FMS, if the score is 7 or higher it suggests OI, which can benefit from treating with a high salt and water intake and medium pressure (20–30 mm) compression stockings which are at least mid-thigh high. Wear the stockings whenever you are upright for extended periods (but not during sleep). This simple low-cost combination can have a dramatic benefit.

A Simple "Poor Man's Tilt-Table Test" for Orthostatic Intolerance

Developed by Dr. David Bell, an excellent and very caring CFS researcher, this test is easily done in the office and requires only a blood pressure cuff—and a good nurse to catch the patients before they pass out.

The test is relatively simple.

- Check the blood pressure and pulse several times during a ten-minute interval while the person is lying down.
- Then have the person stand quietly (with a blood pressure cuff on) without moving or leaning on any object for thirty minutes, or as long as tolerated. Check the blood pressure and pulse every few minutes. If the person feels like he or she is about to faint, the test is stopped and considered a positive test.

This is called a poor man's tilt-table test, and Dr. Bell finds that most people with CFS flunk this test, showing one of the following three common abnormalities while standing:

1. A drop in systolic blood pressure (the top number) of more than 20 points.

2. POTS—the heart rate increases at least 25 beats per minute (bpm) over the resting heart rate.

3. Narrowing of the pulse pressure. The pulse pressure is the difference between the upper number of the blood pressure and the lower number. For example, a normal person with a blood pressure reading of 120/70 would have a pulse pressure of 50. It is actually this difference between the upper (systolic) and lower blood pressure numbers (diastolic) that circulates blood. If the pulse pressure drops below 18, it is abnormal, and not enough to help blood circulate properly to your brain and other tissues.

Patients should be tested in the late morning or early afternoon with no unusual activity prior to testing. Large meals and large volumes of fluid prior to testing should be avoided. It is reasonable to restrict salt for a few days before the test.

KEY TREATMENTS FOR POTS/NMH

These simple treatments can markedly improve function and they can be combined as helpful:

1. **Increase salt and water intake.** I know. You are already drinking like a fish, but you are also peeing like a racehorse. This occurs because one of the hormone deficiencies is antidiuretic hormone (DDAVP-vasopressin—the "anti-peeing" hormone), which leaves you dehydrated. In addition, salt is the sponge that holds water in our body. You need to eat large amounts of salt, sometimes even licking sea salt. You can simply do this from the palms of your hands. If you notice improvement, you will know that your body was craving salt. You will sometimes find that in an attempt to be healthy, many of you are restricting the amount of salt you take in. That misguided advice is a good recipe to crash and burn.

2. **Wear compression socks.** It is remarkable how much improvement many people will see by simply using medium pressure (20 to 30 mm) compression stockings. They should use ones that go to at least mid-thigh, but if you can't wear those, then knee-high ones will still be fairly helpful. You should wear them during the day when you are active (not when you are lying down for extended periods). Although low cost, these first two treatments are very helpful. Wearing something that constricts the abdomen, such as a corset or a girdle, may also be helpful.

3. **Improve adrenal function.** This is a critical part of our holding on to salt and water. As discussed in earlier articles, some will benefit from prescription low-dose hydrocortisone (do not go over 20 milligrams daily). In addition, natural adrenal support with Adrenaplex or Adrenal Stress End is very helpful for optimizing adrenal function.

4. **Increase sympathetic/adrenaline tone.** The medication midodrine (ProAmatine) can be fairly helpful after six weeks of use; I give 5 to 10 milligrams two to three times daily. Do not use the medication after 5:00 p.m., or when lying down, as it can drive blood pressure too high. Lower the dose or stop if it causes too high of a blood pressure or shakiness. I will occasionally increase the dose to a maximum of 10 milligrams three times daily, with the last dose at 4:00 p.m. The blood pressure should be checked after a week or two on the medication to make sure it is not going over 150/88.

5. **Take Desmopressin (DDAVP).** This is an antidiuretic hormone or "anti-peeing" hormone. It is made in the hypothalamic pituitary area and is also commonly suppressed in CFS/FMS. When this hormone is low, holding on to water is like trying to keep water in a bucket full of holes. Usually I give one or two tablets (0.1 milligrams) in the

morning, and give it six weeks to work. If people are waking up frequently during the night to urinate, I may also give one or two at bedtime to control this so they can sleep. With higher dosing, it can alter the salt balance in the body, so your physician may consider checking electrolyte levels every so often.

I also consider giving 0.1 milligrams of fludrocortisone (Florinef). This is a prescription synthetic adrenal hormone, which helps the body hold on to salt and water. Because of this, it can help in POTS. Although more helpful in those under twenty years old, it may also be helpful in those with a chronically racing heart rate.

Both of these hormones can cause headaches in a small percentage of people by shifting fluid balances too quickly. If this happens, I stop them until the headaches pass, and then resume with just a quarter tablet a day. Then I slowly increase the dose as is comfortable. These two hormones can be used together, and they can be synergistic.

6. **Increase serotonin and dopamine.** Fluoxetine (Prozac), sertraline (Zoloft), and dextroamphetamine-related medications (Dexedrine, Adderall, or Ritalin—do not go over 20 milligrams a day to avoid addiction) have all been shown to help autonomic dysfunction.

7. **Change diet.** Some people find that a gluten- and milk-free diet is also helpful. These changes can dramatically help CFS/FMS in general.

Other Helpful Treatments

1. Many physicians use beta-blockers such as Propranolol (Inderal). These may be helpful, but unfortunately in CFS/FMS, I find they are more likely to aggravate fatigue. They are, however, worth using if you feel better. If using with the ProAmatine, consider 25 milligrams of atenolol (Tenormin) a day instead.

2. Ivabradine (Corlanor) is a selective sinus node blocker. Basically, it slows down the heart rate without triggering the fatigue of beta-blockers. Its main downside is that it is about $15 a pill. Of those who tolerated it, 44 percent found 5 milligrams decreased both heart rate and fatigue after six months, although the benefits were likely seen much more quickly. Lower doses of 2.5 milligrams once or twice a

day usually worked better than higher doses. The main side effect was a transient brightening of vision.

3. Pyridostigmine (Mestinon) can help in refractory cases. Its main side effect is diarrhea, so I am more likely to try it in people who have constipation. It doesn't help many people, but in a few very severely ill cases, it has been a life changer. I suspect this small group has antibodies to a brain chemical called acetylcholine triggering their CFS/FMS.

In addition, the Dynamic Neural Retraining System at www.dnrsystem .com may also be very helpful for fibromyalgia in general as well as orthostatic intolerance. See Part Four for more information on this. This program is especially important if you have trouble tolerating most treatments.

For those of you who would like very in-depth information on orthostatic intolerance, check out "General Information Brochure on Orthostatic Intolerance and Its Treatment" by Johns Hopkins professor Peter Rowe (my favorite OI researcher), available at www.dysautonomiainter national.org/pdf/RoweOIsummary.pdf.

Thyroid Intensive Care

The thyroid gland, located in the neck, is the body's gas pedal. To summarize what we discussed in Chapter 2, it regulates the body's metabolic speed. If the thyroid gland produces insufficient amounts of thyroid hormones, the metabolism decreases and the person gains weight. Other symptoms of hypothyroidism include intolerance to cold, fatigue, achiness, confusion, and constipation (though diarrhea from bowel infections is common in CFS/FMS).

The thyroid makes two primary hormones. They are:

- **Thyroxine (T4).** T4 is the storage form of thyroid hormone. The body uses it to make triiodothyronine (T3), the active form of thyroid hormone. Most synthetic thyroid medications, such as Synthroid and Levothroid, are pure T4. These synthetics are fine if your body has the ability to properly turn them into T3. Unfortunately, many people with CFS/FMS find that their bodies do not have this ability.

- **Triiodothyronine (T3).** T3 is the active form of thyroid hormone. Although in some life-threatening illnesses the body appropriately makes less T3, research suggests that when CFS/FMS occurs, the body may not be able to adequately turn T4 into T3, or it may need much higher levels of T3.

TREATING AN UNDERACTIVE THYROID IN CFS/FMS

What treatment will work best often depends on what is causing your thyroid levels to be inadequate. Common causes of underactive thyroid hormone in CFS/fibromyalgia include:

- **Hypothalamic dysfunction.** Your thyroid gland may be fine, but it is not getting adequate stimulation from the hypothalamus and is basically asleep. In this situation, simply taking a mix of T4 and T3 (see below) at the dose that feels best may be adequate. As the CFS resolves and hypothalamic function recovers, it is often possible to wean oneself off the thyroid hormone.
- **Hashimoto's thyroiditis.** In this autoimmune process, your body's immune system attacks and damages the thyroid. This can be diagnosed by a blood test called an anti-TPO antibody. If the anti-TPO antibody is elevated, you likely have Hashimoto's thyroiditis and may need to take thyroid supplementation for the rest of your life.
- **Inadequate conversion of T4 to active T3.** In this situation, which is common in fibromyalgia, patients often respond best to treatment with pure T3 hormone.
- **T3 receptor resistance.** In this situation, your body is making adequate amounts of thyroid hormone but the areas that it stimulates are very slow to recognize the thyroid hormone's presence. Basically, it's like the cells are hard of hearing when the thyroid hormone signals them to make energy. Because of this, it takes a very high level of pure T3 hormone to get a normal response. But when people find the optimal dose, it is like a light switch goes on in their body.

T3 RECEPTOR RESISTANCE

The T3 receptor resistance problem often resolves after six to twenty-four months on the high-dose T3 treatment as the body heals from fibromyalgia and/or chronic fatigue syndrome. So if a person is feeling well on this treatment, and then over time starts feeling worse, that often means it is time to start weaning down the T3 hormone dose.

Given the multiple causes of thyroid insufficiency in CFS and fibromyalgia, let's discuss how to best treat these problems.

Generally, I begin with a thyroid approach I outlined in Chapter 2. Simply using desiccated thyroid (Armour or Nature-Throid) can help considerably. Again, it should be adjusted to what feels optimal, as long as the free T4 blood test does not go too high (too high being in the upper 20 percent of the normal range or higher). It is not a problem if the free T4 blood test actually goes too low. This is because the T3 component of the desiccated thyroid can actually suppress the T4 blood level, which actually can be a good thing. It is part of how the receptor resistance noted above is overcome.

If people don't respond to the desiccated thyroid, then I will often stop the thyroid treatment and switch them over to the pure T3 hormone called liothyronine (Cytomel). If a person simply has difficulty turning the T4 hormone made by the thyroid into the active T3 form, usually the optimal dose is between 5 and 35 µg of Cytomel daily. If they don't respond, I consider an approach developed by the late and excellent Dr. Broda Barnes and Dr. John Lowe. This involves giving a therapeutic trial of high-dose Cytomel, 80 to 120 µg daily. This is enough to leave most healthy people hyperthyroid if their cells were not deaf to the thyroid. So, this treatment should only be done by holistic physicians familiar with the protocol.

There is one thyroid blood test called a reverse T3 that does help point to the need for high-dose T3. In periods of severe energy crisis, the body actually converts the T3 hormone into an anti-thyroid called reverse T3. This tells the cells to go into hibernation, so the body can conserve energy. This can be seen, for example, during times of famine or severe illness.

But sometimes the body gets stuck in this mode in people with CFS/ FMS. In those cases, the reverse T3 is often high normal or elevated. Then slowly raising the liothyronine T3 dose can be helpful. In the people I treat, I have them do so with the caution that if they feel too hyper (like they drank too much coffee), then the dose is too high. As T3 is fairly short acting (its main effect lasts four to six hours), they can try splitting the dose and taking it three to four times a day.

Everybody is different. Some people do best taking the entire dose in the morning and others need to divide it through the day. Others find that they feel better getting a sustained-release T3 hormone from a compounding pharmacy. Treatment is based totally on what feels best to the person. Lab testing, except for checking the reverse T3 to be sure that it is coming down, is totally useless once you go over 35 µg of T3 daily. All you will see is a low free T4 and TSH. The free T3 level will be high, normal, or low—totally dependent on when you draw the blood relative to when you take the thyroid dose.

This will leave your standard physician very confused and, if you draw the blood soon after the dose, very alarmed. So if the blood tests have to be drawn, I have people not take their dose of thyroid until after the blood draw that day.

But when it works, it is dramatic. When people find the correct dose, what I routinely hear them say is that it's like somebody turned on a light switch and that they felt like they finally had blood flowing in their arms and legs for the first time in years.

For the high-dose T3 protocol, worrisome abnormal heart rhythms or heart attacks, although quite rare, can be seen. If the person is feeling too stimulated, the dose is too high. So again, I recommend this sometimes life-changing protocol only be used by physicians familiar with its administration.

THE PROBLEM WITH THYROID TESTING IN FIBROMYALGIA

In addition to what we've discussed above, it is important to realize that in most people with fibromyalgia, their TSH testing will actually go low when they are on the optimal dose of thyroid. This will often alarm their regular physician, who will lower the dose, often causing the person to go from feeling well to crippled again.

The TSH goes low when your thyroid is normal because the hypothalamus controls TSH levels, and it is malfunctioning in FMS. When lecturing at a major worldwide fibromyalgia medical conference, I had the pleasure of speaking with Dr. Gunther Neeck, the world's leading researcher on thyroid in fibromyalgia. I asked him a simple question. "Is TSH reliable in fibromyalgia?" His simple answer was "Absolutely not!"

The bottom line? Thyroid dosing in fibromyalgia needs to be adjusted based on the dose that feels best, while keeping the free T4 blood test from going above the 80th percentile of the normal range for safety.

Testosterone Intensive Care

By and large, the information in Chapter 2 addresses reproductive hormones including testosterone in CFS and FMS, and not only for men. But there are two considerations for fibromyalgia:

- For those needing narcotics for pain, narcotic use will routinely lower testosterone levels in both men and women, worsening pain. Low testosterone equals increased pain. This cycle contributes to the need for ever-increasing doses of narcotics in some people. Because of this, any pain patient who needs chronic narcotic pain medications should have their testosterone levels kept at an optimal level—using only bioidentical testosterone. This not only decreases pain but also improves healing and overall well-being.
- Testosterone has important benefits in CFS/FMS. Though it can take six to twelve months to see the full effects, sometimes people start improving in a few days to weeks. Here are benefits of optimizing testosterone levels:
  - In women with fibromyalgia, a study done by Dr. Hillary White of Dartmouth University showed that giving natural testosterone decreased pain, even if their testosterone levels were normal.
  - Fibromyalgia and CFS are associated with decreased red blood cell levels. In fact, most people with CFS/FMS are anemic despite having normal blood tests. Testosterone supplementation is a highly effective way of increasing the red blood cell levels.
  - Testosterone can improve libido, which is low in 73 percent of CFS and fibromyalgia patients.
  - Testosterone increases bone density, therefore decreasing the risk of osteoporosis. People with fibromyalgia are at greater risk for loss of bone density.
  - Testosterone improves mood and decreases depression.
  - Testosterone increases muscle strength and decreases fat levels.
  - Low testosterone is associated with an increased risk of high cholesterol, angina, and diabetes in men.
  - CFS has been associated with a possible decrease in the heart's ability to pump blood, and testosterone improves heart function.

Reproductive Hormones and Fibromyalgia

In women being treated for CFS/FMS, it is important to be aware that using the SHINE protocol will routinely result in your periods becoming irregular for six to twelve months—whether or not you take estrogen. This occurs in part because your hypothalamus cycles back to its normal rhythm as it starts to heal, and this controls the timing of your cycle.

Pregnancy and CFS/FMS

Women often worry about getting pregnant with CFS/FMS. The good news is that most people with CFS/FMS do very well with pregnancy—and even after the pregnancy, given the proper support.

Most of you will actually feel much better during your pregnancy. It is after the pregnancy that you'll need both nutritional and hormonal support to prevent the CFS/FMS from recurring. I do recommend that, if possible, you follow the treatment protocol discussed in this book for a year before getting pregnant, so you can stop the medications and other treatments that would not be appropriate during pregnancy, without losing the benefits.

After pregnancy, as soon as the baby is weaned, it is often important to resume bioidentical progesterone and other treatments.

Some treatments that can safely be continued through the pregnancy include:

- The Energy Revitalization System vitamin powder (excellent for pregnancy)
- Iron, Vectomega, and magnesium supplementation. These support healthy pregnancy as well
- Diphenhydramine (Benadryl) for sleep
- Thyroid and hydrocortisone treatments

Although most people with CFS/FMS do not have problems with infertility, it is more common in this population than in the non-CFS/FMS population. The good news is that there are many effective natural treatments for infertility. Because they are not expensive, however, they do not get the attention that in vitro fertilization gets. (For more information on natural treatments for infertility, you can email me at fatiguedoc@gmail.com for an article on this.)

Wishing you a happy and healthy pregnancy, baby, and life.

Growth Hormone

Inadequate levels of growth hormone (GH) may be an important factor for some patients with CFS/FMS who do not respond to the rest of the SHINE protocol. It can be detected with a blood test called an IGF-1 level.

Because these injections are expensive and can have side effects (e.g., carpal tunnel syndrome), I prefer to have patients first do SHINE, as most people won't need these injections. The top three things that naturally increase your body's own production of GH are sex, exercise, and deep sleep. I happily recommend all three.

PROLACTIN

Prolactin is synthesized and stored in the pituitary gland, and it is best known for stimulating milk production after childbirth. Unlike other hormones, which are usually low in people with CFS/FMS, prolactin levels are sometimes mildly elevated.

This is because the hypothalamus normally suppresses, instead of stimulates, prolactin production, and the hypothalamus is often dysfunctional in people with CFS/FMS. To make sure that no (benign) pituitary tumor exists, however, I may order a magnetic resonance imaging (MRI) scan in patients who still have elevated prolactin levels after four months of treatment with the SHINE protocol. The MRI generally shows that everything is normal. Some medications, such as antipsychotic medications and risperidone (Risperdal), can also elevate prolactin levels, as can high-dose melatonin.

Most important, when I see an elevated prolactin, it suggests that the neurotransmitter dopamine is low, and then I am more likely to use treatments that raise this neurotransmitter.

As you can see, many problems can occur when the body's glands do not function properly. The good news is that most can be effectively treated. In my experience, this often results in dramatic improvement. It is important, though, to treat the whole person, not simply the hormonal problems.

15 *Infection*
Intensive Care

BFF Summary

1. There are literally dozens of infections implicated in CFS/FMS.
2. I treat virtually everybody who comes to me with CFS/FMS for candida overgrowth.
3. If their history is suggestive (foul-smelling gas, bloating, and diarrhea that persists despite antifungal treatment), I treat for SIBO and also do stool testing at Genova Diagnostics for parasites. I find that parasite testing at most standard labs is inadequate.
4. Next I consider viral infections, especially if the illness began after a viral infection or chronic flu-like symptoms are present. I prefer to consider antivirals first because they are much safer than long-term antibiotics. These are the three main antiviral protocols I consider:
   A. A combination of 500 to 750 milligrams of famciclovir (Famvir) three times a day plus 200 milligrams of celecoxib (Celebrex) twice a day can be very helpful after four months, especially if the Epstein-Barr or HSV-1 IgG viral tests are very high. Simply being elevated just says that the person had the infection in the past, and 95 percent of the healthy adult population are positive for these tests.
   B. If the cytomegalovirus (CMV) or HHV-6 (human herpesvirus 6) IgG antibody levels are very elevated and the person doesn't respond to famciclovir (Famvir), I consider 900 milligrams of valganciclovir (Valcyte) a day for six months.
   C. Work by the infectious disease specialist John Chia suggests that enteroviruses (e.g., Coxsackievirus) are active in a very high percent of cases of CFS and fibro-

myalgia. A supplement called Equilibrant can be very helpful in these situations. Regular lab testing is not helpful. I treat this without doing the lab testing.

5. Next, I consider antibiotic-sensitive infections:

   A. For Lyme disease and coinfections, I do not find most testing to be especially reliable (although it can point in helpful directions). I find that most labs are either almost always negative and others almost always positive. Because of this, I consider it reasonable to treat empirically based on symptoms and simply see if the person improves.

   B. If taking antibiotics for an extended period, it is critical that the person be on antifungal support as well.

   C. Simply treating with the antibiotics without treating the hypothalamic circuit breaker is far less likely to work.

   D. If somebody has a history of being allergic to three unrelated antibiotics, this suggests that it was not an allergy, but rather flaring your symptoms from killing off an antibiotic-sensitive bacteria that was contributing to the CFS/FMS.

   E. Also, when a person reports that they took an antibiotic for a week or two and their CFS/FMS improved markedly while they were on it, it simply makes sense to put them back on that antibiotic for an extended period.

Infections

For those of you with CFS/FMS, welcome to the Infection of the Month Club. Many of you have noticed that there seems to be a regular flow of new infections that get blamed for CFS and fibromyalgia. I have watched this occur over and over in the last forty years, with literally dozens of different infections being blamed as "*the* cause." So let me start by simply stating the obvious: CFS/FMS is generally not occurring from a single infection—but rather most people have many infections that are dragging them down.

Immune dysfunction is an integral part of CFS/FMS. In fact, some people use the name CFIDS, or chronic fatigue and immune dysfunction syndrome, instead of CFS.

Because of the immune dysfunction, people with CFS pick up many "hitchhiker" infections. In addition, there are many viral infections—such as infectious mononucleosis (EBV or Epstein-Barr virus), HHV-6 (human herpesvirus 6) and other herpesviruses, CMV (cytomegalovirus), herpes zoster (aka chickenpox and shingles), and others—that are never entirely cleared from our body once we have them—and most people have had these infections by the time they're twenty years old. For these viruses and others, the body often finds it easier to simply lock up the last remaining bugs in little jail cells where they stay for the rest of our lives unless our immune function goes down, in which case there is sometimes a jailbreak. Then we have what is called viral reactivation.

Unfortunately, although testing is very good at picking up most acute first-time infections, it is very unreliable at diagnosing chronic infections. So deciding whether to treat for infections in CFS/FMS is best based on symptoms and response to treatment rather than simply relying on the testing.

The good news? It is not necessary to track down and kill every infection. Almost all of these infections are what are considered opportunistic infections. By definition, this means that they cannot survive when your immune system is healthy. Because of this, once you have cleared out a few key infections and helped your immune system to heal, it knows how to get rid of the rest of the infections.

An easy way to understand what is going on with infections in fibromyalgia is to think of them like a pack of little yapping dogs. Perhaps Chihuahuas. Any one of them, your healthy immune system would just shrug off and kick away. But if you have a pack of six of them jumping on you, you're in trouble. The job here is not to fight all the dogs. If we simply chase off three of them, your immune system can get rid of the others. It doesn't necessarily matter which three you chase off, but the biggest dog in the pack is the candida, so we go after that one first.

There are certain infections where the organisms are, simply put, massive in size. For example, by way of comparison, if a virus was the size of the period at the end of this sentence, a candida (fungal) thread could be the size of a house. And some parasites would be even larger. We will teach you how to knock out these big bad bugs so your immune system can take care of the little guys.

There are literally dozens of infections implicated in CFS/FMS, and the most important ones to deal with fall under four categories:

1. Candida/yeast infections (discussed in Chapter 3)
2. Antibiotic-sensitive infections (e.g., Lyme disease)
3. Viral infections
4. Parasites

In addition, in some cases, it is not the infection itself but your body's reaction to it that causes your symptoms. Evidence is suggesting that the immune system has trouble shutting down after eliminating some infections in CFS/FMS. This then causes it to exhaust itself, setting up a scenario for infections with common, and often benign, organisms.

I would like to start with going after the simple infections. Then we will discuss the more complex area of viral infections followed by Lyme disease and its coinfections. Then, for those of you that are interested, the next chapter will have a more in-depth and technical discussion of what is happening with your immune system.

Step 1: Kill Off Candida

How to do this was discussed at length in Chapter 3. This is the most important infection to treat in CFS and fibromyalgia, as doing so takes a massive strain off of your immune system, freeing it to fight other infections. To recap simply, almost everybody with CFS and fibromyalgia should be treated for candida. There is no test that I consider reliable. Nasal congestion, sinusitis, intermittent mouth sores, or symptoms of irritable bowel syndrome (gas, bloating, diarrhea, and constipation) suggest that candida is present.

I treat with a combination of the Pearls Elite probiotic, a natural antifungal such as Caprylex or Lufenuron, and 200 milligrams of fluconazole (Diflucan) a day for a minimum of six weeks. I use a compounded Sinusitis Nose Spray (by ITC Compounding Pharmacy) for at least six weeks at the same time as the fluconazole, to kill the candida and toxin-producing bacteria in the nose and sinuses.

When this infection clears, so will many of your other CFS and fibromyalgia symptoms. If the sinus congestion or gut symptoms recur, I will repeat treatment with another six weeks of the antifungals. Because of the immune dysfunction, some people with CFS/FMS need to take treatment long term.

Yeast/Candida Questionnaire
The total score for this section gives the probability of yeast overgrowth being a significant factor in your case. If you answer yes to any questions below, mark it off, then add up your total score and put it below the questions.

50 _____ Have you been treated for acne with tetracycline, erythromycin, or any other antibiotic for one month or longer?

50 _____ Have you taken antibiotics for any type of infection for more than two consecutive months, or shorter courses more than three times in a twelve-month period?

5 _____ Have you ever taken an antibiotic—even for a single course?

25 _____ Have you ever had prostatitis or vaginitis?

5 _____ Have you ever been pregnant?

15 _____ Have you taken birth control pills?

15 _____ Have you taken corticosteroids such as prednisone, Cortef, or Medrol?

15 _____ When you are exposed to perfumes, insecticides, or other odors or chemicals, do you develop wheezing, burning eyes, or any other distress?

20 _____ Are your symptoms worse on damp or humid days or in moldy places?

20 _____ Have you ever had a fungal infection such as jock itch, athlete's foot, or a nail or skin infection that was difficult to treat?

20 _____ Do you crave sugar or breads?

10 _____ Does tobacco smoke cause you discomfort (e.g., wheezing, burning eyes)?

Total: _____

If 70 or higher, candida overgrowth is likely in those with CFS/FMS, sinus, or irritable bowel problems.

STEP 2: KILL OFF BOWEL PARASITES

Although we often think of parasites as just a problem encountered when we are traveling, infection by giardia, blastocystis, amoebae, and numerous other bowel parasites is common in the United States. In fact, in my initial study, one out of six people with CFS/FMS had a parasite, and parasites have been shown to be one of the many causes of CFS/FMS.

In real life, I find that 5 to 10 percent of people with CFS/FMS and intestinal symptoms will have a parasite.

DIAGNOSING BOWEL PARASITES
I generally do stool testing in people with severe and smelly gas or chronic diarrhea, especially if this persists after treating the candida and SIBO (see

below). I also check for parasites if their illness began after traveling overseas or with diarrhea.

Most standard laboratories are clueless about how to do proper stool testing for parasites and will miss the vast majority of these infections. Testing has to be done at a lab that specializes in parasitology. Unfortunately, these are not usually covered by health insurance. These include the following labs:

- **Parasitology Center Inc.** Parasite testing is what they do. Especially for those on a limited budget, this is where I would send the stool specimen (www.parasitetesting.com). I would order the comprehensive stool analysis test (CPT 87177). This offers the information I find most helpful.
- **Genova Diagnostics.** This lab has a wide array of holistic tests (www.gdx.net). Some of the panels can be quite extensive and therefore costly. I find simply doing the bacterial culture and sensitivity and parasite testing to be most cost-effective. This is the main lab that I use for this, sending the second sample to the Parasitology Center when I am very suspicious of parasites.
- **Diagnos-Techs and Doctor's Data.** These are specialty labs that can also be helpful.

When getting the stool sample, remember it has to be a loose, watery stool (i.e., one that takes the shape of the specimen container). This is important to wash the parasite off the bowel wall and into the stool sample where it can be seen. Taking one or two bisacodyl (Dulcolax) tablets the night before is helpful, if you don't routinely have loose stools. At the same time, if you have chronic diarrhea, collect a second stool specimen to test for a special bowel infection called *Clostridium difficile*, which makes a toxin that can also trigger CFS/FMS. The stool test for *Clostridium difficile* toxin, fortunately, can be done well at any lab, making it more likely to be covered by insurance. The sample for *Clostridium difficile* (which is often simply called *C. diff.*) needs to be taken to the lab within two hours or frozen. The other samples for the parasites are sent to one of the labs above and the directions will be included in the specimen kit that you order from the lab (with your health practitioner's prescription) before collecting the specimen.

Treating Bowel Parasites

Common parasites include giardia, blastocystis, and amebiasis. The appropriate treatment for bowel parasites depends on which organism is causing the problem. Some doctors will consider some parasites to be nonpathogenic. This means they don't necessarily cause bowel problems unless a person has immune dysfunction. Because people with CFS/FMS have immune dysfunction, I find it important to treat *all* parasite infections—and people often feel considerably better when the parasite is eliminated. In addition, when a parasitic infection is suspected but no parasites can be found in the lab testing, I sometimes consider treating the person empirically with 1,000 milligrams of nitazoxanide (Alinia) twice a day for ten days. This covers a large number of bowel infections. Warning: This medication is quite expensive, so check to be sure it is covered by your prescription insurance plan.

Treatment for each parasite is quite different, and unfortunately the treatments continually change, as many of these medications have disappeared from the American market (for lack of profitability). For others, the drug companies have raised the price from a few dollars to as much as $1,500 a treatment. Often these now very expensive medications can be found cheaply at compounding pharmacies instead.

Because of this, we are not listing the treatments for each parasite in this book, and instead refer you to your holistic physician if they are present.

Step 3: Kill Off Viral Infections

There are many viruses that have been implicated in CFS/FMS. The most important are:

- **Famciclovir (Famvir) sensitive.** This antiviral kills EBV (Epstein-Barr virus) and HSV-1 (herpes simplex virus, such as the one that causes cold sores). Both of these have been significantly implicated in CFS/FMS.
- **Valganciclovir (Valcyte) sensitive.** These include CMV (cytomegalovirus) and HHV-6 (human herpesvirus 6).
- **Coxsackie B viruses.**
- **Retroviruses.** Most of these remain unidentified, but are in the same family as AIDS. Testing is pretty useless for these, but effective empiric treatment is available.

- **Other viruses.** There are probably more viruses that we don't even know exist than the ones we have identified. We will discuss approaches to going after these. It is possible that viruses that affect the gastrointestinal tract may join this list in the future. COVID-19 is now becoming another major CFS/FMS trigger.

TESTING

The standard tests for these viruses include an IgM antibody, which usually only goes up in the first two to three months after the *initial* infection. Because in CFS/FMS these infections represent viral reactivation, and generally not the initial infection, this test is fairly useless. Meanwhile, the IgG antibody tests for these viruses will be positive in over 90 percent of healthy adults, as this test simply shows that you had this infection in the past. Therefore, a positive IgG antibody test by itself is also relatively meaningless.

This is why seeing most infectious disease doctors, with some rare but notable exceptions including Dr. Nancy Klimas, Dr. John Chia, Dr. Joseph Brewer, and Dr. Susan Levine, is usually just an exercise in frustration and a waste of time. They have no idea what to test for or how to interpret the tests in CFS/FMS.

Viral Testing in the Suspicious Cases

Here are the viral tests that I check in people with the symptoms in the next section or with persistent symptoms despite treatment:

1. HSV-1, HHV-6, CMV, and EBV IgG antibodies (I don't check IgM).

2. Total IgG antibody levels along with IgG 1–4 subsets to look for further evidence of immune suppression. This is discussed below under immune function.

On the other hand, research is suggesting that very high levels of the IgG antibody may suggest viral reactivation. Because of this, if the IgG antibody for the HSV-1 (herpes simplex virus 1), HHV-6 (human herpesvirus 6), or CMV (cytomegalovirus) is greater than 4 (or 1:640 or greater, which is another way these tests may be reported), I am more likely to suspect a reactivated viral infection that needs treatment, especially if the person is not feeling adequately improved with other treatments by four to six months.

EBV (Epstein-Barr virus)—the virus most commonly responsible for mononucleosis ("mono")—tests are more complex. A sample of results in twenty-eight healthy people by Dr. Nancy Klimas, one of my favorite CFS infectious disease researchers in the whole world, found that the median (kind of like average) result for each of the following tests was:

- EBNA (EBV nuclear antigen): 235 (levels over 600 are in the top 25 percent of the population, and therefore suggestive).
- VCA (viral capsid antigen) IgG: 186 (levels over 517 are suggestive).
- EA (early antigen)—10.7 (levels over 18 are suggestive).

We are just starting to also check Coxsackie B viral titers. See below for treating elevated levels (which can be anything at or over 1:80).

Again, these tests are not absolute. When combined with the symptoms below, they may be helpful in determining which antiviral to begin with. Also remember: Over 90 percent of the healthy population are positive for these tests, so a positive test by itself means nothing.

Instead, I use the presence of very high levels in the tests and/or the symptoms below to decide whether to use an antiviral.

Symptoms

I am more likely to suspect an important underlying viral infection if:

1. The person's CFS/FMS began with a severe flu-like illness and symptoms persists despite SHINE.
2. The person has pure CFS with predominantly flu-like symptoms, with debilitating fatigue and little or no pain, or with low blood pressure symptoms (NMH/POTS; see Chapter 14).

Antiviral Treatments

Antivirals can be helpful in about 25 to 50 percent of CFS patients. This level goes much higher if the symptoms above are present. For all of these, you can see initial flaring with treatment, called the Herxheimer reaction. This is a good sign, confirming that the treatment is killing a bug that is causing you problems, but pushing through the flaring will not speed healing. It will delay it. So stop the treatment till the flare passes, then start with a teeny tiny dose and work up slowly as is comfortable.

Absence of your symptoms flaring does not mean that it will not help. Here's how I begin:

Famciclovir (Famvir) Plus Celecoxib (Celebrex)

This is what I begin with in most people. Famciclovir (Famvir) at a dose of 500 to 750 milligrams three times a day was modestly effective. Excellent research by the surgeon Dr. William "Skip" Pridgen and virologist Carol Duffy, PhD, has shown that adding 200 milligrams of celecoxib (Celebrex) twice daily dramatically increases the effectiveness.

I found this interesting. In my first edition of *From Fatigued to Fantastic!* way back in 1995, I noted that most ibuprofen-type anti-inflammatory medications were useless for fibromyalgia, with the exception of celecoxib. I noted at that time that I had no idea why this drug worked in fibromyalgia.

It turns out that celecoxib has significant antiviral properties, which augment those of the famciclovir.

The main side effect of famciclovir is the Herxheimer reaction, so start slowly with a low dose and work up as is comfortable. The main side effect of celecoxib is indigestion or acid reflux. If side effects will occur, they usually happen in the first few days. It takes about four months to see the benefits of this combination, but often it is much quicker.

Overall, this is much better tolerated than the valganciclovir (Valcyte), so I begin with famciclovir plus celecoxib. Famciclovir used to cost over $10,000 a year. Now, using the GoodRx phone app, you can get it for $65 a month.

Valganciclovir (Valcyte)

If people do not respond to the famciclovir plus celecoxib, have suspicious symptoms, and have CMV or HHV-6 IgG titers over 4 (or 1:640 or higher), I consider the valganciclovir. This used to cost $24,000 a year, but using the GoodRx app, it can be found for $250 a month.

The dosing I use is 900 milligrams twice a day for three weeks, followed by 900 milligrams once a day for twenty-three weeks. It is effective against CMV, HHV-6, and EBV viruses. It can take four months to see the benefits, and some people will initially have a die-off reaction where their CFS/FMS symptoms worsen for the first few weeks to months of treatment as dead virus parts are released into their system.

For both of these antiviral protocols, it takes four months to see if it is going to work and I consider six months to be the treatment course. We are finding that many people need to continue treatment past the six months to maintain the benefit.

Coxsackievirus and Other Enteroviruses

Enteroviruses are a group of viruses that predominantly affect the digestive system but can also affect nerve and muscle tissues. Polio is perhaps the best known member of this family, but numerous other usually benign viruses in this family are fairly common. They usually cause short-term infections and go away. These include the enteric cytopathic human orphan (ECHO) and Coxsackie B family of viruses. When the immune system is altered, as in CFS/FMS, they may become chronic, often making a home in the digestive tract.

Dr. John Chia of Torrance, California, is an academic-trained infectious disease specialist and researcher. He became interested in CFS/FMS when his son was crippled with the illness. Looking for a cure, he found that over 83 percent of people with CFS/FMS have enteroviruses on stomach biopsies, compared to only 20 percent of the healthy population. But only a very few labs in the country know how to do the proper staining to look for these infections. He does find special viral neutralization testing done only by ARUP Laboratories to be helpful, but not those done by most other national labs.

Unfortunately, getting your local lab to do the proper testing is both difficult and expensive. Although he recommends getting the proper blood testing, or doing the proper stomach antral biopsies, these are difficult to get unless you are seeing him in his office; otherwise, the blood testing is quite unreliable.

Fortunately, being Chinese American, he combines familiarity with, and an open mind to, both Western medicine and Chinese herbals. He found that the Chinese herb oxymatrine (extracted from the root of *Sophora flavescens*) has significant immune modulating effects. It has been shown in studies to also be effective against the hepatitis virus, so it does not appear to be specific to just enteroviruses.

Dr. Chia has combined this along with several other herbs, nutrients, and shiitake mushroom extract to create a product called Equilibrant (www.equilibranthealth.com). He begins people on just one-eighth of the tablet daily, raising the dose slowly as is comfortable. He recommends that people with severe gastritis (heartburn) or neurologic symptoms go espe-cially slowly, as killing the infection in the stomach (parietal) cells may initially cause ulcers.

Over several months, he raises the dose to three to six tablets daily. What I have seen in a very severe refractory case was that the person's CFS dramatically improved after two months on three tablets a day. Dr. Chia also considers two months to be a fair trial of the treatment once the per-son reaches three tablets a day.

So, although he would only recommend doing the treatment if the testing is positive, there is an argument to be made for simply treating empirically in refractory cases of CFS/FMS. Especially:

- If the illness started with respiratory and/or gastric/intestinal symp-toms.
- If the person has tenderness below the right rib cage, in the solar plexus, or in the right lower abdomen, where immune tissues called Peyer's patches can be found.
- As the treatment is relatively low cost at $1.50 per day for three tablets and fairly safe.
- As it may benefit the Th1/Th2 immune imbalance seen in CFS/FMS.

But again, I start with a low dose and work up slowly as is comfort-able. I have people stay on three to six tablets a day for three months to see if it helps, as both a diagnostic and therapeutic test.

RETROVIRAL INFECTIONS

Dr. Dietrich Klinghardt is a fascinating and cutting-edge researcher. About thirty-five years ago, when I began following his work, his concepts were so radical that I thought they could not be true. But time after time, he has been right. He is simply twenty to forty years ahead of everybody else.

For example, a few trailblazing researchers (such Dr. Mark Sivieri) and I have recently begun exploring the connection between immune and autonomic dysfunction. Although I have been patting myself on the back for making this connection, I found out recently that Dr. Klinghardt's PhD thesis forty years ago was on, you guessed it, the connection between immune and autonomic dysfunction.

He is now finding dramatic results in CFS, fibromyalgia, and a host of other conditions by using a combination of herbals that suppress the activation and reproduction of retroviruses. Retroviruses are a family of viruses that actually insert themselves into human DNA and make up 5 to 10 percent of the healthy human genome. This means that they are not so much infections as part of how our genetic makeup developed. Most of the time, these are kept turned off unless needed.

Dr. Klinghardt is suspecting that many environmental factors, including the overt increases in environmental electromagnetic frequencies (radio, TV, internet, cell phones, etc.) may inadvertently turn these viruses back on.

As an aside, most of these human-made frequencies do not resonate with human cell frequencies. So, they would not be expected to be a problem. But the ones that do can be an issue. They can disrupt and confuse our body's own internal communication systems. It would not be hard to have public safety research done to see which frequencies need to be avoided (this would be easy to do, and simply require adaptation when systems are upgraded in the future). But sadly, I suspect that what is occurring is that this research, and effective discussion about the topic, is blocked by companies with major financial interests.

For more information on retroviruses, Dr. Klinghardt's lecture to physicians on this topic "Retroviral Infections as Causes of Chronic Diseases" can be found at www.acimconnect.com/webinars/retroviral-infections-as -causes-of-chronic-diseases. Another article by him, "The Role of Retroviruses in Chronic Illness—A Clinician's Perspective," can be found at www.klinghardtinstitute.com/wp-content/uploads/2018/05/IHCAN -Dr-K-article-HERV-05.1.pdf.

Regarding some of his concerns on electromagnetic frequency pollution, I generally do not begin with avoiding those, unless the person is having electromagnetic sensitivities. I find it best not to get overly worried about everything in the environment, especially those we can't yet do anything about, but rather to give our bodies what they need to thrive in the modern milieu.

What I want to focus on here is the herbal protocol that he is recommending. The list below also gives the different websites where these can be found. The cost is about $100 to $200 a month, and it may take up to three months to determine effectiveness.

Treatment

Results may be seen with even just the first two treatments below. The first five are the most important supplements. Go slow and start with a low dose. These are powerful treatments and may cause a Herxheimer "die-off" reaction.

1. **Cistus incanus tea.** Drink 6 to 8 cups a day, but work up to this amount slowly. (Some can only tolerate a tablespoon at first.) Brew the same leaves three times using new water each time to extract all the potent polyphenols. Dr. Klinghardt recommends bringing the leaves to a gentle boil, putting the lid on, and simmering for five minutes. If this is too much work, just pour boiling water on the tea and steep for five to ten minutes in a teapot or press pot. Just keep the lid on as it steeps to prevent the therapeutic oils from evaporating.

    An excellent tea to use is from Ki Science (www.kiscience .com/product/cistus-incanus-infusion), but this ships from Europe. The one from BioPure (www.biopureus.com/product /cistus-incanus-tea-100g) in the United States is also good. It costs $25 for 174 servings. Biokoma, Natvita, and Polana are also good sources.

    Sweeten it with a stevia from a whole leaf. A study showed this to be very effective against Lyme and other infections (even more than the prescriptions), but it has to be a brand of stevia that has all of the leaf components (most don't). Use ones from Ki Science, Equinox Farms, BioPure, or Nutramedix.

2. **Baikal skullcap.** This is called the leader among herbs for retrovirus. Dr. Klinghardt uses ½ teaspoon of Baikalin powder two times a day (www.biopureus.com/product/baikalin-powder).

3. **Broccoli sprouts.** Fresh sprouts are best, and two-inch-long sprouts have optimal properties. A dose is 2 tablespoons chopped fresh twice a day for dramatic improvement. You can sprout your own—there are many options on Amazon for organic seed—or buy the sprouts at Whole Foods and Sprouts. Just be sure that they are fresh and not moldy on the bottom. *These must be chewed.* This may seem a small thing, but this is an important treatment. The active component of the sprouts is sulforaphane, and the sprouts must be chewed to activate

this. If you are unable to find or grow your own, Dr. Kling-hardt recommends taking three capsules of BioPure Broccoli Sprout twice a day (www.sophianutrition.com/products/broc coli-sprout-capsules-90-capsules). This costs $184 a month, but other brands may not have the sulforaphane precursor.

4. **EN-V tincture.** This is a combination of six herbal extracts blended with one of BioPure's signature liposomal products. Take 2 to 3 droppers twice daily. The cost is $48 per 2 ounces (www.biopureus.com/product/en-v).

5. **Pantethine.** Take 1,000 milligrams twice a day.

6. **Selenium.** Buy the form selenomethionine or selenocystine. Take 400 micrograms one or two times day.

Dr. Klinghardt has clinics called the Sophia Health Institute, in both Seattle, Washington, and Marin County, California. They also treat Lyme disease.

SHINE for Post–COVID-19 CFS/FMS

As we have discussed, many different infections can cause you to "trip a circuit breaker" and develop post-infectious CFS and fibromyalgia.

Coronaviruses, including the one that causes COVID-19, also put people at high risk for this. Initial data from the World Health Organization suggests that, in mild cases, the average recovery time from COVID-19 is about two weeks from the onset of symptoms. This extends to three to six weeks for very severe cases.

So if you are having persistent severe fatigue more than two months after you started experiencing COVID-19 symptoms, especially difficulty sleeping, you likely have postviral CFS/FMS. You're not alone.

A 2009 study published in *The Journal of the American Medical Association* found that 40 percent of 369 Chinese SARS (severe acute respiratory syndrome) survivors reported a "chronic fatigue problem," while 27 percent met the diagnostic criteria for CFS.

Another Canadian study, by the sleep expert Harvey Moldofsky, also found that a high percentage of people who had SARS also had persistent fatigue and other symptoms suggestive of fibromyalgia. Running a sleep study in a subset of these, he found that the changes were the same as those classically seen in CFS and FMS. This suggests that the fatigue following these viruses is simply another form of postviral CFS/FMS. Which is very good news.

Why?

Because these respond very well to the SHINE Protocol. In fact, decades of research for CFS/FMS may be the cavalry that comes to save the day.

Fortunately, for post–COVID-19, there is unlikely to be persistent viral infection, as is the case with some other viral infections. COVID-19 simply tripped the hypothalamic circuit breaker. Which now needs to be turned back on.

The key focus initially should be to:

1. Optimize sleep.

2. Optimize adrenal function. Other hormones should also be optimized, but the adrenal glands are the most susceptible. Looking for orthostatic intolerance will also be important.

3. Optimize nutritional support. The keys here would be optimizing zinc and vitamins C and D, along with overall high-potency nutritional support. This can be done easily with the Energy Revitalization System and Smart Energy System. This can also optimize immune function, making people less susceptible to future viral infections.

As you can see, there are a number of antiviral treatments. Higher cost does not necessarily mean more effective results, and it is best to tailor therapy to each individual case.

A Powerful Natural Immune Booster

In addition to these prescription antivirals, a natural treatment that may be helpful in markedly augmenting immunity in CFS is thymic protein A, marketed under the brand name ProBoost. Although not a hormone, thymic protein A is an excellent natural immune stimulant and mimics the natural hormone produced by the thymus, the gland that stimulates the immune system. I find it to be extraordinarily effective in fighting common acute infections of any kind that seem to pop up, and I recommend that it be in everyone's medicine cabinet. In fact, whenever my kids would get a cold, the first thing they'd say is, "Dad, where's the white powder [the ProBoost]?"

Although taking it for one to three days will quickly work with most acute viral infections, for augmenting immunity in CFS, one packet three times a day for three months is needed. In one study, this dropped EBV IgG levels by 70 percent after three months in CFS patients.

Available without prescription at www.endfatigue.com.

Step 4: Antibiotic-Sensitive Infections, Including Lyme Disease

These are infections that improve when the person takes an antibiotic, suggesting a hidden infection. If any of these six conditions are present, I recommend antibiotic treatment:

- An ongoing temperature elevation over 98.6°F—even 99°F, as most people with CFS/FMS have a low temperature.
- Chronic lung congestion.
- A history of bad reactions to several different antibiotics (people misinterpret this die-off reaction as an allergic reaction—but being "allergic" to several unrelated antibiotics but not to other medications is quite unlikely).
- Scabbing scalp sores—for these cases, the antibiotic azithromycin (Zithromax) has been found to be helpful.
- A history of vertigo lasting over three months (in which case I suspect Lyme disease, which can irritate the nerve serving the middle ear balance centers). Dizziness and disequilibrium without a feeling of spinning in a circle is common in CFS/FMS and does not count as vertigo.
- A history of CFS/FMS symptoms markedly improving while on antibiotics in the past (in which case I give the antibiotic that helped them).

Unfortunately, there are no reliable tests for most of these antibiotic-sensitive infections, whether they be mycoplasma, Lyme disease, or a host of others.

Lyme disease is especially problematic, as there is *no* gold standard test. I suspect that well over half of the people who have Lyme infections have negative tests, and conversely, if you use some holistically oriented labs to check Lyme tests, it seems like almost everybody comes back positive for one of their tests. For the most common lab, I've only seen two people test negative for their infection panel over the last several decades. This leaves me concerned that the test may be overly sensitive, being positive even when Lyme is not present. It would be helpful for researchers to do their test panel on ten healthy people to see how many test positive.

This all creates enormous confusion, as CFS/FMS symptoms are similar to those of Lyme disease. Because of this, many people desperately looking for an explanation for their symptoms, who have found one of the holistic Lyme tests to be positive, cling to this diagnosis. Often, they actually do have Lyme. This is understandable, as some doctors continue to abusively state or imply to the person and their family that if the generally useless tests that most doctors order are negative, then the patient must be crazy.

Many do feel better on antibiotics, and take this as confirmation that they have Lyme disease. But it is helpful to remember that doxycycline family antibiotics also help with the central sensitization even in the absence of infection. So improvement with doxycycline simply means that the doxycycline is helpful, and not necessarily that there is an infection. But it is suggestive. And Lyme is horribly underdiagnosed by standard medical physicians.

Indeed, many excellent physicians who specialize in treating CFS/FMS feel that the large majority of CFS/FMS patients have Lyme disease. On the other hand unfortunately, the majority of CFS/FMS-illiterate physicians only believe a Lyme infection is present if a test called the Western blot is positive—ignoring that this test has clearly been shown to be negative in a very large percentage of those with Lyme disease.

I suspect that the truth is somewhere in the middle.

Given all of the above, we simply do not know for sure how many people with CFS/FMS also have Lyme disease. If you have a history of tick bite associated with a bull's-eye rash (erythema migrans) and have fatigue or pain, I consider it absolutely reasonable to treat for suspected Lyme disease, even if the tests are negative. But the majority of people with Lyme disease never noticed their rash. So instead I use the clinical symptoms below to determine when to give an antibiotic trial. Simply put, it is possible to help people get well, even while acknowledging that we don't know if Lyme is present or not.

The approach I currently recommend (until we have better testing) is to simply acknowledge that the testing used in CFS/FMS patients for antibiotic-sensitive infections in general is unreliable. The research shows that these infections are common in CFS/FMS and must be treated. And the research also shows that many patients improve when given antibiotics such as azithromycin (Zithromax) or doxycycline—even if testing is negative.

Given this situation, it is reasonable for physicians to use their clinical judgment and treat with antibiotics when appropriate, adjusting treatment based on clinical response, or even the testing available, even if there is no test to confirm the type of infection.

Recovering from Lyme Disease

Lyme disease, and the associated coinfections, are far more common than most physicians suspect. But both standard and holistic Lyme testing is of questionable reliability. Because of this, I treat based on symptoms, then I use how people respond to treatment to guide the use of antibiotics.

But regardless of what infection triggered your circuit breaker, the antibiotics by themselves will not be enough. It is critical to use the entire SHINE protocol as well to recover fully.

Especially important? After one or two months of use, many people find that they initially got better on antibiotics and then got worse as the antibiotics flared candida overgrowth. The response is to continue to increase antibiotics. This is kind of like chasing a drug high and doesn't work in the long term. It's better to continue the antibiotics but to treat for the candida at the same time, while incorporating the rest of the SHINE protocol.

TREATING LYME AND OTHER HIDDEN ANTIBIOTIC-SENSITIVE INFECTIONS

People with the symptoms discussed above seem to be more likely to have infections that respond to special antibiotics. The antibiotics most likely to affect these organisms are the following:

- **Doxycycline or, preferably, minocycline.** These are usually prescribed at dosages of 100 milligrams twice a day. These two antibiotics are in the tetracycline family. These antibiotics should not be given to children under eight years of age because they can cause permanent staining of the teeth.
- **Azithromycin (Zithromax).** Take 250 to 500 milligrams a day. These antibiotics are in the erythromycin family. Azithromycin tends to be fairly well tolerated. I begin with this antibiotic if the person has scalp or skin sores or scabs.

- **Ciprofloxacin (Cipro).** This is usually prescribed at dosages of 500 to 750 milligrams twice a day. This antibiotic has a wide range of effectiveness against a large number of organisms. Cipro has an additional benefit for men, as it also treats any hidden prostate infections, as does doxycycline and sulfamethoxazole/trimethoprim (Septra). You should not take oral magnesium or any supplement containing magnesium within four to six hours of taking ciprofloxacin or you may not absorb the antibiotic as completely.

  A small percentage of the population has a genetic defect that prevents them from breaking down Cipro. In this group, taking Cipro can actually trigger FMS, and this family of antibiotics should be avoided if you are related to someone who developed fibromyalgia after taking ciprofloxacin. Flaring with ciprofloxacin is most often because it triggers candida rather than the genetic defect, but it's better to be safe than sorry.

If you do have low-grade chronic temperature elevations, be sure that you monitor your temperature during treatment. If your temperature drops with the antibiotic, it suggests that you do have one of these antibiotic-sensitive infections and that the antibiotic is helping. This would encourage me to continue the antibiotic trial—even if it takes up to eighteen months to see an improvement in your symptoms.

If a person is clearly better after six to eight weeks, I keep repeating six- to eight-week cycles until the symptoms fully resolve. It may take several years of treatment for the infection to be totally eradicated. To put this in perspective, this is how long children often take antibiotics for acne—which, unfortunately, if not taken with antifungals, can lead to yeast overgrowth and possibly trigger CFS/FMS. You should therefore take a good probiotic such as Pearls Elite once a day. I'll usually add Lufenuron 800 milligrams every Monday, Wednesday, and Friday and sometimes add 200 milligrams of fluconazole (Diflucan) twice each Sunday (one day a week) as well.

Often, people also get what is called a Herxheimer reaction as the antibiotic-sensitive organisms die off. Again, this is a very good sign, because it means the antibiotic is killing something contributing to your CFS/FMS, but it does complicate treatment. Many people mistakenly confuse these with an allergic reaction. These symptoms can be severe and can last for weeks. When this occurs, I stop the antibiotic, let the die-off reaction subside, and then resume the antibiotic at a much lower dose (e.g., 25 milligrams of minocycline every other day) and work the dose up slowly. Trying to play macho and pushing through the symptom flare is a very bad idea. It actually delays healing, instead of speeding it.

Covering Lyme and coinfections is the topic for an entire book. As many books have been written on this, I am simply covering the key antibiotics. But using the entire SHINE protocol along with treatment by a Lyme literate physician (these can be found, along with a wealth of information, at www.ilads.org) can dramatically improve outcomes.

Fortunately, using the entire SHINE protocol along with the antibiotics often results in improvement being seen within three to four months of antibiotic use, and persisting when the antibiotics are stopped. This makes SHINE especially important in those with chronic Lyme infections.

Would You Give up Alcohol for Four Months to Get Rid of Lyme Disease?

Although it's too early to tell, there is some promising research being done using a medication called disulfiram (Antabuse). This medication causes people to throw up whenever they drink alcohol, so it is used predominantly in alcoholics to prevent drinking.

Interestingly, a test-tube study done in 2016 by Venkata Raveendra Pothineni and colleagues at Stanford found disulfiram to be a more effective treatment for Lyme disease than any of the other recommended drugs.

So Dr. Ken Liegner tried it. The first person he treated was symptom-free after four months and was able to stop the medication. He has treated over thirty people since then, and has found that many patients can stop the medication after four to six months and continue to stay in remission. It may be effective against both Lyme disease and infections caused by the bacteria *Bartonella* (including cat scratch disease).

I am only considering using it at this time in very resistant cases of Lyme. This is because, although the medication is very safe for people who are simply taking it for alcoholism, I am hearing worrisome reports of people developing neuropathy (nerve pain) when taking it for Lyme disease. Because of this, it is more reasonable to start with a very low dose and raise it very slowly. If numbness or tingling or pain in the hands or feet occur, I would stop it.

Because of potential Herxheimer reactions, it is best to start slowly. The medication comes in tablets that are 250 milligrams and 500 milligrams. Starting doses are usually 67.5 milligrams or 125 milligrams every three days, with increasing doses every two to four weeks if well tolerated. The full dose for an average adult is 500 milligrams daily.

Some Protocols for Lyme and Coinfections

There are numerous approaches that are being successfully used. In addition, many coinfections exist with and complicate Lyme disease. These also need to be addressed and treated. How to do so is actually a whole book in itself, but here are some excellent starting places.

In people with the most severe environmental sensitivities (see Chapter 19), Lyme disease and its coinfections are especially important to consider. When the sensitivities and severe anxiety are present, the Lyme coinfection *Bartonella* is suspect. This whole area is far too complex to even try a do-it-yourself approach. Instead, look for a Lyme literate physician at www.ilads.org.

Suspect *Bartonella* if you have:

- Intense sensitivity and reactivity
- Intense anxiety with emotional instability and mood swings
- An uncomfortable weird feeling of vibration over parts of the spine
- Bell's palsy, inflammation of the other cranial nerves or optic nerve, or meningitis
- Pseudoseizures or other very unusual neurologic sensations

There is no especially reliable testing for *Bartonella*, with diagnosis being based on symptoms and response to treatment, in combination with the available testing.

Treatment typically includes the antibiotics rifampin, sulfamethoxazole/trimethoprim (Bactrim/Septra), azithromycin (Zithromax), and clindamycin.

The herbal supplement A-Bart or Bar-1 can be helpful for both diagnosing and treating *Bartonella*. More information on this can be found in the book *Toxic: Heal Your Body from Mold Toxicity, Lyme Disease, Multiple Chemical Sensitivities, and Chronic Environmental Illness* by Neil Nathan, MD. Dr. Nathan has found Banderol and Houttuynia to be particularly beneficial for *Bartonella*.

Lee Cowden, MD, has developed a series of herbal tinctures that can be helpful for Lyme disease and *Bartonella*. Dr. Dietrich Klinghardt, discussed above regarding retroviral infections, also has protocols for treating Lyme disease. For those with severe refractory CFS/FMS, he is using quinacrine (Atabrine) with some success. This is an old antimalarial. Its main side effect is that it can turn the skin, nails, and urine temporarily yellow about one to two weeks after treatment. This is not jaundice, but comes from the medication being yellow, and usually resolves a few weeks after treatment, but can persist for up to four months. He has quinacrine compounded at CareFirst Specialty Pharmacy in 100-milligram capsules ($102 for forty capsules). He gives a loading dose the first day of 200 milligrams every fifteen minutes for a total of 800 milligrams. He then gives 100 milligrams three times a day for ten days. If they are tolerated well and it is helping, he may continue it for several months. He finds that even lower doses of 50 milligrams twice daily for two weeks can be helpful. Dr. Klinghardt then considers multiple rounds if well tolerated, with longer pauses between rounds as the person stays improved.

The bottom line? Look for a Lyme literate physician at www.ilads.org. Take antifungals while on the antibiotics. And be sure to apply the entire SHINE protocol to dramatically increase the antibiotics' effectiveness.

Treatable Evidence of Immune Dysfunction: IV Gamma Globulin

As we discuss in the next chapter on addressing immune dysfunction, there are a wide and dizzying array of immune system changes in CFS/FMS. Especially important are inventories of a key part of our defense system called IgG antibody. This is made up of four parts called IgG1–4.

You can think of this like the army, navy, air force, and marines of our body's immune system. Work by Dr. Mark Sivieri has shown that a very large percentage of people with CFS/FMS have their IgG1 and/or IgG3 antibody stocks depleted. To me, this is suggestive of chronic infections that need to be addressed. Other researchers are also showing that this is tied into both small fiber neuropathy pain and orthostatic intolerance (POTS/NMH, see Chapter 14).

In fact, infusions of intravenous gamma globulin have been shown to help in these cases of CFS/FMS, small fiber neuropathy, and orthostatic intolerance. Because they are quite expensive (over $80,000 a year), they need to be covered by insurance. After about six months, about half of our sickest patients find that it helps significantly, making this an important missing link tying together various pieces of the CFS/FMS condition.

Bowel Bacterial Infections (SIBO)

Another antibiotic-sensitive infection deserves special mention. If IBS or spastic colon symptoms (gas, bloating, diarrhea, constipation, or a sulfur smell to your gas) persist after treatment for yeast and parasites, consider treating for small intestinal bacterial overgrowth (SIBO). This is common in CFS/FMS and is aggravated by low thyroid.

The diagnosis can be confirmed by doing what is called hydrogen breath testing for SIBO. Most often, I do not bother with this. Instead, I simply ask, "Does your gas smell particularly bad, especially a sulfur odor?" If yes, this comes from bacteria in the small intestine splitting the sulfur off of undigested proteins. Although candida can cause you to make enough gas to fill up several weather balloons each day, it usually does not have this distinctive smell.

SIBO occurs when bacteria migrate upstream from the colon (large intestine), where they belong, to the small intestine. Normally, the bowel contractions that move food downstream also wash bacteria out of the small intestine. If these normal contractions are weakened, as occurs with an underactive thyroid, SIBO is more likely. Often, simply optimizing thyroid hormone levels can help. If needed, research has shown that treating spastic colon/SIBO empirically with 550 milligrams of the antibiotic rifaximin (Xifaxan) three times a day for ten days can result in improvement. This antibiotic is quite expensive, so if the treatment is not covered by insurance I will sometimes substitute 500 milligrams of neomycin three times a day for ten days.

An excellent natural alternative for SIBO is called Ultra MFP Forte. I give this mix of herbs twice a day for one bottle (one month). This often knocks out the SIBO infection without the antibiotics. If the sulfur smell to the gas returns, I repeat the treatment and make sure thyroid function is optimized.

Prostatitis

Although women tend to be the ones plagued with bladder infections, men also have problems to deal with. It is very common for men with CFS/FMS to have prostatitis, an inflammation or infection of the prostate that is usually seen in men between the ages of twenty and fifty. There are two main types of prostatitis:

- **Bacterial prostatitis.** This is an acute or chronic infection in the gland that causes prostate swelling and discomfort, and in which a bacteria can be found by doing a culture. Although normal bacteria are the most common causes, some bacteria transmitted through sexual contact can also cause prostatitis. This is unusual in CFS/FMS, but is the only thing that most doctors look for in younger men who are having prostate symptoms.
- **Nonbacterial prostatitis or prostadynia.** This is a condition that causes you to feel swelling of the prostate with no detectable infection. This is a general irritation of the prostate that causes a burning sensation with urination, urinary urgency, and urinary frequency, without any infection or swelling of the prostate. This can come from a number of causes including, I suspect, yeast or other infections in the prostate that cannot be cultured. Chronic spasm or tightening of the muscles of the pelvic floor can also aggravate the prostate. Dietary factors include excessive consumption of caffeine, alcohol, and spicy foods. Sitting for long periods while traveling (for example, as a truck driver) can also cause irritation of the prostate.

The symptoms of prostatitis can come and go and be mild or severe. They include:

- Pain or tenderness in the area of the prostate. It is also common to have burning on the tip of the penis.
- Discomfort in the groin and, occasionally, lower back pain.
- Urinary urgency and frequency with pain on urination, especially when you have stool in the rectum.
- Pain with ejaculation.

In some cases, there is a slight discharge from the penis. If the discharge is cloudy, it is most likely bacterial, and you'll need to go to your doctor for antibiotics. Your doctor will probably also check to make sure that the discharge is not indicative of a sexually transmitted disease before beginning treatment. In CFS/FMS, most often the slight discharge is associated with prostadynia and not something they will treat.

In CFS/FMS, for severe cases, I will often prescribe a six-week course of a sulfamethoxazole/trimethoprim (Septra DS) or ciprofloxacin (Cipro) family antibiotic followed by extended periods of fluconazole (Diflucan), sometimes for as long as one year. To help relieve prostatitis and prostady-nia symptoms while taking antibiotics, you may also wish to take 500 milligrams a day of the bioflavonoid quercetin.

In addition, it is important to relax your pelvic floor muscles. This can easily be done by simply relaxing the anal sphincter as when you are having a bowel movement. When you're sitting on the commode, see how far you can let this muscle relax without stool coming out. Then repeatedly let that muscle relax throughout the day. Have a little reminder, such as whenever you look at your cell phone, to take a few seconds to let the muscle relax. That will often break the cycle.

In Summary

Many infections can cause or be caused by CFS and FMS. These are usually associated with immune system malfunction. Personally, I find that testing for most infections is both expensive and often not reliable. I would balance this by saying that many excellent holistic physicians find some of these panels to be critical for the treatment. They are likely right, but I am more comfortable treating clinically based on symptoms instead of relying only on the testing.

Still, there are a few tests that I consider worthwhile. These include stool testing for parasites (done only at a few labs specializing in parasitology) and IgG antibody blood testing in select cases for EBV, HSV-1, HHV-6, and CMV viral infections.

Beyond these, I prefer to treat empirically based on symptoms—that is, without testing. If you have lung congestion and/or recurrent temperatures over 98.6°F, scalp scabs, vertigo, or a history of repeated "allergic" reactions to multiple antibiotics, or if your CFS/FMS improved with antibiotics in the past, your doctor may be able to effectively treat you with antibiotics.

If you have chronic flu-like symptoms or if your illness began with a flu-like infection, and your blood tests show very elevated CMV or HHV-6 IgG antibodies (at 1:640 or higher, or over 4), I consider antiviral treatment with famciclovir/celecoxib (Famvir/Celebrex) or valganciclovir (Valcyte), but usually only if symptoms persist after treating with the rest of the SHINE protocol.

Fortunately, there are now physicians around the country who can expertly guide you through these therapies (see page 317). Our new understanding of how to diagnose and treat the infections found in CFS and fibromyalgia offers exciting new hope!

Healing Your Immune System

Addressing the infections above, and using the SHINE protocol in general, takes a major load off the immune system. This by itself can lead to effective healing in many cases. But in some, the chronic infections and associated symptoms persist and other avenues need to be explored.

One fascinating study using tuberculosis vaccine to treat fibromyalgia is underway at Harvard. We are starting to consider this in a few of the more severe cases we treat, but it will be several years before we know if this is helping clinically.

But there is another option as well: balancing Th1 and Th2.

TIRED OF CHASING ENDLESS INFECTIONS?

The next chapter is based on a guest article written by Sam Yanuck, one of my favorite immunology experts. A heads-up: It is very technical, so I have put his article in an appendix section at the end of the book. For those of you who like or need to keep it simple, it is okay to just read (or quickly browse through) this chapter. At the end of this chapter, you will find a simple quiz that will determine what you need to do to rebalance your immune system. But for those of you who would like a highly technical overview of the immune system in CFS/FMS, including its role in severe sensitivity reaction, I think you'll find the article in the appendix to be excellent.

16

Healing Your Immune System: Balancing Th1 and Th2

BFF Summary

This chapter is somewhat technical. So for those of you who like or need to keep it simple, it is okay to skip to the very end of the chapter. On page 244, you will find a simple quiz that will determine what you need to do to rebalance your immune system.

---

*A*recent National Institutes of Health (NIH) conference had a heavy focus on picking off a few of the hundreds of infectious and immune "ripples" in the great big pond that makes up CFS and fibromyalgia. Those of you who follow the research have seen reports on countless studies looking at immunity and infections in CFS/FMS. For many, it gets overwhelming. It is like having one hundred little dots of information with nothing tying them together.

So in this chapter, and for those who like Dr. Yanuck's technical article in the appendix, we are going to connect the dots for you. This will give you a context to evaluate new research as it arrives. More important, it will help you better understand what is going on with CFS/FMS and what you can do to help.

To make this area simpler to understand, let's look at some of the key things that occur in our body's immune "defense" systems in CFS/FMS:

- An initial infection occurs, making the immune system go on active alert.
- For some reason, in CFS/FMS the immune system is unable to turn off after the initial infectious threat is dealt with. So the body acts as if this infection is chronic. Because of this, it starts to exhaust itself after a few months to years. The immune system begins by being overstimulated and then exhausted. If this is not taken into account, it makes understanding the conflicting research very confusing. But no worries. With the quiz at the end of the chapter, we will tell you in simple terms what needs to be done.

Most of you will find that simply skipping straight to the quiz at the end of this chapter, or leafing through the chapter just letting certain things catch your eye, will be the way to go. But for those of you who are science geeks like me, you will find that Dr. Yanuck's article in the appendix ties things together very well.

Technical Review

Two key parts of our immune system are called:

- **Th1 helper cells:** Th1 cells orchestrate the immune system's response to invading pathogens like viruses and bacteria. Th1 cells make interferon gamma that drives the virus-killing activity of other immune cells like macrophages and natural killer cells. Interferon gamma also promotes the activity of a tool called RNase L inside cells that have been infected with virus particles. RNase L is like a special pair of scissors that recognizes foreign DNA in infections, and snips it into tiny pieces so it can't reproduce. It is especially helpful against a host of viral infections. If the Th1 helper cell response is diminished, the antiviral immune response can become disorganized, like a sheriff that doesn't shoot straight. If the sheriff starts to shoot up the town but doesn't kill the actual criminals, that's when inflammation can become a problem.
- **Th2 helper cells:** Th2 cells promote several useful immune functions. They help B cells make antibodies. They drive mucous production, so you can expel things like pollen from your sinuses. And, where Th1 responses help you kill pathogens small enough that one cell could eat them (bacteria and viruses), Th2 cells help you kill bigger things, particularly parasites. When all is well, the Th2 response helps you quiet down

inflammation after an infection or injury. When you have too much Th2 response, it becomes harder to kill viruses and bacteria, the production of mucous can be greater, and reactions to foods and the environment can be worse. Then, despite the abundant Th2 response, inflammation persists.

So the body generally keeps a balance between Th1 and Th2.

What the research is suggesting is that our Th1 responses can become diminished or weakly functioning, and that our Th2 systems go into overdrive (called Th2 dominance). This makes it very difficult for our body to fight intracellular infections such as viruses, candida, and antibiotic/tetracycline-sensitive bugs such as Lyme, mycoplasma, and chlamydia (along with numerous others). Meanwhile, with Th2 being in overdrive, we see an increase in allergic responses.

Our body's central command is constantly sending out signals telling our defense systems where to focus resources and how much of these go to the Th1 versus the Th2 system.

It is important to remember that, just as we have developed antibiotics and other tools in the millennia-old battle between infections and humanity, the bugs have been doing the same. These viruses and other organisms, which mostly hide out inside the cells and which are killed by the Th1 response, have learned a new trick. They mimic the molecules (such as interleukin 10) that wake up the Th2 immune response, while turning off the Th1 response that would otherwise keep the bugs in check.

So they can simply hide out in the cells and reproduce, while sending your defense system off on a wild goose chase. Smart little buggers.

But much as I respect them, when they are infecting people and causing problems, it's time to get rid of them. So, with the Th1 response being suppressed, people can no longer keep old infections dormant. You then can see "jailbreaks" of a number of different viruses. This is commonly seen even in healthy people who get shingles. In that situation, the chickenpox virus from their childhood makes a jailbreak out of just one single nerve cell. In fibromyalgia, these jailbreaks can occur throughout the body.

This is called viral reactivation. Current research is suggesting that the key infections involved would be enterovirus (e.g., Coxsackie), Epstein-Barr virus, herpes simplex 1 (which causes cold sores on the lips), cytomegalovirus (CMV), and human herpesvirus 6 (HHV-6). Interestingly, HSV-2 (genital herpes) does not seem to be a key player, although some people will flare their CFS/FMS when they get outbreaks. In these cases, the person should be on 500 to 1,000 milligrams of valganciclovir (Valcyte) a night over the long term. Suppression with lysine is not a good idea because it can cause drops in growth hormone.

Another problem when the Th2 system becomes overactive is that the Th1 response can no longer keep fungal infections, especially candida, in check. This puts a major strain on the immune system. Candida is also known to inhibit Th1 response as a survival strategy, making the Th1 deficit worse.

The only defense that the body has left against these intracellular infections is RNase L. RNase L does not kill these infections, but it stops them from reproducing while it waits for Th1 defenses to come and kill them. And waits . . . And waits . . .

But because the body has been tricked by the infection, the Th1 cavalry never comes.

So, although important research is looking at each of the dozens of different components of the immune system and how they are affected, expect this to be of minimal value in the next decade or two, because it is quite complex. Some of the researchers are not yet realizing that these changes are ripples off the main problem and are chasing smoke from the fire. They also do not always realize that different subsets of CFS/FMS will show different patterns, or that there may be initial overactivation followed by exhaustion of immune system components.

Interestingly, the tuberculosis vaccine seems to stimulate or wake up the Th1 system, and it is currently being tested in a Harvard study for fibromyalgia, after having caused a dramatic improvement in childhood diabetics. This study should start to have data available in about two years.

So, often underlying the chronic infections present in CFS and fibromyalgia is an imbalance in various components, especially the Th1 and Th2 responses. Its complexity is enough to make most PhDs' [possessive] heads spin. For those of you with a yet more technical bent, though, I have invited one of my favorite immunology experts to give an overview of what is occurring. If you find it complex (you will), it is okay to simply scan through and pick out the parts that you find most pertinent.

Here is a simple quiz that will tell you if you need to rebalance the Th1 and Th2 responses. It will also guide you on the use of two supplement mixes developed by Dr. Yanuck to do so.

Easily Balance Your Immune System

Here is where I would begin: with balancing out the two key arms of the immune system called Th1 and Th2.

Just want the bottom line of what to do and how to tell what you need? Dr. Yanuck's simple quiz below will show you in a simple way how to determine what is needed and how to balance these with two supplement mixes.

Ready to take the quiz? The first page is for you. I included the second page in case you would like to share this entire quiz with your holistic health practitioner, or in case you yourself are interested in the more technical information.

If your score in the left-hand column is:

8 or higher, take one capsule twice a day.

14 or higher, take two capsules twice a day.

Over 18, take three capsules twice a day of Pure Encapsulations' Th1 Support formula. This will help support your Th1 response.

If your score on the right-hand column is:

8 or higher, take one capsule twice a day.

14 or higher, take two capsules twice a day.

Over 20, take three capsules twice a day of Pure Encapsulations' Th2 Modulator to help calm down your Th2 response.

If there's no response in a month, it's reasonable to increase the dose by a third. It can take three months to observe a useful effect starting to happen. Once a person has been doing well for a solid three months, it's reasonable to see if the improvement can be sustained at a lower dose.

This can help you get to the root cause of your immune problems.

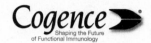

Cogence Brief Immunological Assessment

Please CIRCLE the number that reflects whether the statement applies to you:

0 = Does not apply | 1 = Rarely applies | 2 = Sometimes applies | 3 = Applies | 4 = Strongly applies

Th1 Polarization Support Factors						Th2 Modulation Factors					
Chronic inflammation	0	1	2	3	4	Childhood asthma	No=0		Yes=3		
High stress level	0	1	2	3	4	Childhood intestinal problems	No=0		Yes=3		
Autoimmune disease flares	0	1	2	3	4	Childhood ear infections	No=0		Yes=3		
Tendency to intestinal problems	0	1	2	3	4	Tendency to asthma or other lung issues	0	1	2	3	4
Current intestinal problem	0	1	2	3	4	Active or medicated asthma	0	1	2	3	4
Catch colds that are going around	0	1	2	3	4	Active or medicated other lung problem	0	1	2	3	4
Stay sick longer once you get sick	0	1	2	3	4	Tendency to sinusitis	0	1	2	3	4
Get cold sores	0	1	2	3	4	Headache in forehead, cheek, face	0	1	2	3	4
Tendency to bladder infections	0	1	2	3	4	Current sinus problem	0	1	2	3	4
Current bladder infection	0	1	2	3	4	Produce copious nasal mucous	0	1	2	3	4
Tendency to sinus infections	0	1	2	3	4	Mucous in stool	0	1	2	3	4
Current sinus infection	0	1	2	3	4	Allergy to environment (pollen, mold, etc.)	0	1	2	3	4
Tendency to respiratory infections	0	1	2	3	4	Food sensitivities/reactions	0	1	2	3	4
Current respiratory infection	0	1	2	3	4	Tendency to IBS, SIBO, Dysbiosis, etc.	0	1	2	3	4
Chronically elevated viral burden	0	1	2	3	4	IBS, SIBO, Dysbiosis, other GI currently	0	1	2	3	4
Age: add 2 points for every 5 years over 50						Chronic Stress	0	1	2	3	4
Total of the numbers you circled plus any for age						Work with toxic chemicals	0	1	2	3	4
						Age: add 2 points for every 5 years over 50					
						Total of the numbers you circled plus any for age					

Number of days with symptoms of autoimmune flare in the past month ____ in the past week ____

Number of days with symptoms of inflammation in the past month ____ in the past week ____

Can be body inflammation (aches & pains, body fatigue, GI symptoms, etc.) or brain inflammation (mental fatigue, brain fog, etc.)

Reproduction of this instrument is permitted, provided it is reproduced in full, with images and copyright information intact.

Clinician Section

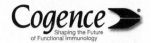

Have patients fill out the first page of this questionnaire at the start of each visit. This provides a mechanism that helps you track the patient's progress.

Clinician Interpretation Section

Th1 polarization support may be useful based on scores:

≥ 8 = 1 cap bid   ≥ 14 = 2 caps bid   ≥ 18 = 3 caps bid

Labs suggesting the need for support of Th1 response:

CBC hallmark: monocytes ≤ 6%. TGFβ >3000. Low normal Natural killer cells absolute or %. Viral IgG's higher than 5x the range for EBV, CMV, HSV-1, HSV-2, HHV-6, Parvovirus. EBV EA any elevation. High salivary cortisol. Chronic susceptibility to infection of any kind suggests the need for Th1 support.

Innate immune system support may be useful based on Th1 polarization scores:

≥ 8 = 1 cap qd   ≥ 14 = 1 bid   ≥ 18 = 2 bid

Labs suggesting the need for support of innate immune response:

WBC's <5 & TGFβ >3000 suggests the utility of at least 1 bid

Other indices:

NK % in lower ⅓ of range. Neutrophils ≤ 48%.

Monocytes ≤ 6%. Increased viral or bacterial burden.

Th2 down-regulation may be useful based on scores:

≥ 8 = 1 cap bid   ≥ 14 = 2 bid   ≥ 20 = 3 bid

Labs suggesting the need to down-regulate Th2 response:

CBC hallmarks: Eosinophils ≥ 5%, or Basophils ≥ 2%.

Low CD8 count and/or high CD4/CD8 ratio. Stool parasite.

The presence of asthma, environmental allergies, or any eosinophilic GI disorder strongly suggests Th2 dominance and the utility of dampening excessive Th2 response.

Addressing inflammation:

A baseline dose of substances intended to dampen NFkB and inhibit inflammasome formation, at appropriate concentrations, is 2 capsules 2x per day, for anyone whose goal is to influence inflammatory activation. Some people may need higher doses, to offset factors that are driving more inflammation. Generally, clinicians should consider using doses that yield few or no days per month of aches and pains, fatigue, brain fog, fluctuating weight that suggests inflammatory fluid retention, or other symptoms suggestive of chronic inflammation.

Addressing autoimmune flares:

The goal should be to inhibit the NFkB-STAT3 axis, with the goal of zero flare days for a given week or month. If the patient is having fewer flare days with each subsequent time they fill out the questionnaire, you're on the right track with dosing. If the number of flare days has increased since the patient's previous visit, increasing doses may be needed.

For patients not yet using NFkB-STAT3 inhibitors, (new patients, example), it is useful to consider the following doses:

Number of flare days per month:

≥ 10 days = 3 caps tid (some patients will need 4 caps tid)

≥ 6 days = 3 caps bid   ≥ 2 days = 2 caps bid

For patients in ongoing care, each patient will likely have two different dose levels:

1) The dose that quiets down flares

2) The dose that keeps them quiet between flares

The first dose is usually higher than the second dose. It's useful to instruct patients that this is their "flare dose," which they can go to when they feel a flare coming on. This is often the dose you start with to help them quiet down initially.

Once the case is ongoing and flares are occurring much less frequently, they can use the lower dose. You can determine the lower dose by having the patient gradually decrease the dose and observe if they do well at each reduced level (no flares). If the patient has a flare, you've gone too low.

17 | *Nutrition Intensive Care*

BFF Summary

1. Begin with the Energy Revitalization System and the Smart Energy System. This one drink and two pills a day can give outstanding nutritional support and dramatically increase energy after one month.

2. Most people with CFS/FMS do best with a high salt and protein intake and avoiding sugar. Beyond that, eat the diet that leaves you feeling the best, while keeping it fairly whole and healthy. Many find a ketogenic diet improves symptoms.

3. Take Recovery Factors (www.recoveryfactors.com). This has resulted in dramatic benefits, usually seen in one to two weeks. See the dosing and other information on the website.

4. For four to six months, consider adding 200 milligrams of coenzyme Q10 a day, 500 milligrams of acetyl-L-carnitine twice a day, 500 to 1,000 milligrams of NAC a day, and one capsule of Vectomega a day. I add iron if the ferritin blood test is under 60.

5. A subset of people feel markedly better on a gluten- and dairy-free diet. I usually don't begin with this because it is a nuisance for people to do, but it can make a big difference. Lauren Hoover-West's website (www.nowheatnodairynoproblem.com) can guide you on how to do this while still enjoying your food.

6. Genetic testing for methylation is not very reliable, and most healthy people are positive. A guest article by Dr. Neil Nathan discusses how to tell if you have methylation issues and how to address them.

7. B12 shots (tiny needles, like insulin syringes) in the form of hydroxocobalamin, given in 3,000-microgram (3-milligram) doses a few times a week, can result in dramatic improvement for a significant number of people. After fifteen doses, sometimes just giving yourself the injection once a month is enough to maintain benefit.

---

*O*ptimizing nutrition is critical to optimal energy production, and it doesn't have to be difficult. Begin with the information in Chapter 4. For many, simply taking a morning drink combining the Energy Revitalization System and Smart Energy System will result in a significant improvement after four to six weeks.

Overall Nutrition for CFS/FMS

Most people with CFS/FMS find that they feel best with a high-protein, low-carbohydrate diet. Additional salt intake benefits those with CFS/FMS, and unless you have high blood pressure or heart failure, it is safe to add the amount your body craves.

People with CFS/FMS often ask if they can drink alcohol. I tell them yes, if it doesn't make them feel worse. Some people with CFS/FMS, especially when candida is severe, feel lousy when they have any alcohol, although it's not hurting anything. In these cases, I don't have to tell them not to drink, as their body has already done so. For everyone else, up to two drinks a day is okay.

Same for caffeine. Caffeine can aggravate the symptoms of low blood sugar often seen in those with adrenal fatigue. In those who don't have this problem when they drink caffeine, one or two cups of tea or coffee a day are okay if not taken too late in the afternoon. Otherwise, they can aggravate insomnia. The problem is when people start using the caffeine as an energy "loan shark," drinking four or more cups a day to function. That's when it starts to drag you down.

Why Do People with CFS and Fibromyalgia
Need More Nutritional Support Than Everybody Else?

In addition to eating the standard American diet (often appropriately abbreviated as SAD), with half of its calories being stripped of nutrients, people with CFS/FMS have additional problems:

1. They crave sugar more than most people because of the low adrenal function, candida, and increased thirst (what I call "drink like a fish, pee like a racehorse" syndrome).
2. Because of increased bowel infections, people with CFS/FMS have decreased nutrient absorption.
3. Because of the illness, they have increased nutrient needs, such as B12, magnesium, iron, essential fatty acids, and other nutrients.

FOOD SENSITIVITIES

This is a common problem, which can severely limit people's diets with CFS/FMS. Read the section on food allergies on page 274.

Jump-Starting Your Body's
Mitochondrial Energy Furnaces

Each cell in your body contains structures called mitochondria, the tiny furnaces that produce energy by burning calories. Many problems, including some viral infections, can suppress these, so it is critical to go to the heart of the problem and optimize our body's energy furnaces.

Let's begin our discussion of Nutrition Intensive Care with nutritional support that directly increases energy production.

The Consequences of Severe Mitochondrial Dysfunction

People with fibromyalgia and CFS have almost 20 percent less energy in their muscles than normal, and they have trouble using oxygen effectively to make energy. To get an idea of what this means, think of taking a 20 percent pay cut. Ouch. A large number of clinical findings common in CFS/FMS can be explained by mitochondrial furnace malfunction:

- **Hypothalamic suppression.** Particularly severe changes in the hypothalamus have been seen in genetic mitochondrial dysfunction syndromes.
- **Brain fog.** Mitochondrial dysfunction can cause decreases in levels of neurotransmitters in the brain, specifically low dopamine and acetylcholine, and possibly low serotonin.
- **Sensitivities and allergies.** Decreased ability of the liver to eliminate toxins and medications could also contribute to sensitivities to medications and environmental factors, as well as food sensitivities.
- **Post-exertion fatigue.** Low energy production and accumulation of excessive amounts of lactic acid in muscles could inhibit recovery after exercise.
- **Poor digestion.** Mitochondrial dysfunction could also contribute to bowel-related problems along with the lack of digestive enzymes and buildup of unhealthy gut infections.
- **Heart dysfunction.** Research shows a decrease in heart function in CFS and fibromyalgia, which also contributes to the symptoms. This is not caused by a problem with the heart itself but rather with its energy production.

Thus, mitochondrial dysfunction might well be the root cause—or at least a contributing factor—of many of the problems seen in CFS/FMS.

IMPROVING MITOCHONDRIAL FUNCTION NUTRITIONALLY

A key question is whether anything can be done to make your cellular energy furnaces work better. Fortunately, the answer is a resounding yes!

High-dose B vitamins, magnesium, and malic acid are especially important. These are already included in the Energy Revitalization System vitamin powder. Ribose is also critical and is available separately as SHINE D-Ribose, or combined with five other energy-raising herbals in the Smart Energy System. This combination gives an outstanding foundation for everyone, making it easy and affordable (discussed in Chapter 4).

But there are a few other nutrients that are especially important for those with CFS/FMS.

OTHER KEY ENERGY NUTRIENTS

Other key energy boosters include:

- **Coenzyme Q10.** Take 200 milligrams of coenzyme Q10 each morning. Take it with a meal containing some fat or oil, so you absorb it. A special note: Most cholesterol-lowering drugs deplete coenzyme Q10 and in my experience can cause and worsen fatigue and pain. Anyone taking cholesterol-lowering medications (called statins) should also take 200 milligrams a day of coenzyme Q10.
- **Acetyl-L-carnitine.** This is not needed in day-to-day fatigue but is important if you have CFS or fibromyalgia, where muscle biopsies show that it is routinely deficient. Carnitine is found in animal flesh (think *carni*vore), and any brand is fine as long as it is pure acetyl-L-carnitine. Although you may not see a marked effect, in CFS/FMS it helps lay the foundation for your getting better and may even help you lose some of the weight you have gained. Take 500 milligrams twice a day for four months.
- **NAC (N-acetyl-cysteine).** Take 500 to 650 milligrams a day. Glutathione deficiency is a critical part of CFS/FMS, as it is the key human antioxidant. If taking glutathione by mouth, the only brand I recommend is called Clinical Glutathione by Terry Naturally. But in most cases of CFS/FMS, I simply give the NAC that is turned into glutathione by your body. The Energy Revitalization System vitamin powder contains 250 milligrams, so after four months of supplementing, many people can stop the additional NAC.
- **Omega-3 fish oils.** This has numerous health benefits. A special form called Vectomega allows one pill to replace seven regular 800-milligram fish oil pills. I simply have people take one each morning. This both decreases inflammation and helps mood and dry eyes.

Although there are literally dozens of other nutrients that help in some cases, for most people the Energy Revitalization System vitamin powder, Smart Energy System, and coenzyme Q10 are key for long-term use. The others are usually only needed for about four months.

Recovery Factors: A Powerful New Tool

A SOLUTION FOR UNEXPLAINED COMPLEX SYMPTOMS

Many people have trouble adapting to the modern-day environment. Like canaries in the coal mine, we are the first ones to show the effects of these growing problems.

Ready for a solution?

A recent study I completed showed that most people had a marked improvement within six weeks—usually within a week or two. The study report can be seen at www.recoveryfactors.com.

BACKGROUND

Recovery Factors was developed as a unique nutritional support supplement for severely malnourished people. But something fascinating happened.

Serendipitously, it was found that using this supplement for malnourished people in Africa resulted in other remarkable benefits. This included dramatic improvements in fatigue, post-exertion malaise, brain fog, and pain. Having heard about this, a few researchers in the United States who treated very complex conditions decided to try it.

What happened was nearly miraculous. People who had been hopelessly nonfunctional improved dramatically. When they ran out of this unique therapy, their symptoms came back and the people taking it were desperate to get more. So Dr. Gaetano Morello and I decided to do a research study—and the benefits were remarkable!

This unique and very safe natural nutritional supplement has been used for over a decade in countless people with malnutrition. Derived from animal serum proteins, it contains all twenty amino acids the human body requires for growth and regeneration (not just the nine essential amino acids that are sometimes considered a whole protein), in a dipeptide and tripeptide form. But I have never seen a protein supplement do anything like this!

It is natural and has been very well tolerated, despite people with these symptoms frequently being sensitive to other treatments. It contains no gluten, soy, GMO, dairy, or other products that people frequently have sensitivity to.

SAFETY AND PURITY

Recovery Factors has been used in countless thousands of people for well over a decade with no major problems being seen. The product is derived entirely from porcine blood components (i.e., from pigs). This is a special unique herd that is raised humanely and in a very clean and healthy environment, as they are raised specifically for heart valves for human valve replacement surgery. It is predominantly a unique purified serum protein.

WHY IT WORKS

The simple answer? We don't know. What we do know is that Recovery Factors helps a vast array of people with diverse conditions, suggesting more foundational levels of support within the body.

Meanwhile, many people have found their lives dramatically improved on it.

We do have some guesses about how it works, and we are researching those. Our suspicion is that it helps rebalance immune function. But as scientists, we have learned to first see what is and then work to understand why.

Peptides are more easily absorbed and more bioavailable than amino acids (the usual building blocks of proteins). "Protein" is a general term given to everything made from polypeptide structures, but it is very different from source to source. By way of analogy, amino acids are like random words. This unique mix is like a book written from these words. How they are combined makes all the difference in the world.

The porcine immune system is in many ways very similar to humans, which is why guinea pigs are often used in research. Their very strong immune system, though, is what allows them to wallow in mud without getting sick. One remarkable thing we saw in our study is that protective antibodies (e.g, IgM, total IgG, and IgG subsets) increased an average of about 14 percent.

As Carl Sagan said, "The beauty of a living thing is not the atoms that go into it, but the way those atoms are put together."

THE BOTTOM LINE?

There are numerous ways that Recovery Factors may be working to help your body. We are currently doing research to study these further. But in the interim, while we figure it out, the research is showing Recovery Factors to be dramatically helpful—helping healthy people feel healthier and helping some of the sickest of the sick recover their vitality.

Below is information from Emile Kok, the person who developed the supplement. He has over a decade of experience using it with thousands of people.

Dosing Protocol

Based on what we have seen, the first three days of taking Recovery Factors are pretty important, with a lot of changes going on. The product is easily used up during that period, given how much is going on in the body, so we recommend the following protocol:

Day 1 to 3: Take four tablets three times a day (twelve tablets per day) for three days.

Day 4 to 5: Take note of your overall condition. If no relief is experienced, then take note of your energy levels; if the energy levels are improved, then continue the same dosage for days 4 and 5; if there is no energy improvement, increase the dosage to five tablets three times a day for days 4 and 5 (fifteen tablets per day). Increased energy levels are the usual barometer that the person has taken enough; it is possible that it is all used up in the body and there isn't enough excess for increased energy levels.

Day 6: Take four tablets twice per day (eight tablets per day). If relief is not already felt by then, it is simply going to take longer, so you need to be patient. For most people there should be some sort of relief at this point. One to two bottles will certainly be enough to tell you if it is going to help you.

For maintenance, the vast majority of people do best with the mid-range dose: four tablets twice a day. See the information in the "Dosing" section at www.recoveryfactors.com for some dietary modifications that will also help during the first few days of use.

Timing

It is recommended that you take the Recovery Factors first thing in the morning on an empty stomach and again around three o'clock in the afternoon. For a small number who have too much energy at night or suffer from mild anxiety, take it with lunch.

Recovery Factors Study Results

The full study can be seen at www.recoveryfactors.com, but here is a quick summary.

60 percent of people improve considerably. For that group, the *average* improvement was:

Energy: 69 percent

Sleep: 54 percent

Pain: 38 percent

Overall well-being: 69 percent

Cognition: 60 percent

Anxiety: 35 percent

Gut function: 55 percent

Protective antibody levels went up an average of 14 percent.

It was very well tolerated, with improvement seen within one month of being on the supplement. Incredibly remarkable results for a single nutrient!

People's Experience

Whether one is nonfunctional or a top athlete, the effect of Recovery Factors is dramatic. For many years we have seen people from all walks of life with vastly different conditions all benefit from use of the product. People with no health conditions or ailments also benefit in numerous ways, including:

- Lifting of moods
- Improved sleep
- Improved digestion
- Increased physical and mental energy

- Improved strength and endurance
- Improved recovery from any kind of physical, emotional, or mental stress
- Improved levels of focus and concentration
- Improvement in people with skin condition (varies depending on the condition and the person—from 100 percent elimination to only mild benefit in some cases)
- Balancing or vast improvement in people with hormone imbalance
- Gained muscle in people with muscle wasting
- Deep sleep for the first time in years in people with erratic sleep
- Improved coping in people struggling to detox or in withdrawal

This is just a sample of the various things that people have seen with the supplement. The experiences in very general terms are as follows:

Day 1

- The first day people sleep deeply and very well, waking up refreshed.
- Energy levels for most people improve within a few hours; the three o'clock slump is not happening anymore.
- Concentration levels improve within a few hours for most.
- Strength and endurance levels increase from the first dose—we have seen athletes (such as cyclists, swimmers, and weightlifters) break personal records after their first dose.

Day 2

- There seems to be an increase in nitric oxide levels as many impotent men have woken up with erections the next day for the first time in many years.
- Overnight recovery seems improved from general fatigue levels with generally better sleep than normal on the first night and, therefore, greater clarity, mood, and energy levels.
- There is usually a shift in digestion. Many people go to the toilet a few times the next day; those with constipation tend to find some relief.
- Recovery from anything stressful the previous day is vastly improved—especially muscle soreness levels being much lower than normal.

Day 3

- For some people strong symptoms associated with their condition diminish anytime from this point on.
- Digestion issues tend to be vastly improved by this point.
- Continued general recovery to higher levels.

Day 4

- The first three days seem to have a lot of smaller activity going on, but generally by the end of day 3 and beginning of day 4, there is a pretty big shift in general immune function and pain levels. This is especially noted with people who take the advice of increasing the dosage for the first three days and who take the product regularly during these three days.
- Overall feelings of general well-being seem to improve after the first three days.
- Moods tend to become more stable.
- Energy levels are good and people tend to feel a bit stronger and have more mobility.

One common observation regarding Recovery Factors is the rate of growth of hair and nails and the improvements in the condition of the skin. One user said: "My hairdresser says that my hair grows about 50 percent faster than anyone else's hair that he cuts. I also trim my nails every two to three days because they grow so fast." This has been echoed time and time again by people who take the product. Although it can help even top-tier athletes, the most dramatic benefits are seen in those people who are nearly nonfunctional.

THE STUDY

By the time this book is in print, I expect that the study will have been published. You will be able to see the results at www.recoveryfactors.com. Here is one of the first reports I got back from somebody in the study who had been on it for about two weeks:

The supplement has been one of the most positive things for me
in years. I've had increase in energy and that underlying fatigue it
has helped noticeably.

—Jason K.

Most people are reporting back that it is helping quite dramatically.
They are already asking where they can get more. Recovery Factors appears to be a major breakthrough for those needing nutritional intensive
care. I recommend combining it with the Energy Revitalization System
and Smart Energy System for an incredibly powerful nutritional support
foundation. Available at www.recoveryfactors.com.

Gluten- and Dairy-Free Diet

No discussion of nutrition in CFS/FMS would be complete without addressing the topic of gluten (e.g., wheat and bread) and dairy sensitivity.
Although many if not most people do fine with these foods, there is a
significant subset that find these foods to be a major trigger for their symptoms. This is why you find the words "gluten-free" so prominently dis-
played on many foods.

So why has bread gone from being the staff of life to the stuff of allergies?

There are many theories, and no clear answers. For a more detailed
discussion on the rise in dietary intolerances, see Chapter 19. But here are
a few thoughts I find especially interesting:

- Part of the increase in food sensitivities in general comes from a
  mix of:
  - The removal of the enzymes found in food during food
    processing
  - Dysbiosis (overgrowth of unhealthy organisms, especially
    candida) in the intestines causing leaky gut
  - Adrenal fatigue
- Many people with gluten sensitivities find that they can eat bread
  in France and Italy. Why this is the case is unclear. It suggests that

chemicals used in growing the plants or making the processed foods are more the culprit than the gluten itself. But for now, we are only guessing.

• In a similar vein, many people who are dairy intolerant can tolerate dairy from overseas herds.

So I suspect that a large part of the problem is due to some or even many factors associated with modern farming and food processing.

Although a very small percentage of people with gluten sensitivity have celiac disease, if you note that you may have sensitivity to wheat, you should be tested for this illness. This is most easily done by checking the transglutaminase IgG and IGA antibody test. Most people with gluten sensitivity will be negative for this test, but it is important to check. The test will not be reliable if you have been eating gluten-free for more than several weeks.

Unfortunately, I do not find any other tests for wheat sensitivity to be adequately reliable. The best test is simply to eliminate gluten and dairy products for one month. This has dramatically improved symptoms in a fair number of very stubborn cases of CFS and fibromyalgia.

If you find you do have these sensitivities, please don't go on a long-term gluten- and dairy-free diet on your own. You're likely to simply have a nutritionally inadequate diet that is no fun. Instead, I highly recommend Lauren Hoover-West's website (www.nowheatnodairynoproblem.com) and book *No Wheat No Dairy No Problem Cookbook*. These will give you a wealth of information on how to do this easily, while keeping eating incredibly enjoyable. A nutritionist and chef, Lauren Hoover-West has appeared and cooked on ABC News Live in Chicago and ABC Sacramento, and she has cooked for four US presidents. She does phone consultations, and I highly recommend her—she is a great resource for people with these food intolerances.

Methylation Issues

For those in search of relief, methylation has gotten a lot of attention lately. Although this is a significant issue in some people, the problem is that the genetic testing is poorly understood. The results come back showing positive for "methylation defects" that are present in the majority of healthy people. This means they are not so much defects as variations, so I don't bother with this test.

In this chapter and at the protocol at the end, we discuss tests that can be helpful. But it is reasonable to simply treat and look for clinical response as well.

I have asked Dr. Neil Nathan, one of my favorite CFS/FMS experts and a key methylation expert/researcher, to write a section that can add clarity to this often confusing area. More on methylation and other areas critical to CFS/FMS (including a discussion of the cell danger response) can be found in his book *Toxic: Heal Your Body from Mold Toxicity, Lyme Disease, Multiple Chemical Sensitivities and Chronic Environmental Illness*.

Rebooting Methylation

By Neil Nathan, MD

While methylation is important and methylation dysfunction commonly accompanies all chronic illness, it has been receiving, understandably, an increasing amount of attention lately. However, some practitioners have placed an undue emphasis on diagnosing and treating methylation, which has skewed our understanding of the role that it plays. I'm hoping this article can help put this whole concept into perspective.

Methylation is simply the biochemical process of adding a methyl group to a molecule. This reaction is critical to hundreds of important biochemical reactions in the body, especially in the making of the antioxidant glutathione.

The most common symptoms of methylation deficiency are fatigue, cognitive impairment, pain, and insomnia. These are symptoms that can occur from many other causes in CFS and fibromyalgia.

I had the privilege of hearing Dr. Rich Van Konynenburg, a key methylation researcher, speak in 2007 on what he felt was the underappreciated role of methylation as a causative factor of CFS. I was so intrigued by the logic and simplicity of his ideas that when I got home from the meeting, I immediately placed fifty-one people with ME/FMS/CFS on the five supplements that he described as a "simplified methylation protocol."

Essentially, this consists of taking hydroxy B12, a tiny dose of 5-methyl tetrahydrofolate (5-MTHF), and several other supplements to support methylation chemistry. After several months, 70 percent of my patients had improved, 20 percent of these markedly.

Working with Dr. Van Konynenburg, we received funding for a more elaborate clinical study, and we entered thirty people with ME/CFS/FMS into a study for nine months. Instead of tests of methylation genes, we looked at methylation chemistry using the blood test from Health Diagnostic Laboratory. These did show significant deficiencies in methylation chemistry in all of our patients (as Dr. Van Konynenburg had hypothesized), and on treatment over nine months, we saw complete normalization of methylation chemistry in every patient. This included statistically significant normalization of both glutathione and SAMe, which are crucial metabolites of methylation.

In addition to the testing improving, 77 percent reported improved energy, 65 percent improved sleep, 73 percent improved mental clarity, and 54 percent reported a decrease in pain. A remarkable 83 percent of people improved, with 27 percent reporting that they were much better. The average improvement after only six months was 48 percent.

This study was followed by an explosion of interest in methylation.

Methylation appears to be something that needs to be addressed early on in treatment, perhaps for everyone who is chronically ill. But as you might expect, in complex patients it is more complicated than that.

Timing Methylation Correctly

CFS and fibromyalgia are associated with the cell danger response (CDR). One important component of this is that when the cell feels threatened, it *intentionally* shuts down methylation to deprive the affecting microbe of the capability to hijack the body's own methylation chemistry to reproduce. So it comes as no surprise that virtually all chronically ill and inflamed patients, in whom the CDR has been triggered, have measurably low methylation chemistry.

But does that mean we should immediately provide all patients with supplements to maximize methylation? The answer to that question is: *It's all about timing.*

Because the CDR is a protective mechanism, overriding that mechanism before the body is ready to move forward turns out, often, to be counterproductive. (Translation: Patients get much worse.) This is especially true for sensitive patients. In my experience, approximately half of sensitive patients, if given vitamin B12 or folate (usually in the form of 5-MTHF), experience an intense worsening of their symptoms, even when given minuscule doses.*

I would like to emphasize that giving only 200 µg of 5-MTHF improved every patient's ability to methylate. Some practitioners are giving massive doses with the idea that giving more is better. This is rarely true. In my practice, the opposite is far more common. In fact, people often improve when the dose is reduced or stopped.

Some practitioners also recommend that the supplements continue to be used even if they make the patient feel worse. This is not wise. The body is saying that it is not yet ready to begin this area of treatment. But I found that once a patient has eased into treatment of the underlying main issue (usually mold toxicity or Lyme disease), he or she can take methylation supplements comfortably and would benefit later in the course of treatment.

Please keep in mind that the body has many avenues and organs of detoxification, so if methylation can't be started early on, the body can and does utilize other systems to detoxify. Sensitive patients who cannot take methylation supplements yet can begin other treatments, improve, and then initiate efforts to methylate better. Please note that recent research has confirmed that while methylation is vital to metabolism generally, it is one of the least-needed detoxification processes specific for mycotoxins.

It is important to also discuss glutathione supplementation. While there is no question that glutathione is an essential component of health, its indiscriminate use is not always justified. Many people with mold toxicity, for example, get worse when given glutathione in any form. In sensitive patients, glutathione mobilizes mold and other toxins faster than the body can process them, and the patients become more toxic. This is not a reaction that you can override by pushing yourself to ride it out. If you flare with glutathione, it is important to stop it until later when you're on the mend.

I have intentionally emphasized difficulties with methylation and use of glutathione because these difficulties are common in my sensitive patients. I also want to make it clear that the use of glutathione in patients who have stronger constitutions can be quite helpful. Janette Hope, MD, has discussed the use of intranasal glutathione being of great help in treating patients with mold toxicity. Many patients have felt immediately better using oral or intravenous glutathione as well.

---

* See Chapter 19, "Sensitive to Everything?"

So start slowly, and if your symptoms flare, stop the glutathione and/or 5-MTHF treatments until later.

While I believe that methylation is indeed important (heck, I helped put it on the map), I urge patients and physicians to put its value into perspective and to always look for the greater context in which we view treatment.

I trust this section by Dr. Nathan has been helpful. Below, I am adding some of the details of how to approach it.

Methylation Protocol

Based on work of Neil Nathan, MD

Begin with the SHINE protocol. Address infections, including Lyme and mold toxins, if present. Then if you're not better, optimize methylation. It is important to start slowly, and stop the treatments, or lower to a comfortable dose, if your symptoms get worse on them.

Start with much lower dosing than recommended and begin one treatment at a time. If well tolerated, you can continue increasing the dosing to the recommended level, slowly adding the next treatment. If your symptoms worsen, stop the offending treatment. When the flare resolves, you can try resuming a dose that was well tolerated:

1. **Optimize electrolytes.** Increase your magnesium (present in the multivitamin), potassium (can get in avocados, bananas, or coconut water), and salt.

2. **5-MTHF folate.** Take 200 milligrams a day. You can take one quarter tablet of 800 μg FolaPro daily.

3. **The Clinical Essentials multivitamin.** This contains the recommended amounts of 200 micrograms of 5-MTHF and 12.5 milligrams of pyridoxal 5 phosphate (P5P) per two tablets. Side effects will usually occur from the 5-MTHF within three days if they are going to occur, but I find this to be unusual with the multivitamin.

4. **Perque Activated B12 Guard (hydroxocobalamin).** Take 2 milligrams (2,000 micrograms) under the tongue once daily.

5. **Phosphatidylserine.** Take 100 milligrams each night.

If this protocol is going to help, the benefits usually begin by two months.

Testing

If not better by eight weeks, consider doing the methylation panel by Health Diagnostics Lab (approximately $300, which tests glutathione, SAM, SAH, and folate metabolites; not covered by insurance) to then tailor the treatment protocol.

Screening may consider testing histamine levels (usually covered by insurance):

1. An elevated histamine is seen with poor methylation. A low histamine suggests that the person is over-methylating. In those cases, using the MTHF folate can worsen symptoms. Approximately one-third of people who are bipolar, schizophrenic, or have OCD are over methylators with low histamine and should not be on the protocol. It can flare their psychological symptoms.

2. For treatment, the results of MTHFR genetic testing are not especially significant. So *don't panic*. Why? MTHFR genetic testing does not add much helpful information for treatment, as the majority of the healthy population (approaching 100 percent) has some "defects"— more accurately called variations. The MTHFR testing is most helpful for prevention, if one is looking to create a program tailored to one's metabolic strengths and weaknesses. But I find it tends to be grossly over-interpreted, leaving many people unnecessarily, and incorrectly, frightened.

THE IMPORTANCE OF VITAMIN B12 INJECTIONS

Some people have trouble absorbing vitamin B12 and getting it into the brain where it is critically needed. Because of this, we have a very high amount of vitamin B12 in the Energy Revitalization System vitamin powder (500 µg). Some people with CFS/FMS benefit from even higher levels by injection. These may help regardless of the vitamin B12 level. Many dosing regimens are used.

In people who are not responding to other treatments, I will often begin with 3,000 µg of B12 by subcutaneous injection twice a week. It can be given even more often or at a higher dose. After ten injections, people will know if it is helping, then they can take it at a frequency that feels best.

Some will take the injections daily, some monthly, but many find twice a week is optimal for maintenance.

Intravenous Nutritional Therapies

A very powerfully effective treatment that I have found for treating chronic fatigue syndrome and fibromyalgia is the use of intravenous (IV) nutritional support. Especially important is the magnesium, which when given via IV opens up blood vessels to tight muscles, flooding these starved areas with nutrients and washing away the toxins. You'll find that when your holistic doctor administers these injections, you'll feel a warm flush in the areas that have been most significantly affected by your illness.

I recommend that, if you have a holistic physician to give them and you can afford them, all patients with CFS/FMS receive these IV therapies at least once a week for six weeks and then as needed. Along with ribose and the other supplements I've recommended (which should be continued while on the IVs), the IV therapies can dramatically jump-start some of your body's systems and can markedly shorten the time it takes to begin feeling better. Many physicians refer to these therapies as Myers' cocktails. If you have a physician who is willing to give nutritional IVs, I strongly recommend that you have them.

18 *Exercise Intensive Care: Exercise as Able*

BFF Summary

1. As is true with any disabling disease, including cancer, it is important to walk or even exercise as able to avoid deconditioning. Nobody would dream of implying that this makes cancer any less real.
2. In the same vein, anyone who implies that CFS/FMS does not warrant treatment because people need to maintain conditioning as able should get the same attention as those who would imply this is the case for cancer—which is essentially that they be ignored. Seriously. They are not worth your attention or time.
3. Walking is the best exercise. Do as much as you comfortably can while still feeling good that day and better the next day. If you feel wiped out the next day, you did too much. Rest a few days and then cut down by 20 percent.
4. Using devices and apps like Fitbit can help.
5. After ten weeks on the SHINE protocol, your energy production will usually start to increase, allowing you to increase your walking by fifty steps every few days.
6. If you are too weak to walk, reconditioning by walking in a warm water pool can help, as the buoyancy makes this easier. Be sure that orthostatic intolerance (see Chapter 14) is also addressed.

Reconditioning During
CFS/Fibromyalgia Treatment

Let's finish up the SHINE intensive care protocol with exercise *as able*. The key words here are "as able."

Although exercise seems a simple topic to discuss, I know for many of you it has been a difficult one to implement. Post-exertional fatigue is a common part of CFS/FMS, but it doesn't even begin to express what you have experienced. Post-exertional fatigue means that people may be bedridden for several days after exercise. Meanwhile, some idiots out there still imply to your physician that this isn't a real disease, encouraging them to just tell people to exercise more. I know sometimes it makes you feel like screaming.

But here's the simple truth: When being treated for any debilitating illness, including cancer, reconditioning is a critical part of getting well. The difference is that no researcher who studies cancer-related fatigue with exercise is idiotic enough to imply that this means the cancer is not real.

Fortunately, even most researchers looking at exercise therapy in CFS/FMS recognize that this is a real and severe illness. And it's okay to simply ignore the ones who don't.

What You Need to Know About the PACE Exercise and Cognitive Behavioral Therapy Study—and Controversy

Ignore it.

There has been an enormous amount of controversy about this study, which looked at cognitive behavioral therapy and graded exercise in CFS. It showed that both of these were helpful. The study results say nothing about whether the disease was real or other physical measures helpful, but some physicians and some in the media tried to use the study to imply that CFS is not real and that health insurance should not cover other treatments.

This resulted in a firestorm of controversy.

As discussed earlier, exercise and coping skills help in any chronic disease including cancer. This doesn't, of course, make the illness all in people's minds. And you can, of course, draw your own obvious conclusions about people who would say otherwise.

So, for people who use this kind of data to try to invalidate CFS? Ignore them, too.

So, let's get to what you need to know, so you can recondition despite your CFS/FMS. Because of the body-wide energy crisis seen in CFS/FMS, most of you have found that you are unable to condition beyond a certain point. This is because it takes energy to store energy in the muscles, which is what conditioning is. And the energy crisis in this illness has limited your ability to make this energy.

Most physicians are not aware of this. Instead, they usually push you to exercise, and you spend the next two days in bed feeling like you have been hit by a truck!

The good news is that as you do SHINE, you will find that your body starts making the energy needed to condition. You will then be able to exercise more and more—and it will actually leave you feeling better and stronger.

For most CFS/FMS patients, the words "exercise as able" do *not* mean starting with jogging or going to the gym. Instead, doable exercises include walking, gentle yoga, and tai chi, to name just a few. For those too ill to do the above, beginning to recondition in a warm-water pool may allow you to condition to where you can begin a walking program after a while.

The key to a successful exercise program is not to overdo it. As Lisa Davenport, an excellent fibromyalgia advocate, tells people, "Get yourself a pedometer [now an app on your phone], a good pair of walking shoes, a yoga mat, and a positive attitude. Start slowly and take one day at a time. Increase the intensity and duration of your program with caution. Every day will not be the same. Record your accomplishments in a journal and be proud. You will be pleasantly surprised at the number of steps you can accomplish and the increase you will see in your strength and flexibility. Self-empowerment is all you need to get started."

I'd like to thank Lisa for reminding me of the importance of reconditioning as people get well from fibromyalgia. I used to call this the SHIN protocol. Lisa added the E for "exercise" to make it SHINE!

Here are a few tips to help you get started:

1. Begin with light exercise like walking. Consider warm-water walking in a heated pool if regular walking is too difficult.
2. Walk to the degree that you feel "good tired" afterward and better the next day. If you feel worse the next day, stop for a few days and then cut back.
3. Walk only as much as you comfortably can (or start with five minutes). Then increase by one minute every other day as is comfortable. When you get to a point that leaves you feeling worse the next day, cut back a bit to a comfortable level and continue that amount of walking each day.
4. After ten weeks on the SHINE protocol, your energy production will usually improve considerably, and you'll be able to continue to increase your walking by one minute every other day.
5. When you get to one hour a day, you can increase the intensity of the exercise. Again, listen to your body and only do what feels good to you. You'll know the difference between how "good pain" feels versus "bad pain" or crashing. Overall, "no pain, no gain" is stupid. Pain is your body's way of saying, "Don't do that!"
6. Do consider a Fitbit exercise device and app. It makes it more fun to be able to see your endurance go up. Set it to track the total number of steps you walk a day. You may not notice an extra fifty steps a day without it, but increasing by fifty steps a day will get people up to the magic six thousand to ten thousand steps a day in six months. And this isn't just an excellent level for those with fibromyalgia. It is an excellent level for anyone, as it equals three to five miles a day.
7. Unless it is cold, and the cold flares your pain, I recommend you get your exercise by walking outside, so you can get sunshine—your key source of vitamin D. Many people with CFS/FMS, or chronic pain in general, are vitamin D deficient. Vitamin D from sunshine (or supplements) will help improve immune function and will also decrease pain, along with the risk of hypertension, diabetes, and cancer.
8. When it's cold outside, wear woolen long underwear. A cold breeze can throw muscles into spasm. So can sweating during the walk if you're overdressed. Woolen long johns will soak up any sweat and wick it away from your skin. Meanwhile, don't forget a scarf and hat.

Even without CFS/FMS, anybody put on bed rest will decondition very quickly. This happens even to extremely fit astronauts when they go into a weightless environment for a few weeks. So even though overdoing it has taught you hard lessons, the magic balance can leave you conditioned without crashing.

And remember: As you do the SHINE protocol, energy production will increase, allowing you to condition.

You now have learned the basics of the SHINE protocol and know the keys that you need in order to recover. Welcome to getting your life back!

Don't Panic

I sometimes get panicked calls from people who recovered from their illness, only to have it come back years later. Don't worry if that happens. Simply take care of these three things and it will go right back away:

- Make sure you are still taking the Energy Revitalization System or Clinical Essentials multivitamin. These should be used long term as your body really needs these nutrients.
- Improve your sleep. If sleep starts getting worse again, it is usually from some severe stress. I simply adjust the sleep medications so they are getting eight hours again, and look for the new physical and situational stresses and take care of them. For example, was there a new infection? Did the person go back to doing what made them sick in the first place? Forgetting to say no to things that feel bad and only choosing the things that feel good?
- Check if the candida came back. This is common in many people every few years, especially after the holidays when sweets are hard to resist. You can tell because the nasal congestion, gas, bloating, diarrhea, or constipation are often recurring as well. I have the person simply cut back on the sugar and repeat a six-week course of fluconazole (Diflucan) plus a natural antifungal.

Then they go back to feeling great again.

Now you know the secret, so you don't have to worry or panic.

---

19 *Sensitive to Everything?*

BFF Summary

So many people with fibromyalgia are incredibly sensitive to *any* treatments. This makes figuring out how to treat them quite the challenge. Here's how to begin:

1. Consider mast cell activation syndrome. No testing is needed. It is better to try the treatments below and see if they help. They tend to be well tolerated and often work within a week or two. Give six weeks to see the full effect. So simply try the following:

   A. Quercetin: Available from any health-food store. Take 500 milligrams twice a day.

   B. Antihistamines: Take loratadine (Claritin) or any over-the-counter, non-sedating oral antihistamine in the morning and diphenhydramine (Benadryl) at night.

   C. Montelukast (Singulair): Take 10 milligrams at bedtime.

2. When your computer goes on the fritz, the first thing tech support tells you to do is reboot. Simple techniques can help you hit the reset button on your brain and immune system. A simple acupressure technique called NAET (www.naet.com) can eliminate food and other sensitivities, rebooting your immune system. And a simple exercise can help you reboot your nervous system (vagal nerve). I also highly recommend the Dynamic Neural Retraining System (DNRS) by Annie Hopper, which you can do at home. Once you do these, you're much more likely to be able to tolerate other treatments, and you will feel dramatically better. I will discuss these in more detail in Part Four on the

mind-body connection. These can be dramatically helpful with your sensitivities—and CFS/FMS symptoms in general.

3. Consider mold toxins if:

   A. You do not respond adequately to the SHINE protocol.

   B. You have severe environmental and treatment sensitivities, including sensitivity to light, sound, smells, and even electromagnetic fields.

   C. You have severe anxiety or depression.

   D. Electric shock sensations (*not* numbness or tingling in the extremities, which are present in 44 percent of people with fibromyalgia), ice pick–like pains, vibrating or pulsing sensations running up and down the spinal cord, odd tics and spasms, or seizure-like events.

   E. The sensitivities do not go away with treatment for mast cell activation.

Addressing mold toxins is not to be undertaken lightly, as it can be fairly pricey to get rid of mold in your home or work environment. The good news? If your illness began before you moved into your current home or work environment, then it may simply be a matter of clearing the persistent mold toxins from your body, using low-cost binders. A urine test ($400 to $700, not covered by insurance, but not necessarily critical for treatment) can help tell if you have elevated mold toxins and guide treatment. It often takes twelve to eighteen months to see improvement, but it may occur more quickly. Start very slowly with the toxin binders we discuss, increasing the dose as is comfortable.

So many people with CFS/FMS are incredibly sensitive to any treatments, especially to medications but sometimes even to herbals, nutrients, their environment, and sometimes even cell phone and other electromagnetic frequencies (EMF). This makes it tricky to treat individuals.

So, how can you take the treatments you need if you react to them? Although this sensitivity does make treatment more complex, the good news is that you can bypass this problem.

In this chapter, we will discuss some of the major triggers for severe environmental and treatment sensitivities, including multiple chemical sensitivity (MCS). We will begin with mast cell activation and resetting your vagal nerve, as these are easy, low cost, and often highly effective.

When problems persist, that's the time to consider looking for and treating mycotoxins (mold toxins) and the Lyme coinfection *Bartonella*. If you are considering these, I strongly recommend reading the book *Toxic* by my friend Dr. Neil Nathan. He is one of the most gifted and experienced CFS/FMS physicians, particularly in this area of study.

Ready to start with some simple fixes? Read on . . .

Mast Cell Activation Syndrome

Mast cells are our body's first responders when making contact with things in the outside world. If they meet something in the environment that concerns them, they can pour out over two hundred chemicals. The most prominent of these is histamine. This is one reason why antihistamines are a mainstay of treating allergies.

Just like our immune system in fibromyalgia can be on overdrive in general, in some people this is also occurring for their mast cells. These guardians then have an itchy trigger finger, seemingly reacting to things at random.

"Random" is the key word here, and this helps distinguish mast cell activation from regular allergies and sensitivities. One day you may have no reaction to something, but you react excessively to the same trigger on other days. So, no problem eating an ear of corn one day. But the next day, you may have the sudden onset of flushing, nausea, diarrhea, sweating, or palpitations.

Interestingly, most of the brain's histamine is located in the hypothalamus. Also, mast cells are also found in the pituitary and other glands. Because of this Dr. Theoharis Theoharides, one of the main researchers on mast cell activation, theorizes that this may be a major trigger for many people with CFS/FMS. The mast cells may then be a major trigger for microglial cells pouring out inflammatory factors (central sensitization) even in response to minimal stress.

TESTING

Testing is usually not helpful for this condition. As about half of fibro folks with sensitivities have mast cell activation syndrome and treatment is simple, it's better to simply try these and see if they help.

TREATMENT

I usually begin in the following order:

1. **Quercetin.** This bioflavonoid is a cousin to vitamin C. It helps stabilize the mast cells, kind of like calming down and soothing a crying

baby. I start with 500 milligrams once a day. If your main sensitivities are to foods, take it about thirty minutes before major meals so it can be in place when you eat. This simple supplement can often be very helpful, is low cost, and can be found in any health-food store. After a few days, you can increase to 500 milligrams (or even 1,000 milligrams) two to four times daily.

2. **Montelukast (Singulair).** Take 10 milligrams at bedtime. This prescription asthma medication is only thirty cents a day using the Good Rx phone app, and most physicians will be comfortable letting you try it.

3. **Loratadine (Claritin).** Take 10 milligrams in the morning. If this over-the-counter medication makes you drowsy, you can use it at bedtime or try 10 milligrams of cetirizine (Zyrtec). Doses over 20 milligrams or more are likely to be sedating. If you have any other side effects to these medications, it is likely caused by the binders or fillers rather than the medication itself. In that case, try a different brand or have it made by a compounding pharmacy without the fillers. If this medication helps, consider 12.5 to 50 milligrams of diphenhydramine (Benadryl) at bedtime.

4. **Acid-blocking medications.** Some people will get additional benefits by adding 150 milligrams of ranitidine (Zantac) twice a day, 20 milligrams of famotidine (Pepcid) twice a day, or even 150 to 300 milligrams of cimetidine (Tagamet) twice a day. These acid-blocking medications are actually also antihistamines. Do not use the other acid-blocking medications (called PPIs). They will not help here and are quite toxic long term.

Cimetidine, famotidine, and ranitidine have the additional benefit of modifying immune function quite dramatically in ways that can be beneficial, especially against Epstein-Barr virus. In fact, I have seen cimetidine knock out acute cases of Epstein-Barr (mono) in less than twenty-four hours. This tip was taught to me by Dr. Jay Goldstein.

The downside is that they turn off stomach acid production as well, and your body needs stomach acid to digest your food. The cimetidine can be the best choice of these three for long-term use in this regard, but see which one works best for you.

These medications may work within days, but Dr. Neil Nathan finds that it may take up to two months to see the full effect.

5. **DAO (Umbrellux).** This supplement taken fifteen to thirty minutes before eating can be helpful, but it costs about a dollar per capsule. DAO contains the enzyme diamine oxidase, which helps break down histamine. Starting with one capsule taken thirty minutes before a meal, you can increase the dosage to two to three capsules before each meal.

6. **Cromolyn (gastrocrom) ampoules.** Taking one ampoule (100 mg/5 mL) before each meal can be quite effective for histamine reactions from food, but this is often not covered by insurance. With the Good Rx app, they are about a $1.60 per ampoule.

7. **Low histamine diet.** In persistent severe cases, consider a low histamine diet. Information can be found online, but this is quite a nuisance and I rarely use it.

Dr. Theoharides is now exploring the possibility that intranasal curcumin and luteolin (a bioflavonoid related to quercetin) may also be especially helpful. The highly absorbed form of curcumin found in Curamin or CuraMed by Terry Naturally may have similar benefits as the intranasal.

Food Sensitivities

Many people find that they have a number of food sensitivities. They find themselves limiting their diet, and then sometimes find themselves becoming sensitive to the few foods they could eat. They find that they over time have painted themselves into a corner where there is nothing left to eat.

THE CAUSE

There are three main things that trigger food sensitivities:

1. Incomplete digestion of proteins because of too little stomach acid or digestive enzymes.
2. Leaky gut from infections, especially candida, and other causes. Anti-inflammatory arthritis medications such as ibuprofen are major triggers.
3. Adrenal fatigue.

Our digestive system is one of the main borders between ourselves and the outside world. Because of this, our immune system patrols our gut pretty aggressively. When we are eating food, especially proteins, the border guards check to make sure that these have been broken down to their component amino acids before being absorbed into the body.

You can think of proteins as being long sentences made up of letters called amino acids. The letters by themselves have no meaning, but are important building blocks that the body uses to make a wide array of necessary things. But if you absorb a long string of letters (i.e., an incompletely digested protein) into your blood, your body has to treat it like an outside invader. Then you develop sensitivities to the food.

Therefore, if your digestion does not completely break down the food, or if your border patrol is not doing its job and letting in incompletely digested food (called leaky gut), your body will react. Normally, this reaction is tempered by a healthy adrenal gland. When your adrenal gland is fatigued, however, you then have the perfect triad for developing food allergies.

When you limit your diet, you then get large amounts of just a few foods. Your digestive system is made to break down a wide array of foods, and if your diet is limited, you are more likely to have incomplete digestion of those few foods, and then you get sensitive to them as well.

SENSITIVITY VERSUS ALLERGY

Medically, these are two very different things. Allergy is when one specific part of your immune system is triggered (e.g., IgE antibodies and histamine). Sensitivities reflect a more generic term for your body and immune system reacting adversely to something.

Most people have food sensitivities and not food allergies. Sadly, most physicians are unfamiliar with food sensitivities and often believe they don't exist.

FOOD ALLERGY TESTING

Most food allergy blood tests are, in my opinion, worse than useless. A study done by Bastyr Naturopathic College showed that if you have three tubes of blood drawn and send them to the same lab (fibbing and writing different names on the three tubes), your results will each come back showing you to be allergic to about twenty to thirty foods. But each lab result will show a totally different mix of food allergies—even though all three tubes were drawn from you at the same time.

I would note that one lab founded by Dr. Russell Jaffe (www.elisaact .com) seems to have avoided the problems with the results being random.

If people have already had them done, I tell them to ignore the results of these tests, especially if they were IgG antibody tests. The exception would be if *only* IgE testing was done. This would be clearly shown on the lab report. In that case, most people have no positive results. If something shows positive, it is a true food *allergy* and that food needs to be avoided, but this test will not look for food *sensitivities*.

My preferred approach to testing? Muscle testing (see below) in the hands of somebody experienced in the technique can be very reliable.

An elimination diet is most reliable, but a nuisance. You can find a kinder and gentler elimination diet at www.vitality101.com (search on "Rapp elimination diet").

Eliminating Food Sensitivities

Although allergy shots can be very effective for inhalant allergens like pollen, they're not very effective for food sensitivities. But there is a technique that is gentle yet very powerful called the Nambudripad Allergy Elimination Technique (NAET; see www.naet.com).

NAET uses muscle testing called applied kinesiology to test for sensitivities. My first reaction as a scientist was that there was no way on earth this testing or treatment could possibly work. In fact, until my early forties, I suffered with severe hay fever (ragweed allergy). I met an NAET practitioner who said that she could get rid of it in twenty minutes. Being an all-knowing doctor, I told her, "Leave me alone. That voodoo can't help me."

A few weeks later, when I was especially miserable, she said, "Stop being a nitwit and let me treat you." Twenty minutes later, my hay fever was gone, never to return.

One of my mentors, Dr. Janet Travell, used to say, "First, see what is going on before you need to understand it. Otherwise, you will never see anything unexpected." As a physician, however, we are unfortunately more likely to follow Winston Churchill's quote: "We often stumble over the truth. Fortunately, we get up, brush ourselves off, and quickly walk away before any real harm is done."

Keeping both of those thoughts in mind is part of what got me into trouble as a physician. Instead of closing my eyes to what happened, and then quickly walking away, I flew to California to meet Devi Nambudripad, MD, PhD, RN, DC, Lac. Despite all the letters after her name, I found her to be brilliant, with no ego. I studied her technique and was so impressed that I went back home to Annapolis and married the woman who had used it to eliminate my hay fever.

Years later, I came to work one day and my wife was helping a five-year-old girl with autism. I had never heard this child string more than two words together. That day, though, she was running around the office and chatting up a storm with everyone. My wife had desensitized her to one nutrient group that day, and some aspects of her autism seemed to go away.

I spoke with other NAET practitioners who found this to be a common occurrence in those with autism. Our foundation then funded, and I was chief investigator on, a study using NAET to treat autism. By the end of one year, twenty-three of the thirty children with autism were back in regular school as opposed to zero of the thirty in the control group.

We published this study, and a large double-blind placebo-controlled study is currently underway. For those of you who know any children with autism, you can find information on how to enroll in the study at www .naet.com.

NAET is very simple. The practitioner does a test looking for muscle weakness in response to each food. If present, the practitioner stimulates acupressure points along the spine, and the next day the food sensitivities to that food group are often gone.

I told you it's hard to believe, but it works brilliantly. The mechanism is not clear, but it seems to reset the immune system so that it no longer sees that food as an enemy. Kind of like hitting the "restore factory settings" on your phone when it goes on the fritz.

If the child is having behavioral problems, the NAET can be combined with applied behavioral analysis (ABA), a treatment which believes that desired behaviors can be taught through a system of rewards and consequences.

NAET practitioners can be found at www.naet.com, though most are not on the website, so you can do a search online for people in your area. If you find one on the website, they are more likely to be more experienced.

I have seen NAET by itself eliminate CFS/FMS in some people with severe sensitivities.

To prevent the food sensitivities from coming back, it is important to take a good plant-based digestive enzyme (CompleteGest) and something to enhance stomach acid (e.g., a vinegar-based salad dressing) with larger meals; eliminate gut candida and other infections; and address the adrenal fatigue.

Simply put, an easy and rather remarkable treatment.

Neurologic Triggers

Our psyche and brain functions are intimately intertwined. For people with the most severe sensitivities, who cannot tolerate natural or prescription therapies, addressing these would be the place to begin. Many of you are empathic, and most of us have been through severe trauma from the illness itself, and often other trauma predating the illness. This has reprogrammed our brain's response to the environment.

In Part Four, we will address this in much more detail. But for sensitivities, it is especially important to reset the vagal nerve and limbic systems. There are many tools that can powerfully do this, but two of my favorites are:

- **Rebalancing the vagal nerve and autonomic system.** This may sound like a complex mouthful, but it's actually quite simple. We will describe an easy basic technique you can do for free at home that will get you started.
- **Rebalancing the limbic system.** A home DVD course called the Dynamic Neural Retraining System by Annie Hopper has had profound benefits for many people. See more on this in Part Four or at www.retrainingthebrain.com.

Part Four will also offer many other tools that you will find very helpful. I would do these before proceeding with the rest of the information in this section. These can dramatically improve pain, orthostatic intolerance, immune function, and mood as well as helping the sensitivities.

Molds and Mycotoxins (Mold Toxins)

Dr. Ritchie Shoemaker, author of *Mold Warriors*, initially formulated the concept that molds and mycotoxins affected sensitivities. Ritchie is so bright as to be almost unintelligible in his complexity. His work has been synthesized and simplified by Dr. Neil Nathan, author of the exceptional book *Toxic*. If you decide to explore mold toxin treatment further, I highly recommend reading this book.

I'd like to say a little more about Dr. Nathan. I spent the first two decades of my medical profession synthesizing the seminal work of giants in healthcare. Their work was so cutting-edge that medicine still has not caught up with them. These included especially:

- **Dr. Janet Travell:** The godmother of understanding muscle pain, she was the White House physician for Presidents Kennedy and Johnson, and a professor of medicine at George Washington University.
- **Dr. William Crook:** He developed our understanding of candida and yeast overgrowth.
- **Dr. William Jefferies:** A professor of endocrinology at Case Western Reserve medical school, he gave us our understanding of adrenal fatigue.

These three stand out among the dozens of experts whose work is synthesized to create the SHINE protocol.

Then I had the pleasure of meeting Dr. Neil Nathan. He took my work, and that of dozens of other experts, and has now synthesized all of these to take our understanding to a whole other level. I consider him to be one of my most respected experts in treating fibromyalgia and other complex illnesses of modern life. Therefore, I highly recommend his work, but it is still quite complex, so I am going to aim to simplify it. My apologies, Neil, if I'm simplifying it down too far.

I will be discussing this area at length, because there is a significant subset of people with CFS/FMS who will simply not recover without treating mold toxins and who improved dramatically when they do, especially when they combine it with the methylation protocol treatment (see page 258).

WHAT ARE MOLD TOXINS?

Most species have ways to defend their territory. For example, humans have all kinds of weaponry. But molds can't move to directly attack other molds, so they focus on chemical warfare. When other molds are present, they can expel toxins into the air to keep other species away.

About three-quarters of people are genetically able to eliminate these toxins are therefore not very sensitive to them. You can have a number of people in the same home or office environment who are doing fine, while you may be sick as a dog.

The problem with mold toxins is that they tend to be fairly small molecules. The body tries to get rid of them by attaching them to bile in the liver and dumping them into the gut, but then they get reabsorbed right back into the bloodstream. Because of this, people can't get rid of them.

WHEN TO SUSPECT MOLD TOXINS

This is not a diagnosis to entertain lightly. At work, it means leaving that building. If it is in your home, mold remediation can cost tens of thousands of dollars.

Dr. Nathan states very simply that until the molds are eliminated from the home, work, and car environment, the mold toxin treatments are unlikely to help. But he finds these treatments to be very helpful for those with persistent CFS and fibromyalgia despite other treatments, and especially in those who are unable to tolerate treatments because of sensitivities. His book *Toxic* goes into more detail on home and urine testing and overall treatment and symptoms, but here are some considerations that may make the treatment more accessible.

Consider mold toxins if:

- You do not respond adequately to the SHINE protocol.
- You have severe environmental and treatment sensitivities, including sensitivity to light, sound, smells, and even electromagnetic fields.
- You have severe anxiety or depression.
- You have electric shock sensations (not numbness or tingling in the extremities, which are present in 44 percent of people with fibromyalgia), ice pick–like pains, vibrating or pulsing sensations running up and down the spinal cord, odd tics and spasms, or seizure-like events.

- The sensitivities do not go away with treatment for mast cell activation syndrome.

Dr. Nathan has found that given the above, about 80 percent of people will have mold toxin issues and about 20 percent will have Lyme disease or coinfections (especially *Bartonella*).

TESTING

Urine testing for mold toxins costs about $400. It is usually not covered by insurance, but can be very worthwhile. These can be done by mail at the Great Plains laboratory. It is reasonable to check for mold toxins every six months until the results are normal.

When doing the urine test, it is critical that you take one tablet of Clinical Glutathione by Terry Naturally under the tongue twice a day for at least a week before the test and also the day that the test sample is obtained. This pulls the toxins out of the cells so they can be seen in the urine test. If the glutathione worsens your symptoms, you can get the sample that day while your symptoms are flaring, instead of waiting the week. When doing repeat testing, stay off of the binders (see page 285) for the three days before the test.

Blood Tests to Consider

Dr. Shoemaker recommends a wide array of blood tests. He finds that markedly elevated levels of C4a, TGF-beta-1, MMP-9, and leptins and low levels of MSH, VIP, and VEGF all suggest and can give an indication of the severity of your body's reactions. But I am not convinced that these are specific to mold, and they may reflect a larger problem called the cell danger response.

Dr. Nathan agrees that these tests are less specific than the urine mold testing and have less value now that this is available. I don't use them, but many other excellent practitioners do.

Another helpful testing option is a visual contrast sensitivity (VCS). Information can be found at Dr. Shoemaker's website, www.surviving mold.com, and the vision test can be done at a low cost ($15) online. Although the urine test should be the primary test used, the VCS offers a very helpful low-cost way to monitor how your body is doing over time with treatment, while also giving some initial clues as to whether mold issues are present. So it may be one simple screening tool you use to decide whether to explore this area further, then I would use it as a low-cost tool for following how you are doing and treatment. The website also has a wealth of information on surviving mold, including resources for home testing and remediation.

One Person's Experience with Mycotoxin Treatment

I was sick for about four years before beginning mycotoxin treatment. And when I say sick, I mean *sick*. I was fourteen when it began and didn't even know what a mycotoxin was. Fatigued to the bone, so weak I could not walk without assistance, bedridden, daily migraines, brain fog, and sensitive to fragrance, light, and noise.

It wasn't until testing, months after beginning treatment, that the results were accurately reflecting what was going on in my body. The results were insanely high levels of mold and mycotoxins. Over the years, treatment had its challenges. My body at the time was incredibly sensitive and fragile. Sometimes it felt like treatment and healing went at a snail's pace.

The protocol needed tweaking over the years. It was a delicate dance to find the perfect rhythm for my body. After two years of mycotoxin treatment, I began to see gradual change, which felt like the most miraculous healing. I should note that remarkable healing at that time for me meant being able to take short walks or standing for five minutes without feeling faint, or being able to sing or laugh without being in immense pain.

It felt extraordinary and was not taken for granted on my end.

Around this time, I began a program to retrain my brain out of constant fight-or-flight called Dynamic Neural Retraining System. I eventually also used a similar strategy called the Gupta Program. Both helped immensely and I recommend them to anyone overcoming an environmental illness or suffering from being in constant fight-or-flight.

The following three years of treatment I saw somewhat steady healing, but it was not linear. Life happens. Mold reexposure, emotional trauma, and food poisoning happen. And I had to learn to let go and go with the flow. It was around five years from my first mycotoxin test that I had clear results for the first time. In the five months leading up to this test, I felt it in my body. I could feel health, a strength I had not felt before. It felt like, suddenly, parts of me were alive that I had forgotten about. My mind was clear. My body was physically growing stronger. I wasn't having to rest after every outing.

Each day that follows I feel this strength growing in me. Not just physically and mentally, but also spiritually and emotionally. One of the greatest lessons I've learned through this hardship is that every part of my being is connected: mind, body, and soul. When one is sick all are affected. To be the healthiest, most loving and giving human I can be, I must take the time to prioritize health. Health is not something I take for granted now. It's a gift, one that I will cherish and celebrate with all my mind, body, and soul.

—Kaitlin K.

TREATMENT

There are three key parts to treatment if your urine mold toxin test is positive.

1. If it is still present, get the toxin-producing mold out of your environment. This includes home, work, and even automobile heating and AC systems. This is often a difficult and expensive proposition. Many mold remediation companies do not know how to tell even if obvious mold problems are present. Others will see it everywhere even if it's not a problem.

   One approach is doing home "petri dish" testing from www .immunolytics.com. If the results are positive, you will need somebody trained in doing mold remediation. For more information on this, I refer you to Dr. Nathan's book *Toxic*. The testing company may also be able to help guide you.

   But for so many people who are devastated financially by this illness, this simply is not an option. If this is your case, and your mold testing is positive, you may need to consider other alternatives:

   A. If your illness began before you were in your current home, there's a good probability that you left the mold behind, but the toxin-producing molds still have stayed in your body. Then, if there is no obvious mold issue in your current home, an argument can be made for simply treating and seeing if the mold levels start coming down after six to nine months using the binders we discuss below.

B. If you are working outside the home and have not moved to a different office building since your illness began, see if your business can have you work from home or in a different building.

C. If you are renting, consider moving to a different building.

2. Kill any toxin-producing mold that may still be in your body. For this, I recommend 200 milligrams per day for at least three months of the prescription fluconazole (Diflucan) or itraconazole (Sporanox) daily. Most of the people I treat will have already been on this before exploring mycotoxins, but if they were unable to tolerate it because the antifungal severely flared symptoms (the Herxheimer reaction), Dr. Nathan finds that having people on the binders below for several months can stabilize the toxin levels. Then these medications can be retried very slowly.

I also recommend using Argentyn 23 colloidal silver nose spray and a compounded prescription nose spray for at least six months. There is a good argument for using both of them long term. This will kill any mold in your sinuses, which is the main area where they produce toxins. Use one to two sprays of each in both nostrils two to three times daily. The prescription compounded nose spray is Sinusitis Nose Spray from ITC Pharmacy (www.itcpharmacy.com or 888-349-5453). Get the one that includes bismuth and 0.06 percent amphotericin B (30 cc). Your doctor can call in a prescription to ITC Pharmacy for "sinusitis nose spray with bismuth and ampho," and the pharmacy will know what to supply. For long-term use after the six months (or even after two months to lower costs), ask your compounding pharmacist to make a 1 percent itraconazole nose spray. The prescription Sinusitis Nose Spray will also kill problematic bacteria called MARCoNS (multiple antibiotic-resistant coagulase negative staphylococci), which can aggravate your illness. I do not bother doing nasal swab testing for these bacteria, relying instead on the nose sprays to do their job.

3. Use the binders below. Take them about a half hour before eating; this way, they will be positioned like a catcher's mitt where your bile comes out after you eat. They soak up the toxins and pull them out in your stool. This usually takes about eighteen months for the toxins to get low enough for you to start feeling much better, though improvement can be seen more quickly.

As you pull the toxins out of your system, you may actually start feeling worse. This happens because the toxins are getting pulled out faster than your detoxification system can handle them. *Do not try to play macho and tough it out. This will only set back your recovery.* Ease back to a dose where you do not have worsening. You will slowly be able to increase the dose comfortably over time. In the first six to nine months, urine mold toxin levels may actually go up with treatment, as dead mold and also fat cells are releasing toxins for elimination.

Taking one capsule of Klaire Labs' InterFase Plus twice daily can also help kill the yeast and may settle down the flaring of symptoms during detoxification.

Here are the five binders:

- **Cholestyramine (Questran).** Get the sugar-free one by prescription. If you do not tolerate the additives, it can be made by a compounding pharmacy, but this is more expensive and then it will not be insurance covered. Start with ⅛ to ¹⁄₁₆ teaspoon every other day a half hour before meals. Increase slowly as is comfortable to one scoop (4 grams, or 1⅔ teaspoons) two to four times a day. Don't be surprised or concerned if you can't go over 2 teaspoons a day. Some people get well with even a ¹⁄₁₆ teaspoon every two to three days.

    Colesevelam (Welchol) works taken the same way, with the usual dosage being two capsules (625 milligrams each) three times a day. Constipation is the main side effect, so increase your magnesium and vitamin C intake to compensate.
- **Bentonite.** Take 500 milligrams one to two times daily from Premier Research Labs. If poorly tolerated, you can use the Yerba Prima Great Plains Bentonite liquid clay. Start at ¹⁄₁₆ or ⅛ teaspoon taken once daily and slowly work up to 1 teaspoon as is comfortable.
- **Activated charcoal.** Take 280 milligrams (one to three capsules a day) from Integrative Therapeutics. The tablets and powders are messy.

- **Chlorella.** Take one to three capsules (not the pellets) a day, available from BodyBio.
- *Saccharomyces boulardii.* Take one capsule (3 to 5 billion units) with one meal per day, working up to three times a day. This also inhibits growth of other unhealthy bacteria and yeast.

Dr. Nathan likes to begin with the *Saccharomyces* first, as it is best tolerated. When people are comfortable with this, he likes to add in the bentonite clay, starting with one capsule a day.

Some people respond within six months, although it takes most one to two years to start improving. Some people take three to five years to get well. This is when it is especially worth considering urine testing, to reassure yourself that the mold toxin levels are indeed coming down. They usually have to come down into the normal range before people start feeling better.

If you want to tailor the toxin binders to specific mold toxins that show on your test, here is information that Dr. Joseph Brewer, a noted infectious disease specialist, and Dr. Nathan find to be helpful:

- Ochratoxins appear to be bound best by cholestyramine and activated charcoal.
- Aflatoxins and sterigmatocystin are bound by activated charcoal and bentonite clay.
- Trichothecenes (including roridin E and verrucarin A) are bound by activated charcoal. Chlorella and bentonite clay may be helpful.
- Gliotoxins are bound by bentonite clay, *Saccharomyces boulardii* (a probiotic yeast), and N-acetyl cysteine (NAC). Take 500 milligrams of NAC twice daily. Take one capsule with 8 to 10 billion units of *Saccharomyces boulardii*, with one meal per day, working up to three times a day.

What Is Going on in Mold Toxin Illness?

Here is a play-by-play for those of you that are *very* technically oriented. But seriously, it is totally okay to skip this section if you're not.

The most common and problematic toxin-producing molds are the black mold *Stachybotrys*, *Aspergillus*, *Penicillium*, *Fusarium*, *Chaetomium*, *Alternaria*, and *Wallemia*. These then trigger the cell danger response (CDR), causing your immune system to go into overdrive. This can trigger not only increased sensitivities but eventually immune exhaustion.

These immune chemicals, called cytokines, block the body's leptin receptors, causing leptin resistance. Leptin is the hormone that suppresses appetite and tells you that you are full after a meal. This is part of what contributes to the average thirty-two-pound weight gain seen in fibromyalgia. The toxins also prevent the hypothalamus from making MSH (alpha-Melanocyte-stimulating hormone) and VIP (vasoactive intestinal polypeptide). These are critical for regulating your immune, brain, and hormonal systems.

Basically, mold toxins are one of the things that can cause hypothalamic dysfunction that we've talked about earlier.

Meanwhile, the immune system is unable to shut off. This can be demonstrated by measuring the cytokine C4a. The chronic immune activation causes inadequate oxygen to reach the tissues. This stimulates your body to increase the production of VEGF to stimulate new blood vessel formation.

Over time, the drop in MSH and immune exhaustion leaves you set up for infections such as MARCoNS. This nasal infection can make exotoxin A, which can further destroy MSH, while making thick layers of biofilm that keep your immune system and antibiotics from getting to the infections. The EDTA, silver, and bismuth in the nose sprays discussed above melt the biofilms.

A piece of good news? VIP can be measured by a blood test, but you must specify that it has to be done at ARUP Laboratories. Most local labs can send the test to ARUP. Testing elsewhere is likely to simply not be reliable. When your VIP levels are low, this triggers out-of-control immune activation. Compounding pharmacies can make VIP nose spray, which can sometimes quickly improve symptoms.

Dr. Shoemaker also uses other tests that are more often covered by insurance and can be done by most labs. My suspicion is that these tests are not specific to mold, but are the body's cell danger response to numerous stressors. But they do have two benefits:

1. Showing a number of abnormal blood tests helps if you have family members or physicians who don't believe anything is going on, largely because you have been getting the wrong tests for this illness.

2. Over time, you can see that things are improving physiologically, which can occur before physical improvements begin, and this can be very encouraging.

I don't use these tests, because they don't affect my treatment decisions. But they are not unreasonable to do anyway. In many people with CFS and fibromyalgia, the tests will show elevated levels of C4a, TGF-beta-1, MMP-9, and leptins and low levels of MSH, VIP, and VEGF.

For difficult cases, it is very reasonable to make an appointment with Dr. Neil Nathan for him to direct your mycotoxin treatment. As you can see, mycotoxins can be a very complex area. But it also can potentially be fairly simple, letting the toxin binders work in the background for sixteen to twenty-four months while you are addressing the rest of the protocol.

When People with Illnesses Have to Be Their Own Researchers . . .

I have invited Erik Johnson, a strong advocate of the connection between toxic mold and CFS, to offer his powerful experience:

During the famous Lake Tahoe outbreak of "mystery illness" in 1985, I observed that all of the clusters were in "sick buildings." This has been called sick building syndrome (SBS), the cause of which was not yet known. The culprit—toxic mold—had not yet been discovered and entered into the medical literature.

This cluster association between prior mold exposure and the chronic form of illness was so consistent that it seemed prudent to ask whether individuals with the mystery malady had problems with mold prior to the Tahoe Flu virus that passed through in the fall of 1985 through mid-1985. All had a mold story to tell.

To my way of thinking, this elevated the role of mold to "critical cofactor" in development of the Lake Tahoe mystery illness, as was later noted by the 1994 abstract by Chester and Levine,* based on this very same outbreak.

I devised an experimental strategy of "extreme avoidance" of toxic mold, which resulted in recovery so spectacular that CFS doctors considered it unbelievable.

---

* Alexander C. Chester and Paul H. Levine, "Concurrent Sick Building Syndrome and Chronic Fatigue Syndrome: Epidemic Neuromyasthenia Revisited," *Clinical Infectious Diseases* 18, Supplement 1 (January 1994): S43–S48, https://doi.org/10.1093/clinids/18.Supplement_1.S43.

For the purpose of achieving validation, I took volunteers diagnosed with chronic fatigue syndrome on a "CFS Mold History Tour" to the sick buildings where the clusters occurred. The reaction of CFS patients to these locations is consistent and compelling enough to warrant incorporating the toxic mold *Stachybotrys chartarum* into the official CFS definitional criteria as an extreme risk factor for the disease currently known as chronic fatigue syndrome. Considering this is the very first documented clue in the clusters for which this syndrome was coined, it should be included in all studies in which the "chronic fatigue syndrome" terminology is used.

Further information and details can be found at www.moldfactor.com.

—Erik Johnson

Mold at Ground Zero for CFS

The history of Chronic Fatigue Syndrome (CFS) begins in Incline Village, Nevada, in 1985. In the medical history of CFS, each of the concepts applies—failed theories and failed criticism.

One victim, Erik Johnson, told everyone who would listen that mold was a cause of CFS. He came up with his theory at the wrong time in the politics of medical opinion, as an unknown viral cause was blamed instead. Johnson tried repeatedly to get the attention of leading CFS researchers then and now to look at what he knew about mold sensitivity.

Twenty years passed before Erik's mold opinions were vindicated.

—Dr. Ritchie Shoemaker, *Mold Warriors* (Gateway Press, 2005): Chapter 23

20 Losing Weight with CFS and FMS

*I*n addition to the myriad other problems you have to bear, two of our in-house studies found that people with fibromyalgia and CFS have an average weight gain of thirty-two pounds. This occurs because of the metabolic problems present in these syndromes, causing fewer calories to be burned.

It is much easier to lose the weight and keep it off, however, when one understands and addresses the many things that contribute to this problem. Put simply, for people with CFS/FMS, simply altering your diet is not enough to lose weight. A large percentage of you have found that it is impossible to lose weight and keep it off no matter what you do.

There are several ways that CFS/FMS is contributing to your inability to lose weight. Both physical stresses (e.g., infections and nutritional deficiencies) and emotional/situational stresses can result in a metabolic chain reaction that results in weight gain. With effective treatment of their CFS/FMS, most people find that their weight gain stops and that usual weight-loss measures can finally work.

What Caused the Weight Gain?

Let's begin with poor sleep. The expression "getting your beauty sleep" actually has a basis in fact. Deep sleep is a major trigger for growth hormone production. Growth hormone stimulates production of muscle (which burns fat) and improves insulin sensitivity (which decreases the tendency to make fat), while also decreasing fibromyalgia symptoms. Thus, getting the eight to nine hours of sleep a night that the human body is meant to have can powerfully contribute to your staying young-looking and trim. Poor sleep also causes lower levels of the hormone leptin, which regulates hunger.

In addition, as we've noted elsewhere, the hypothalamic circuit breaker that gets suppressed with stress also controls our hormone system. This results in inadequate levels of thyroid and adrenal hormones. The thyroid regulates how many calories you burn—and low thyroid can dramatically trigger weight gain. The adrenal glands are the body's stress handlers. In the beginning of your illness, chronic stress and depression result in elevated cortisol levels, which can directly cause weight gain. Continuing excessive stress may result in exhaustion of the adrenal glands over time.

As it is the job of the adrenal glands to maintain blood sugar levels in the time of stress, adrenal exhaustion can result in episodes of hypoglycemia (low blood sugar). If you get periods where you feel that somebody had better feed you *now* or you're going to kill them, you are likely hypoglycemic and would benefit from adrenal support. The sugar cravings caused by low blood sugar then lead to further weight gain.

Infections can also contribute to weight gain. Clinical experience has shown that fungal overgrowth stirs sugar cravings and leads to weight gain. Although we do not know the mechanism for this, we have repeatedly seen excess weight drop off once this overgrowth is treated and eliminated.

Another major problem is carnitine deficiency, a problem that is present in most CFS/FMS patients. Unfortunately, this deficiency forces your body to turn calories into fat and makes it almost impossible to lose fat. Simply taking supplemental carnitine does not help adequately, however, as it does not transfer into cells optimally in this form. I do recommend that people take 1,000 milligrams of acetyl-L-carnitine daily for four months, as cells can absorb this form easily, leading to energy production and weight loss.

Last but not least, many people with CFS/FMS have insulin resistance—meaning they need high blood levels of insulin to maintain a normal level of blood sugar. Unfortunately, high insulin levels increase your body's production of fat. If weight gain is a problem, check your fasting blood insulin level. To do so, do not eat after midnight, then have your lab check your insulin level first thing in the morning.

If the insulin reading is higher than 10 mIU/mL, especially if your DHEA sulfate and testosterone levels are also high or high normal, your doctor may decide to prescribe the diabetes medication metformin. This improves insulin sensitivity, even in nondiabetics. Metformin can not only help weight loss but also improve other symptoms of CFS/FMS. A recent study showed a marked decrease in pain with metformin in people with fibromyalgia who had insulin resistance.

In females, the combination of high normal insulin, DHEA-S, and testosterone levels suggest PCOS (polycystic ovary syndrome—another cause of CFS/FMS). I also treat PCOS with metformin and very low-dose hydrocortisone (Cortef). It is important to not overdo the carbohydrates that you crave. Be sure to take the Energy Revitalization System vitamin powder or B complex supplements if on metformin; otherwise, it will cause a vitamin B12 deficiency.

How Can You Treat These Problems So That You Lose Weight and Feel Better?

1. Cut down the sugar and simple carbohydrates in your diet and increase your water intake. If your mouth feels parched and you are not taking a medication that causes dry mouth, then you are thirsty and need to drink more water (even if you already drink like a fish).
2. Increase your sleep. Get eight to nine hours of solid sleep every night.
3. Treat low thyroid or adrenal function, if applicable.
4. Treat yeast/candida overgrowth, if present.
5. Get optimum nutritional support. When you are deficient in vitamins or minerals, your body will crave more food than you need, and your metabolism will be sluggish. As mentioned, take 500 to 1,000 milligrams of acetyl-L-carnitine daily along with the Energy Revitalization System vitamin powder.
6. Take the Smart Energy System along with the vitamin powder. Studies show that its components also cause weight loss.
7. Treat insulin resistance, if present.

It is not unusual for people to shed thirty to fifty pounds by simply treating these metabolic factors.

PART FOUR

The Mind-Body-Spirit (MBS) Connection

BFF Summary

1. CFS, fibromyalgia, and day-to-day fatigue are physical processes with physical causes. However, like most illnesses, they also have psychological components that must be treated.

2. If a doctor implies that he or she doesn't know what's wrong with you so you must be crazy, leave.

3. If something does not feel good, that is all the justification you need to say "No!"

4. Emotional traumas, including the illness itself, can trip circuit breakers throughout your brain and nervous system. We will review a number of approaches to resetting the circuits. These can powerfully help immunity, sensitivity, pain, orthostatic intolerance, and more. We will discuss a number of tools, many of which you can do at no cost on your own.

5. Use the trembling technique (discussed in the book *Waking the Tiger* by Peter Levine) to release the muscle memory of the traumas. A technique called the emotional freedom technique (EFT) can help you release the emotional energy. Then as needed, activate the ventral vagal part of your nervous system, which stimulates the feeling of safety.

6. Historically, a number of cultural approaches have been used to activate the ventral vagal. For example, tai chi, meditation and prayer, and pranayama (yogic breathing).

Social activities such as chatting, small talk, or having a meal or a cup of coffee with someone also are important and helpful.

7. We discuss the importance of triggering the "feeling safe" part of your brain, called the polyvagal theory.

Am I Crazy?

After dealing with an insane medical system, people with CFS/FMS, and even those with simple day-to-day fatigue, often come away wondering if they are crazy.

The simple answer?

NO!

At least not any more crazy than anybody else.

Nonetheless, with all that you have been through, let's take a look at this issue in a little more depth.

We have a bad habit in medicine. If a doctor cannot figure out what is wrong with the patient, the doctor brands that person a "turkey." Imagine calling an electrician because your lights do not work. The electrician checks all the wiring, can't find the problem, and says, "You're crazy. There's nothing wrong with your lights." You flip the switches and they still do not work, but the electrician just says, "I've looked. There's no problem here," and walks out the door.

This is analogous to the experience of many CFS/FMS and day-to-day fatigue patients. I apologize on behalf of the medical profession if we've called you crazy just because we cannot determine the cause of your problem. It is inappropriate, abusive, and downright cruel.

To put this in a historical perspective, multiple sclerosis used to be called hysterical paralysis. Over time, neurologists came to their senses. No neurologist in their right mind would still consider calling people with multiple sclerosis hysterical or neurotics. Lupus and rheumatoid arthritis also used to be considered neuroses.

What do these illnesses have in common? As is the case with most immune illnesses (including CFS/FMS), they affect predominantly women. You can get an idea of the medical profession's bias in the situation by simply looking at the medical word "hysteria." This word comes from the Latin *hystero*, which means "uterus." Despite the fact that half of U.S. physicians are female, this medical bias still persists.

Unfortunately, some patients become so frustrated by being told that their CFS/FMS or day-to-day-fatigue is all in their head that they are in a catch-22. They feel that if they acknowledge that they also have emotional issues, just like everyone else, they are validating the abusive doctors who say that their illness is all emotional. Rest assured, however, that extensive research proves that CFS/FMS and day-to-day fatigue are real and physical.

One of many studies that proved that CFS and fibromyalgia are real was our placebo-controlled study. This is because people who received the active SHINE treatment improved dramatically and those receiving the placebo did not. If it was all in your head, the placebo group would have improved as much as the active group. This means that anyone who says it's all in your head is no longer simply a nitwit. Now they are unscientific nitwits. Give yourself permission to be human. You are no more and no less crazy than anyone else.

People often ask if they should get counseling. The simple answer is that, as in any other severe illness, the time to get counseling is if and when you feel like it.

How to Tell If You Are Depressed in Thirty Seconds

Research has shown that there is a very good way to tell if people are depressed. It is as effective as or more effective than many of the complicated depression questionnaires such as the Beck Depression Inventory.

What is this new high-tech technique?

Simply ask the person if he or she is depressed.

Not sure if you're depressed? Here is one more important tip: Ask yourself if you have many interests. If the answer is that you have many interests but are frustrated that you have no energy to do them, then you're probably not depressed. If you have no interests or have lost interest in the things you used to enjoy, then you likely are depressed. And it is good to treat that along with the SHINE protocol.

Depression can accompany any severe illness such as cancer, but we wouldn't dream of telling people with cancer that they were crazy. Whether or not you are depressed, you may consider some type of therapist for emotional support and guidance. Be careful who you choose, however. Make sure "psychotherapist" is one word—not two. Talk to your friends and relatives to find somebody who is good. Your physician may also be an excellent resource.

The Problem with Cognitive Behavioral Therapy (CBT)

Cognitive behavioral therapy teaches people coping skills and can be very helpful for many crippling illnesses, including cancer, multiple sclerosis, and a host of other conditions. The problem occurs when practitioners think that they have to convince the person that the person's illness is not real as part of the CBT. Those practitioners have lost touch with reality and can be quite abusive—even if well-meaning.

Picture the reaction if a CBT practitioner was not only trying to convince people with metastatic cancer that they did not have a real illness but aggressively worked to get legislation passed making it illegal for these people with cancer to get the treatments or insurance coverage they needed and had paid for. This would be considered obscenely abusive, and it is equally inappropriate in CFS and fibromyalgia. On the other hand, many excellent CBT therapists treat their CFS and fibromyalgia patients with respect, helping them cope by giving them the powerful tools that CBT has to offer—without trying to invalidate their illness.

I would note that there is nothing wrong with physicians who say, "I'm sorry I don't know what's wrong with you." They're simply being honest. It is also totally understandable for physicians to not be willing to prescribe treatments they are not familiar or comfortable with. Please simply thank them for their honesty.

But what do you do if you're at a physician who implies "I don't know what's wrong with you, so you are crazy"? My recommendation? Simply tell them: "You may want to look at the research on this illness, and in the future simply let people know you're completely unfamiliar with this disease." Saying this graciously will be much more powerful than being angry. Then walk out the door.

If it makes you feel better, many physicians work in systems where you can go online and rate them. Simply do a search on your physician or on rating physicians to find sites where you can do this.

The Mind-Body Connection in CFS/FMS

I suspect that all illnesses have a psychological component. Although highly stressed executives may have a bacterial infection such as *Helicobacter pylori* or excess acid causing their ulcer, it helps to remove the three telephones from their ear while treating the infection and excess acid.

I find that most people with CFS/FMS are often mega-type-A overachievers, with many having been through a traumatic abusive experience. To some degree, this psychodynamic often applies to day-to-day fatigue as well. We are approval seekers who avoid conflict to avoid losing approval. We often grew up seeking approval from somebody who simply was not going to give it—no matter what. And we take care of everybody except one person—ourselves. Does this remind you at all of yourself?

Being empathic, we also often find ourselves being emotional toxic waste dumps for other people. It almost seems like we attract every energy vampire in town. How do you tell an energy vampire? After an interaction with them, they tell you how much better they feel—and you feel like you were energetically sucked dry.

THE ANTIDOTE

So how do you break the psychodynamic? It's pretty straightforward. In fact, it can be summarized in two letters.

N. O.

Learning to use this wonderful word can free you.

Here's how: When somebody asks you to do something that will take you more than two hours, tell them that you are sorry, but the doctor (that's me) told you that he would wring your neck if you took on anything more. Tell them that the answer is probably no, but you'll get back to them in the next twenty-four hours if you change your mind and are able to. Then walk away.

Most often, when you get home you will feel great, like you have dodged a bullet. Since it was left as the answer being no unless you got back to them, you are now off the hook. If, on the other hand, you feel that you really wish you had said yes, and that it would feel really good to do it, you can always call them and change your mind.

Simple—yet effective.

In general, I encourage you to decide to say yes or no based on how things *feel*, rather than based on what you *think*. Although it is good to do your homework and check into things, once you have finished this, see how things *feel*. If it feels good to say yes, then do so; otherwise, say no.

Why is this? Our mind is a product of our programming as a child. It basically feeds back to us what we were told that we should do to be accepted by and get approval from our parents, our religious organizations, television, and God knows how many other authority figures. Our feelings, on the other hand, reflect our intuition and also let us know what is authentic to us.

So simply remember the wonderful word "no." It is an amazingly versatile word. It is a complete sentence. It can be said graciously or firmly. There is even a great T-shirt that says, "What Part of 'No' Don't You Understand?"

Although this simple guidance will go a long way, for many if not most people with CFS and fibromyalgia, there is more work that needs to be done. The traumas that they have experienced from life and the illness have often tripped numerous circuit breakers. This leaves some systems, such as adrenaline, stuck in cycles of constant overdrive and exhaustion. Many techniques, including retraining the vagal nerve and limbic systems (not as complex as it sounds), can reset and rewire your brain, with dramatic benefits throughout your body.

Let's start with some easy yet very powerful approaches you can do on your own—for free!

A Powerful Secret

We sometimes forget the power of simply smiling. Take a few moments now and simply smile—not necessarily for any reason, just because it feels good. When you do, you may stumble across a secret you've forgotten for a while, but which your heart and soul (or deep psyche, if you prefer) remembers.

That all is truly well. Watch then, as your smile gets bigger.

This is a powerful, and free, tool for healing—and wonderment. It is how a small 1'9" by 2'6" painting became the most well-known piece of art in the world. Play at being your own walking *Mona Lisa*, and watch how your world changes . . .

Smile, and you can feel the healing process begin. Smile a lot, and health will begin to ease out and replace illness.

Then just breathe . . .

Let's do this now: Breathe in very long and deeply, slowly and gently. Be open to drawing in the soft sweet nothingness of life, allowing in the universe's unconditional love and infinite energy.

Take your time and simply notice while you do this. Let the old pain, trauma, and fatigue melt away. You may even discover that the love you'll find can make you cry—with joy—for you'll start to remember and return to yourself.

I invite you to put down this book for a few minutes and let yourself do this. Right now.

Know that this feeling is always here, ready for you whenever you open yourself and let it in.

Are You an Empath?

People ask me, "What's a nice Jewish doctor like you doing in a field like fibromyalgia?" My answer? I got into it the old-fashioned way: I had the illness.

I grew up as a highly empathic child in the family of Auschwitz concentration camp survivors. It almost destroyed me. To survive childhood, I had to go through my "I am a rock, I am an island" phase where I shut down almost all of my feelings.

When I got to medical school, my family imploded. As is often the case with empaths, I mistakenly took on the role of peacemaker in the midst of a psychotic conversation. I came down with a nasty viral syndrome that simply would not go away. After several months, I could no longer function and had to drop out of medical school. As I was paying my own way, this left me homeless and sleeping in parks.

As I described earlier in the book, this was the beginning of my experience with fibromyalgia. And grew into my life goal of making effective treatment available for everyone.

Many of you reading this book will find that you are empathic. You can tell and actually experience what others are feeling. If you don't learn to set boundaries by the using the word "no" as we discussed above, it can lead people into fibromyalgia. If this sounds like you, I happily recommend the *New York Times* bestselling book *The Empath's Survival Guide: Life Strategies for Sensitive People* by my friend Judith Orloff, MD.

The Importance of Feeling Safe

PART 1: THE INTERPLAY BETWEEN IMMUNITY AND THE PSYCHE

An important fact to realize? Our unconscious mind directs our immune system. So, whether or not we feel safe plays a major role in immune function, which plays a key role in CFS/FMS.

Although we were never taught about this in medical school, I learned this by accident. I was paying my own way through medical school by working as a nurse in the children's hospital. I was scheduled to work the burn unit and decided to learn medical hypnosis from my psychiatry professor. I wanted to help the children decrease the pain during their burn dressing changes.

Professor Byron Stinson, who passed away just a few years ago at the age of ninety-four, taught me something interesting. While someone was in a hypnotic state, which accesses the deep unconscious, you could prevent their developing a blister after a severe burn. Usually the dead skin turns white and falls off. But if you gave them the suggestion right after the burn that there was no injury, they simply wouldn't blister.

The burn blister is our immune system attacking an area of perceived injury and invasion.

There is a good reason I am not a surgeon. I have world-class butterfingers. Because of this, it is not at all uncommon for me to injure myself. Using quick self-hypnosis when I burn myself, and giving myself the simple suggestion "heal quickly—no injury," I simply no longer blister.

Much of our immune system's response comes from our psyche's perceiving a threat, real or otherwise. This translates to feeling unsafe. This plays a major role in why the immune systems of people with CFS/FMS are so reactive. There are many techniques that do not use hypnosis that can effectively reprogram how our brains function, resulting in dramatic improvements in health and fibromyalgia with no medications.

So, if you have severe sensitivities, read Chapter 19 and pay especially close attention to the information below.

PART 2: THE DYNAMIC NEURAL RETRAINING SYSTEM (DNRS)

It's time to start looking at mind-body-spirit (MBS) intensive care.

For those of you with severe sensitivities, sometimes seemingly to everything, DNRS is the place to begin. Limbic system retraining can work miracles for people with fibromyalgia.

This drug-free, neuroplasticity-based healing approach to rewire chronic illness patterns in the brain was developed by Annie Hopper in 2008. It was geared to conditions such as chemical sensitivities, chronic fatigue syndrome, and fibromyalgia, and she created it as part of her own healing from these illnesses.

Basically, this program helps rewire the brain's limbic system, a complex set of structures in the midbrain that includes the hypothalamus, along with the hippocampus, amygdala, and cingulate cortex. It has been described as the feeling and reacting brain, and is what forms memories and helps us determine whether we feel safe. It also acts as the brain's anxiety switch.

It is closely integrated with the immune, endocrine, and autonomic nervous system. So, you can see how its malfunction explains so many of the problems seen in fibromyalgia.

Limbic system malfunction can occur from many stressors, including infections, toxic exposures, and traumas. It then becomes hypersensitive, reacting to stimuli that it would usually disregard as not representing a danger. This causes inappropriate activation of the immune, endocrine, and autonomic nervous systems. Over time, this state of hyperarousal can exhaust the immune and other systems.

I would begin by ordering the DVD training program from www .retrainingthebrain.com. Aim to watch these and follow directions for an hour a day. If you can't do that much, even fifteen minutes a day can help. After about two to three months of using this program for an hour a day, many people start to see dramatic improvement. This may be the best $270 you ever spend on fibromyalgia treatment. You may also want to read Annie Hopper's book *Wired for Healing.* These are usually enough. For those who can afford it, she also has five-day boot camps that run about $3,400.

Again, if you have severe sensitivities or respond poorly to other treatments overall, I recommend you do the Dynamic Neural Retraining System.

FEELING SAFE: PART 1

THE POLYVAGAL THEORY

A major part of our brain and nervous system, which controls most of our organs, blood pressure, pulse, and sweating, is called the autonomic nervous system. Historically, doctors have viewed this as having two components:

- **The parasympathetic nervous system.** This has been described as "the old man after dinner." It is a time for resting and recharging. Acetylcholine is the main brain chemical associated with this. Scientists have found this to be the oldest evolutionary part of the autonomic nervous system, found in early and even extinct reptiles.
- **Sympathetic nervous system.** This is the adrenaline system that has been called fight-or-flight. It is activated during perceived threats.

New research is showing that there is a third critical component. The parasympathetic "resting after dinner" nervous system has another major part. It turns out that the vagal nerve is not a single nerve; in mammals, it has evolved to have a branch (called the ventral vagal) involved in being social. *For this to turn on, it is necessary that the person feels safe.* This regulates your heart and lungs, slowing down your heart rate and making it easier to breathe.

Finally, the fourth component is that the "old man after dinner" component of the vagal nerve (called the dorsal vagal) has another function. When put under severe stress that we can't escape from, it puts people into a numb and checked-out space that has been called playing possum or freezing.

Let's look at what happens during a traumatic event. Say a child is being attacked by an alcoholic parent. The first thing that kicks in would be the sympathetic fight-or-flight adrenaline part of the nervous system. But what if you can't run away?

That's when the resting part of the nervous system (the posterior vagal) can actually drop the animal into a playing-possum or frozen state. This is often switched on along with the adrenaline state at the same time, leaving the person's body systems in a numb yet hyper-alert state. This is actually a heroic measure taken by the nervous system. In situations such as child abuse, being robbed at gunpoint, or even rape, your body going into this mode was heroic and lifesaving. Trying to fight back in those settings was not only impossible (your nervous system wisely took the choice out of your hands) but may have cost you your life.

THE PROBLEM?

In more highly evolved mammals, such as humans, it is very hard to shift back out of this frozen/hyper-alert state, and people get stuck. They can stay this way for decades. This is very common in PTSD and also frequently seen in CFS/FMS, and people will feel immobilized but with a racing heart.

The antidote? Turning on the part of the vagal nerve system (the ventral vagal) that is involved in play (between people) and socializing. This, along with the trembling technique discussed on page 309, takes people out of the numb/hyper-alert mode. This can be life changing.

For example, research done by Stephen Porges, the professor who developed the polyvagal theory, has shown that doing some of the treatments below can be dramatically beneficial for kids with autism. They can then become much more social. Peter Levine has found offshoots of this work to be very beneficial for PTSD and other emotional traumas.

HOW CAN YOU TELL WHAT STATE YOU'RE STUCK IN?

Certain symptoms are tip-offs. A constant high heart rate suggests that the adrenaline system is locked into place. This causes it (and you) to exhaust at the same time. When this happens, people are hyper-alert with a racing heart and exhaustion.

Symptoms of the Playing Possum/Frozen Mode

- Sound hypersensitivity: being in noisy places becomes uncomfortable. People then also often have trouble making out speech clearly despite being hypersensitive to sound.
- Flat facial and voice features: We instinctively can tell the difference between somebody whose facial and vocal features are alive versus flat. Think about the college professor speaking in this monotone drone versus one that was animated. Which one left you feeling more engaged?

- Diarrhea
- Depression
- Shut down, depressed or apathetic, or dissociated (feeling disconnected or "not with it")

Symptoms of Adrenaline Overdrive

- Chronically elevated resting heart rates
- Constipation
- Anxiety
- Stress behaviors: angry, aggressive, anxious, fearful (sympathetic fight-or-flight), or withdrawn

Symptoms of Your "Feeling Safe" (Ventral Vagal) Part of the Nervous System Being Shut Down

- Forward head posture (FHP): Looking from the side, your ears should be right above the middle of your shoulders. Each inch forward decreases lung capacity and adds ten pounds of extra work to carry one's head. This stresses the neck muscles and can trigger neck pain and headaches.
- Asthma

The mix of these symptoms suggests that you are stuck in a combined frozen/adrenaline overdrive combination. Turning on the third part of this nervous system is the key to getting unstuck.

FEELING SAFE: PART 2

TURNING ON THE "ALIVE AND SOCIALIZING" PART OF THE NERVOUS SYSTEM

A key to recovery is feeling safe. How many of you, if you really think about it, have noticed that you rarely feel *really* safe? This is the tip-off.

Here are several ways to turn on the "feeling safe" part of the nervous system and wake up from being in the checked-out/hyper-alert mode that you may have been in for decades and that may be triggering a significant part of your fibromyalgia, sensitivities, and inability to handle stress:

1. The Dynamic Neural Retraining System (DNRS) discussed on page 303 is very helpful.
2. The trembling technique (see page 309) can shake off the tight muscles and fascia from the traumas.
3. Singing or playing wind instruments, especially if doing so with others, can be very effective.
4. Pranayama yoga is helpful.
5. Listening to music that has a lot of high-frequency melodies, and less of the low frequencies, can be very helpful.

A study of autistic children with sound sensitivity showed doing this for one hour a day for five days had dramatic benefits. Not only did the sound sensitivity go away, but their ability to make out normal speech improved as did their overall function.

You may find that initially it will leave you a little more fatigued but better able to sleep as your body rests from the chronic adrenaline overdrive. This begins the healing process.

The music used in the Listening Project protocol in the study above is, unfortunately, only available through selected practitioners and at a significant cost. The soundtracks to listen to can be found as samples at https://integratedlistening.com/download-dreampad-music/ in thirty-second to thirty-minute clips. One could simply listen to these and hit replay to get the full hour. See which of these tracks feels best for you.

Another option is to listen to music by Johnny Mathis. Perhaps not as effective, but it contains a lot of these same features and may be very helpful.

In his excellent but quite technical book, *Accessing the Healing Power of the Vagus Nerve: Self-Help Exercises for Anxiety, Depression, Trauma, and Autism*, Stanley Rosenberg offers several tips on both how to diagnose that your "feeling safe" (ventral vagal) is shut down and how to quickly wake it back up.

To tell whether the "feeling safe" ventral vagal is asleep, he does a test that is pretty easy to do called the uvula lift test for ventral vagus function. Open your mouth and use your phone flashlight to look at the back of your throat in a mirror. You will see that funny-looking piece of tissue (called the uvula) hanging there. In a staccato manner, say "ah-ah-ah-ah" repeatedly. With normal function, the uvula should go straight up and down (and tissues on either side of it in the back of the throat should go up and down the same amount on both sides). If the uvula pulls to either side, or the soft tissues on the roof of your mouth go up more on one side of the uvula than the other as you go "ah-ah-ah-ah," it indicates shutdown of the "feeling safe" ventral vagus.

Next, gently squeeze the muscle right on top of your shoulders between your fingers. They should feel equally thick to you. If one side feels thicker, it suggests that ventral vagus inactivity is a problem.

Rosenberg's basic exercise for turning on the "feeling safe" ventral vagal will take two minutes to learn and two minutes to do. For simple traumas, even doing it once can help your system reset. For fibromyalgia, it's reasonable to do it at least once a day for a few months.

Each time you do it, you'll be able to recover more quickly and be less prone to being thrown into freeze mode. A quick look at your uvula while going "ah-ah-ah-ah" may quickly tell you if the basic exercise treatment took.

Here is the basic exercise:

The first few times, do this exercise lying on your back. After that, you can do it sitting or however is comfortable. Begin by interlacing the fingers of both hands while looking at the palms of your hands. Keeping your fingers interlaced, put the palms of your hands behind your head so that they cup the base of your skull.

Then, keeping your head pointed straight forward, with the base of your skull still in the palms of your hands, move (only) your eyes so they are looking as far as you can to the right and keep them that way. You may find that you have to sigh, swallow, or yawn. You may even feel an emotional letting go. This will tell you that the nerve on that side has reset. No need to hold your gaze to the right for more than sixty seconds.

Then, still keeping your head aimed forward, look straight ahead of you for a few seconds. Then repeat the above, shifting your gaze all the way to the left.

That's it. If you had an abnormal uvula lift test, it may now have normalized. You may find that you have increased your range of motion in turning your head from side to side or a change in your breathing pattern. Get up slowly the first few times, as it is not uncommon to have brief dizziness. This is caused by your nervous system relaxing after the release.

Rosenberg finds that this technique can be very helpful for numerous conditions beyond fibromyalgia, including:

- Migraines that occur on only one side of the head (followed by massaging the trigger points associated with your headache's pain distribution)
- Anxiety
- Phobias
- Depression
- Bipolar-manic (this is sympathetic/adrenaline chain activation/depression dorsal vagal "freeze" mode)
- Autism spectrum disorder (begin with the allergy elimination technique called NAET at www.naet.com and the Listening Project tools at www.integratedlistening.com)

Mind-Body-Spirit (MBS) and Pain

How does MBS interplay with pain? Although there are many factors, an especially critical one in CFS/FMS can be understood fairly simply. We have talked about what happens when the nervous system freezes, but in addition, your muscles and the fascia tissue that encases them tighten up like a suit of armor when your body goes into a hyper-alert and numb mode. This mode persists until you do something very critical to reset the system and release the muscles and fascia.

Wondering what that is? It's simple.

You need to "shake it off." Use the trembling technique discussed below, based on *Waking the Tiger*.

In humans, after a severe trauma or even years of trauma, it is critical that the freeze state be shaken off with trembling. People often feel silly when the trembling comes to the surface, so they suppress it, leaving them in the freeze state for decades, with tight muscles and being numb when hyper-alert.

The trembling technique is very simple—and free. Being aware of this, you may find that times come up when you feel like trembling. Simply let it happen. Explain it beforehand to your spouse or family so they don't get frightened when it happens. If you're out in public, it's okay to suppress it. It will come up again later when you are by yourself.

After each wave of trembling, you'll find that your muscles feel looser, and you feel calmer and less numb. Once in a while, you may even have a mental snapshot of the trauma that is being released. Because most of us carry numerous traumas, this may go on over several years, releasing the traumas in layers. But over time, the trembling may last for just a few seconds and be very mild. You'll find that you look forward to them.

This trembling releases both the muscles and the fascia. This tightness is the primary pain trigger in most cases of fibromyalgia.

ORTHOSTATIC INTOLERANCE AND AUTONOMIC DYSFUNCTION

Our autonomic nervous system controls blood pressure, pulse, sweating, and gut function along with numerous other processes. Many of you find that you have trouble with these including low blood pressure. See Chapter 14 for more information on this.

The antidote? Activating the ventral vagus nerve and triggering a feeling of safety.

HEALING PTSD AND EMOTIONAL TRAUMA

Severe traumas triggering post-traumatic stress disorder (PTSD) are all too common in fibromyalgia. This requires a stepwise approach for healing.

COUNSELING
Your first step toward healing should of course be counseling with a mental health professional. Although this lays a helpful and necessary foundation for healing, for most people it is nowhere near enough. This is because although it helps the mind come to terms with things, it does not affect the other key components of the problem. So the next step is to add in the trembling technique.

THE TREMBLING TECHNIQUE
You may want to follow up on the trembling technique by reading Dr. Levine's later book *Healing Trauma*. For those of you with PTSD or other severe traumas, Dr. Levine also has a wonderful approach called the Somatic Experiencing program (www.traumahealing.org). The website can give you more information on this and how to find practitioners. I highly recommend it. After beginning work on your own with the trembling technique, add EFT.

EFT (EMOTIONAL FREEDOM TECHNIQUE)

This technique uses "tapping" and the acupressure system. It makes no sense in our Western model, yet it is dramatically effective for people clinically. It helps them release the emotional energy of old traumas in under twenty minutes. There have been a number of studies published on this.

My wife introduced me to EFT. I would see people with horrible traumas and depressed quiet affects walk into her treatment room. Fifteen minutes later, I would routinely hear intense giggling as the person wondered where their decades of trauma disappeared to. I understood when I finally tried it myself.

Words can't really explain it. You simply need to do it and see for yourself.

Fibromyalgia was treated effectively in a randomized controlled trial of EFT. Roughly one-third recovered completely. Study author Gunilla Brattberg, MD, and Dawson Church, PhD, author of *The EFT Manual*, incorporated these in a new twelve-week program called FibroClear. The details are at https://fibroclear.com/yes/. I invite you to watch EFT videos with Brad Yates on YouTube and do the technique on your own along with the video, though it is more effective working with a practitioner. Search online for one near you. This is also a simple technique for therapists to learn so they can apply it with their clients directly. Both the trembling and the tapping techniques are synergistic and can dramatically enhance the effectiveness of talk therapy. They are fairly low cost and easy to learn. And these three steps are where I would begin.

But what about severe cases that need even more?

Here's a possibility that may sound a bit controversial, but is very hopeful. It involves government-registered research currently underway using MDMA (the street drug ecstasy) in a controlled setting. There is no counseling done during the four to five hours of drug effect. Rather, the person simply is lying in a comfortable position in a quiet room wearing a blindfold and headphones playing calming music.

Doing this, they quickly process their traumatic experiences on their own during the sessions. In the study setting, the psychiatrist running the study is quietly present. In speaking with my friend Scott Shannon, MD, the psychiatrist who is a principal investigator on the study, the preliminary findings are quite dramatic.

Ketamine, which can be given intravenously or intranasally, has also been useful. While the pharmaceutical industry is charging $800 per dose for ketamine (Esketamine) used in treating refractory depression, compounding pharmacists can make the drug in a 10 percent solution for just a few dollars per dose. The main limitation is the requirement to have someone with you to assist in case you have an uncomfortable psychological reaction. These are unusual with MDMA, but more common with ketamine.

As with most illnesses, combining the art and science, treating both the psychological and physical, are what works best for deep and long-lasting recovery.

In Conclusion

Just like treating the body, a holistic comprehensive approach works best for treating the mind and spirit. Begin by learning to set your boundaries by saying no to things that feel bad, so you can start the journey to feeling safe again or perhaps for the first time in your life.

See a mental health professional if you feel this would be helpful. Use the trembling technique to release the muscle memory of the traumas and EFT to release the emotional energy. Then as needed, activate the ventral vagal part of your nervous system, which stimulates the feeling of safety.

Historically, a number of cultural approaches have been used to activate the ventral vagal, for example tai chi, meditation and prayer, and pranayama (yogic breathing). Social activities such as chatting, small talk, or having a meal or a cup of coffee with someone are also important and helpful. Choose to spend the time with people who you feel good being around. And as with any chronic condition, don't talk about your illness unless they ask. Otherwise, after a while friends may get tired of this being the key topic of conversation and may start to disappear. Also, when you are with friends, that is a good time to be shifting your own attention away from your illness.

Improvement of the CFS and fibromyalgia symptoms above combined with feeling safer, feeling more vibrant and more playful, having decreased sensitivities, and having your facial features and vocal tone be more "alive" will tell you that you have shifted into the "feeling safe" part of the nervous system. You will find this leaves you feeling so much better. It also allows the permanent part of your healing process to begin.

PART FIVE

How to Proceed and Resources

How to Proceed—Made Simple

You now have far more expertise than the vast majority of physicians for treating day-to-day fatigue and pain as well as CFS and fibromyalgia. This doesn't mean that you're expected to have my forty-plus years of experience doing so. This part is included in my two quizzes below.

My goal has always been to make optimal health as accessible and easy as possible. With my new consultation appointments taking three hours of my one-on-one time, and millions of people with the illness, this presented a challenge for making effective treatment available to everyone. My answer?

I obtained the first US patent for a computerized physician, so that everybody could get the care they need. I programmed over twenty years of experience into a computer algorithm, which analyzes symptoms and labs to determine the cause of the energy drain and tailors a regimen to each person to address these.

Initially, we charged people $400 to use the program, but we told people they could use it for free if they couldn't afford it. Some 80 percent of people wrote back that they were financially devastated by the illness. So my wife and I decided to make the online program available free to everybody.

This program has morphed into the Energy Analysis Program and Tune-Up Docs quizzes.

For those of you with CFS or fibromyalgia, your first steps will be to tailor a program to optimize your energy production and eliminate your energy leaks. This can be done in ten to fifteen minutes by doing the free Energy Analysis Program at www.energyanalysisprogram.com. This simple quiz can analyze your symptoms and even your key lab tests, if available (but they are not critical). It will then determine the key areas that need to be addressed to optimize energy and tailor a protocol for doing so. This addresses, evaluates, and organizes the key areas discussed in this book, so you don't have to figure it out on your own. You may find that this is all you need to get your life back.

For those you who simply have day-to-day fatigue or pain, do the free Tune-Up Docs quiz at www.tuneupdocs.com (see also Chapter 7).

There are often many things that can help, but you can start to have dramatic improvement with just a few simple steps. For everyone, I would begin with:

1. The Energy Revitalization System vitamin powder plus the Smart Energy System. This single drink and two capsules will usually result in marked improvements after just one month.
2. If you are having trouble sleeping, start with the Revitalizing Sleep Formula and/or Terrific Zzzz.
3. If you're having pain, add in the Curamin. Combining these with the Hemp Select capsules and End Pain can add further benefits. Give these six weeks to see the full effect. Then the doses can often be lowered.

These products can all be found at www.endfatigue.com.

If your symptoms are severe, add in four capsules of Recovery Factors twice a day. This can be found at www.recoveryfactors.com. You will know if this is helping within six weeks, and usually after just five to seven days. The effects are often dramatic.

Then add in the other recommended options from your quiz results. Simply start with the areas that feel most important to you. For the prescriptions, take the printout results to your holistic physician. They will be much more likely to be familiar with these and open to prescribing them.

You can find yourself feeling dramatically better—very quickly!

Finding a Holistic Physician

BFF Summary

1. Don't expect most physicians to be familiar with fibromyalgia. Holistic physicians have far more expertise with this.
2. See the websites below to find a holistic practitioner in your area.
3. I do in-person and phone CFS/FMS consults with people worldwide. For information, email Sarah at appointments@endfatigue.com.

People ask me how they can talk their doctor into giving them the treatments they need. In most cases, the answer is that you can't. Most doctors, appropriately enough, will not do the things that they are not properly trained in. This does not make them bad physicians. If you came to me and said, "Dr. Teitelbaum, I would like you to do a heart bypass operation on me," I would say, "I'm sorry, I am not trained in that, and I can't." If you then gave me a copy of a book called *The Bypass Solution* and a scalpel, well, you still would not want me performing surgery on you. This would not make me a bad physician, and your doctor's not treating you for CFS/FMS or fatigue does not make them a bad physician, either. The best thing to do is to go to a holistic physician who specializes in treating these complex problems.

Most physicians who know how to help fatigue and CFS/FMS patients are considered holistic. These doctors usually have advanced training in using natural therapies and spend a lot of time exploring the scientific literature. They also allow the much longer visits needed to treat these problems.

Unfortunately, most insurance companies will pay well for procedures and surgery but not for a physician to spend time working with the patient. Basically, they often pay less than the physician's overhead for time spent, if you spend more than ten minutes with the person. They also don't cover natural therapies. Because of this, most physicians who can effectively deal with these illnesses cannot participate in insurance. Fortunately, the biggest expense is for lab testing and medications, which are often covered by insurance. So even though the cost to see the physician won't be covered by your insurance, many of the other costs may be.

WHEN LOOKING FOR A PHYSICIAN, CONSIDER THE FOLLOWING QUESTIONS

1. Do they specialize in treating fatigue, CFS, and FMS and recognize these as real and physical conditions?
2. Will they prescribe the medications needed for you to get eight hours of sleep a night?
3. Do they use bioidentical hormones based on your symptoms, even if the tests are normal?
4. Will they treat for candida with Diflucan for six weeks?

If the answer to these four questions is yes, you have a physician who is likely to be able to help you.

Not able to afford a non-insurance-covered holistic physician? Check with your family doctor first to see if they would be open to prescribing some of the recommended treatments. Don't begin by going to them with a list of fifteen things. Pick one or two of them, such as the sleep medications. Most will be open to any of the sleep treatments except perhaps the Ambien. Then at each visit, you can ask them for one or two more.

Most, unfortunately, will not be open to treating infections or hormonal problems that can't be clearly tested for unless you fall in the lowest 2 percent of the population, making the test they use abnormal. Basically, their training has taught them that a size 6 shoe, being in the normal range, should fit everybody, so for infections and hormonal problems you will need a holistic physician. Such a doctor will treat the person and not only the blood test.

A good place to find physicians familiar with treating CFS and fibromyalgia is www.vitality101.com/find-practitioners. This lists physicians who have at least done an eight-hour training course in treating these conditions.

In general, you will find that naturopaths (NDs) are far more familiar with and open to these treatments. More and more states are rejecting the pressure from the medical monopoly and appropriately granting naturopaths the right to diagnose and prescribe. Soon this will be the case in most states. For day-to-day fatigue and pain, I would start here.

Be aware, however, that almost anyone can call themselves a naturopath, so be sure you go to one trained by an accredited naturopathic college.

Find a Holistic Physician

Holistic doctors are much more likely to know how to help CFS/FMS patients. More and more states are recognizing naturopaths' rights to prescribe medications as well as natural therapies. To find a holistic doctor near you, I recommend the following organizations:

- American Academy of Naturopathic Physicians (AANP): www.naturopathic.org. Check here for a list of naturopathic physicians with four-year advanced training.
- American College for Advancement in Medicine (ACAM): www.acam.org.
- The Institute of Functional Medicine Website: www.ifm.org. Click on "Find a Practitioner."

WOULD YOU LIKE A CONSULTATION WITH DR. TEITELBAUM?

I consult both in person and by phone, treating people with CFS, fibromyalgia, and severe fatigue worldwide. My new patient visits are three hours of my one-on-one time, which allows me to prescribe and manage your care.

In addition, I offer ninety-minute "executive tune-ups" by phone for those who would like to optimize their energy and vitality. These visits really can help make fifty be the new thirty.

For more information, email Sarah at appointments@endfatigue.com.

My Favorite CFS/FMS Journalist

Want to stay up-to-date on the newest and most important CFS/FMS research and treatments?

Check out Cort Johnson's work at www.healthrising.org.

He operates this site on a shoestring with support from reader donations. If you're looking to get the most bang for your buck to help people with CFS and fibromyalgia, I suggest people donate to him.

Getting $800 Million in CFS/FMS Research Funding in One Minute; Feel Powerless in Affecting Our Government?

BFF Summary

Want to get CFS/FMS funded the way it should be?
Wish your government represented you, and not only the very wealthy? You can do this in under a minute.

1. Go to www.oneminutefix.org and sign the petition.
2. Share the website and petition with your friends.

This is simple yet powerful. And it really will work!

CFS/FMS is the Cinderella stepchild of modern medicine. People with this illness are often too crippled to make their voices heard. Instead, other health conditions get the research funding, in large part because their advocacy organizations are sponsored by pharmaceutical companies that make billions of dollars in profits yearly treating those illnesses.

Sadly put, money decides how our politicians vote. Before you go blaming them, consider that we have created a system where each politician needs to raise as much as $40 million a year in bribes (which we call campaign contributions) to get a $200,000-a-year job. So it is not surprising that research shows they spend 60 percent of their time sucking up to wealthy corporations. And I suspect most of the rest of their time paying them back.

But what if you could fix it in one minute, and get the $800 million a year in research funding we deserve? You can—easily! There is a simple "one-minute fix" for this problem. And it *can* easily get us the $800 million a year in research funding CFS and fibromyalgia deserve, based on the numbers of people affected and the severity of the illness.

Even though the NIH has now determined that the disease is biological, funding has yet to catch up. Between 2015 and 2018, the agency allocated a yearly average of a little less than $11 million to CFS, which is

a tiny sum for medical research. The agency gave more funding to tuber-
ous sclerosis, a rare genetic disorder that affects fewer than forty thousand
Americans, and to osteogenesis imperfecta, a brittle-bone disease, which
affects some twenty thousand.

By comparison, it spends $3 billion on HIV/AIDS research (which,
like CFS, affects about a million Americans). Dr. Mariela Shirley, an official at the NIH Office of Research on Women's Health, says funding is
determined by the number of researchers in a field, their experience in
competing for NIH funding, and other factors.

One of those key factors is whether politicians care. Here's how you
can make them care. A lot. *And it will take you just one minute and cost you
nothing.*

WHAT IS THE "ONE-MINUTE FIX"
FOR OUR BROKEN GOVERNMENT?

Sadly, research shows that the public's preferences (and thus our country's
well-being) have virtually no impact on how our representatives vote. This
is because approximately 70 percent of the $3 billion yearly needed to win
the presidency or a congressional seat comes from larger donations. This
means our representative form of government no longer functions across a
wide array of issues, including CFS/FMS and natural health funding.

There is a simple solution. We call it the one-minute fix.

Here is our proposal:

Each adult citizen would get to direct $100 per year *of the govern-
ment's money* to the candidates of their choice. People could simply go
online and direct which candidates their $100 yearly allowance would go
to. This would be simple. A box could pop up saying "Hi, you have $88
left for 2021." From a drop-down box, you would click on the candidate(s)
you choose and note how much goes to each. It would go directly from the
treasury to the candidate—and it would cost you nothing. Any candidate
who has registered at any level of government to run for the upcoming
election (or the previous one) would be eligible to receive the money.

This would create a healthy check and balance to the power of large
donors. Politicians on both sides of the aisle will support it because they
want the money. And most would rather work for the public.

The media gets this money in new advertising, increasing the likeli-
hood of their support.

This combination can make it happen, but only if the idea can get attention. Given the above, we are hoping that one hundred thousand signatures on a petition would get the media's and then the politicians' attention. Again, because it serves both. We hope to get these signatures through Facebook and Instagram campaigns—and with your help.

About six million Americans suffer with CFS/FMS or related conditions, and they and their family members are highly motivated to find a cure. So if even just one family member joins them, that is twelve million people with the potential to control $1.2 billion a year in campaign contributions. This is over four times what the entire pharmaceutical industry pays to control our government. I guarantee you it will get the politicians' attention, and they will be falling all over each other to guarantee the proper level of research funding for CFS/FMS.

For those of you without CFS/FMS, wouldn't it be nice to get our government back and have our politicians actually represent *us* instead of a few very wealthy industries?

All you need to do to make it happen is:

1. Go to www.oneminutefix.org and sign the petition.
2. Share the website with your friends and social media network.

One minute of your time could equal $800 million a year of CFS/FMS research funding. Please go to the website right now, sign the petition, and share it with your social media friends. Please ask them to share it, too. Then please come back and continue reading.

Sourcing Supplements

BFF Summary

1. I am very picky about what supplements I recommend—and for very good reason.
2. The brands I recommend can be found at thousands of health-food stores and online.
3. Many can also be found at www.endfatigue.com.

As you've noticed, I'm often specific about what supplements I recommend. I've found that this is necessary for people to get the correct ones that actually work. But almost everything I recommend is readily available at thousands of health-food stores and online sources.

Want to make it easy while also supporting my goal of making effective treatment available for everyone? Start by going to www.endfatigue .com. My website has dozens of supplements, which I've picked from the best companies. We also have great prices, including a large auto-ship discount (for products that allow it). I picked the products based on both the science and what we have found works for thousands of people. And I thank you for your patronage and supporting my work!

Financial Transparency

I consider transparency about finances to be very important, especially for assessing health information. I would love to see it extend to politics and elsewhere as well. In this spirit, I am happy to supply the information below.

As part of my dedication to promoting your health, I have a policy of not taking money from any pharmaceutical company. My royalties for products I've designed, and the fees for consulting I currently receive from natural product companies also go directly to a tax-exempt foundation. This foundation has many goals, including especially supplying the public access to optimal and accurate natural and overall health information, supporting research on natural therapies, as well as addressing issues such as childhood hunger internationally.

I donate my time for the foundation and outreach work, so about two-thirds of my workweek is unpaid or minimally paid.

I support myself and the work I do financially by my work treating people twelve hours a week as a physician and from website sales (www .endfatigue.com) of products from numerous companies that I find especially helpful. These products are readily available from numerous health-food stores and online sources. Purchasing from my website does help support me in the work I do, and I thank you!

I also personally produce two products, SHINE D-Ribose and Dr. Teitelbaum's Smart Energy System, which help support me, my work, and my outreach programs. At the time of this writing, I am also running two studies on a new supplement called Recovery Factors, which has shown dramatic promise for people with fibromyalgia. I will likely also personally be financially involved with that company.

Surviving Prescription Costs

BFF Summary

1. You can save as much as 95 percent by using the free GoodRx phone app (or at www .goodrx.com).
2. Costco also has excellent prescription prices.
3. Most medications charge by the pill, rather than by the amount in the pill. So getting a pill that's twice the strength and splitting it in half can save 50 percent.
4. For those with low income and no prescription insurance, helpful information on patient assistance programs through the pharmaceutical companies can be found at www.goodrx.com/blog/what-are-patient-assistance-programs/.

Sadly, because the pharmaceutical industry largely owns our elected representatives, our free market system no longer works for medications. If you doubt that they own our government, consider this: Our government is the largest purchaser of medications in the world. Virtually every other government in the world uses their buying power to negotiate prices down as much as 95 percent, as do most health insurance companies.

But "our" representatives voted to make it illegal for our government to negotiate prices with the pharmaceutical industry, requiring us to basically pay whatever they choose to charge. Perhaps this has something to do with the pharmaceutical industry being one of the largest campaign donors in the country? I'll leave that for you to figure out. Please read the section on the one-minute fix for how we can solve this (page 320).

But here's how you can save as much as 95 percent right now.

With the pharmaceutical industry basically making up insane prices, many local pharmacies have decided to cash in on the phenomenon as well. Because of this, prices for the exact same pill often vary by over 1,000 percent from pharmacy to pharmacy.

So, if you don't have health insurance to negotiate for you, you are basically on your own.

Unless you know this simple trick. There is a free app called GoodRx that gets you the insurance-negotiated prices. They will also tell you the exact cost that you would pay at the pharmacies near you, and you can show the GoodRx coupon on your phone at the pharmacy to get the negotiated price. You can also print out the coupons and get the prices at www.goodrx.com.

Try it. You'll be amazed.

Another excellent option is to simply go to Costco. Their pharmacy offers some of the lowest prices. Another trick? You don't have to be a Costco member to use the pharmacy. Simply let the person at the door asking for your membership card know that you're going to the pharmacy. They will smile and wave you right in.

For those of you without prescription insurance coverage who have low incomes (common in CFS/FMS), many, if not most, of the medications you'll need may be supplied for free by the drug companies. For more information on this important option, go to www.goodrx.com/blog/what-are-patient-assistance-programs/.

I will note that for me and my family, I virtually always use the generic medications. There are a few cases where some people find they don't work as well, and feel free to go with the brand name if you need to do so and are able to pony up the money.

Another great trick? Unlike most things where you pay more for larger sizes, this is not the case for medications. If milk were a medication, you would pay the same for gallon as for a pint. So if you get a larger size pill and simply break it in half, you save 50 percent. Break it in quarters and you can save 75 percent. So a simple $5 pill cutter can save you big bucks.

A Thought on Costs

Generic Ambien costs about 10 cents a pill versus $3 for the brand name—and works every bit as well. This is the case for most medications when generics are available. Although there are unusual cases where the brand name works better, usually the price difference just reflects drug company profits. Personally, and for my family, I go with the generic options when available. Use the free GoodRx phone app to get the best prices on medications. Otherwise, if you are going in without insurance, you may be charged $300 for the same medication that costs $10 with the app. Costco also has excellent prescription prices, and you don't need to be a member to use their pharmacy.

Also realize that for most medications you pay by the pill, not by the medication strength. So you would pay the same price for a 5- or 10-milligram tablet. This means you can often save 50 percent by simply getting a higher dose and breaking the pill in half.

Would You Like My Brain in Your Pocket?

BFF Summary

The Cures A–Z phone app (free, with an optional $2 upgrade) is a natural owner's manual for your body. It will give you a short and simple summary of how to use the best of natural and prescription therapies to address over one hundred conditions.

Ever wish that the human body came with an owner's manual? Especially one geared toward natural options?

Now it does.

I have spent over forty years researching, writing, and teaching about natural alternatives. In the process, I have critically reviewed tens of thousands of studies and explored the full healthcare tool kit beyond the biochemistry (nutrition, herbals, and pharmaceuticals), including structural, energy, and mind-body-spirit healing.

I have now distilled this lifetime of work into a free phone app (there is a $2 upgrade available). Understanding that pain and disease are our body's way of saying that it needs something, this app tells you what it is. A great way to save forty years of having to scour the scientific literature yourself.

Basically, this app is like having my brain in your pocket—just a lot less messy.

This amazing app gives you the information needed for numerous health conditions summarized in seconds, and the information needed to apply it immediately.

You'll find yourself using this priceless app routinely through the day, looking up hundreds of conditions—from A to Z.

Getting Disability Approved When Needed

Denise Haire handles the disability claims for the 15 percent of people I treat whom we can't get well enough to return to work. She has become a master at this, so I asked her to write this section.

GETTING DISABILITY BENEFITS APPROVED

by Denise Haire

Filing for disability can be a challenge without proper guidance. There are several types of disability benefits that can be obtained, and here's a breakdown of each:

- **SSDI (Social Security Disability Insurance):** This disability benefit is for people that have worked and paid taxes into the Social Security system for years prior to becoming disabled. This benefit does not look at assets.
- **SSI (Supplemental Security Income):** This is a needs-based benefit for those who may not meet the work history criteria for SSDI but who have a qualifying medical condition. Qualifying for this benefit does look at your income and total assets.
- **STD (Short-Term Disability):** This benefit is given through an employer and is paid by a benefits company for a predetermined period of time depending on your employer's plan. This requires a medical condition that impacts the ability to work.
- **LTD (Long-Term Disability):** This benefit is also through an employer and paid by a benefits company if you still need benefits when your STD time frame runs out. For the first two years, you will need to prove that you cannot perform your specific work duties. After the initial two

years, you will be required to prove that you cannot perform any type of employment.

Since employer-sponsored plans can vary from plan to plan, we will focus on Social Security Disability Insurance benefits. However, much of the same information can be applied to the STD and LTD process.

It is important to understand that applying for Social Security benefits can take time and most claims are denied for the initial review. Approval is more likely if you can learn everything you can about the process, the Social Security definitions and descriptions of your medical condition, and the role your functional limitations play in the process.

Your initial step will be to apply for benefits and this can be done online at www.ssa.gov. You will be able to save information and come back to your application, so no need to complete this in one sitting. Be sure to list any medical providers whom you have seen throughout your experience with your illness who you feel will have evidence of your symptoms, your testing history, and hopefully your inability to work.

Social Security will first review your work history to determine if you meet the work criteria based on the date of onset of your disabling condition or when you had to leave work. SSA looks back ten years from the date of onset. To qualify for SSDI benefits, you will need approximately twenty hours per week during this ten-year period.

For any time past your date of onset that you list, you cannot have worked over the substantial gainful activity (SGA) amount or they will consider you employed during that time frame and use this as part of your ten-year look back. Currently, the SGA amount for non-blind individuals is $1,220 per month and for blind individuals is $2,040 per month.

If your work history qualifies for SSDI benefits, your claim will be transferred to a medical review department for evaluation of your medical condition. If you do not meet the work requirements, you will be considered for SSI benefits and will need to undergo the income and asset review before your claim is transferred for medical review. Generally, making under $1,600 per month currently with no assets will qualify for decreased SSI benefits, but the financial review is a complicated process and might be better determined by looking at an online calculator for SSI benefits. Take a look at the website www.disabilitysecrets.com and do a search for "income limits and SSI disability eligibility" for more details. This site is a great resource in general for information regarding filing for benefits.

Once your claim is sent for medical review for either SSDI or SSI benefits, two key factors will be considered. The first is your (in their view) "alleged illness or diagnosis" based on objective evidence. Objective evidence is any testing or assessment that can measure your condition such as blood work, X-rays, CT scans, and MRIs. I will also use accredited definitions as objective measures—for example, the CDC or Institute of Medicine definition of CFS and the American College of Rheumatology definition of fibromyalgia. I will also use SSA's own rulings for CFS and fibromyalgia as objective evidence. These are outlined below for you.

You will need to have evidence in your medical records that shows that you indeed have the alleged conditions that interfere with your ability to work. This should be a combination of tests that confirm your illness and the medical history that shows that you've been trying to get help for your condition. I will provide more details about specific conditions later. If your records are lacking or SSA feels that there are not enough current records, they will request that you be seen by an independent medical examiner. These are physicians that are contracted by SSA but are, in theory, third-party examiners and have no stake in your claim. Additionally, if you list conditions such as anxiety or depression on your application but do not list any mental health providers for records, SSA will send you for a psychological independent medical review. For any independent medical exam, request a copy of the practitioner's report before your appointment through the SSA contact. This will more likely give you a chance to receive a copy within a reasonable time frame, while waiting until after the appointment can take several months to get a response.

The second determining factor is your functional capacity level or your physical and mental limitations. You will need to be able to show that the condition you have limits your ability to function either physically, mentally, or both to a degree that does not allow you to work. This is typically the more challenging thing to prove. Most practitioner visit notes do not include information regarding functional capacity, so be sure you are discussing your limitations with your providers and that they are documenting this for you. For example, if you can only perform simple tasks like making a snack or you need to take breaks to perform simple household chores, have your physicians document this. Here are some additional examples:

- Fatigue keeps me from concentrating and focusing on any type of paperwork, including forms. I need help with this type of work.

- Fatigue interferes with my ability to stand or walk for more than a few minutes before I need to take a break.
- Pain keeps me from sitting at a desk for longer than ten to fifteen minutes because it worsens the pain in my back, head, and neck.
- I can only manage one activity per day or week like an appointment or church and then I have to rest.
- I am homebound most of the time except for very short trips to the grocery store, about ten to fifteen minutes.
- I rely on my family for driving longer distances or I rely on my family for driving any distances.
- I need assistance getting into and out of the car because of my muscle pain and weakness.

Be sure your physician fills out a functional capacity form, such as the one that is used by SSA, to determine limitations. A form like this completed by your physician, or several physicians if possible, will be helpful for providing functional information to SSA.

The hope is that the functional information that is provided is consistent with the medical evidence and alleged illness. The more consistency that you can show, the stronger your claim will be. This will require communication with your providers so they are on the same page if they are completing a functional form for you. You don't want one form to show one level of limitations and another form to show a completely different level. Make sure your physicians understand the degree of your limitations and your complete medical condition. For example, if you have post-exertional fatigue and malaise that requires several hours or even days of rest after a trip to your doctor's office, it is important that all of your providers completing this form are aware of this. I recommend having your doctors send you a copy of the form to review before it is sent to SSA. Even better would be if they allow you to complete the form and they can review and sign it if they agree.

Other things that have no medical weight but can be helpful to help show your functional limits are listed below. Unless you clearly meet one of the SSA blue book listings, you will be denied during the initial review. Because of this, I typically recommend that supporting information for functional limitations is saved for the first level of appeal, but this is ultimately up to you. Otherwise, my thought is that it will be overlooked.

- **Personal letters:** These can be written by family members, friends, employers, coworkers, etc. Anyone who has seen your change in abilities can write a letter for you. This does not require any medical information but merely what changes the person has observed prior to your illness and then after. They will want to address how the illness has changed your abilities or how it has affected your life. Even a change in social life is taken under consideration, so have someone include this information as well.
- **Daily journal:** Try to keep a daily journal of your activities to include for your appeal to show exactly what your day entails. This will give the SSA examiners a better picture of exactly what you can and cannot do.
- **Activity forms:** I've included an example of an activity form to include as part of your claim. Again, this is likely better to include as part of your first level of appeal.

To take a closer look at the medical review, let's look at SSA's descriptions of certain conditions. Fortunately, SSA provides descriptions of some illnesses that can be used to help with your claim. SSA has impairment listings that they consider their blue book of impairments. If you meet the criteria for these, medically and functionally, you will automatically be approved.

Keep in mind that you will still need to provide evidence that you meet this description from your medical records. You can view the blue book listing of impairments at www.ssa.gov/disability/professionals/bluebook/Adult Listings.htm. For CFS and FMS, you will likely fall under listings such as 1.00 Musculoskeletal System, 11.00 Neurological Disorders, or 14.00 Immune System Disorders. Each listing details the testing that is required and the functional barriers required. Many times you may not meet a specific listing exactly, but you can prove that your condition is just as disabling as a certain listing. For example, someone with CFS may have some immune dysfunction but will not meet the 14.00 testing criteria, but they can show that their illness with marked immune dysfunction including recurrent infections or infections with long recovery periods are equivalent to impairment listing 14.07 Immune Deficiency Disorders, excluding HIV infection.

For CFS and fibromyalgia, you can also show that you meet the SSA criteria for these illnesses (listed below for you) as well as the CDC definition of CFS and the Institute of Medicine definition of CFS. For fibromyalgia you will want to show that you meet the SSA criteria for fibromyalgia and the

American College of Rheumatology definition. Below I've included a sample letter that supports the existence of a disabling condition based on the SSA rulings.

SSA ruling SSR 14-1p uses the old CDC definition of Chronic Fatigue Syndrome, which states that CFS is the presence of persistent or relapsing fatigue that is of new or definite onset, cannot be explained by another illness, is not the result of ongoing exertion, and is not relieved by rest and results in the substantial reduction in previous levels of activities. Additionally, you must have 4 or more of the following diagnostic symptoms:

- Post-exertional malaise
- Self-reported impairment in short-term memory or concentration
- Sore throat
- Tender lymph nodes
- Muscle pain
- Multi-joint pain without swelling or redness
- Headaches of a new type
- Waking unrefreshed

Other symptoms include:

- Muscle weakness
- Disturbed sleep patterns
- Visual difficulties
- Orthostatic intolerance
- Respiratory difficulties
- Cardiovascular abnormalities
- Gastrointestinal discomfort
- Urinary or bladder problems

Recommended testing based on the SSA ruling SSR 14-1p on CFS includes the following tests, which will show that the infections that are typically associated with CFS are positive and can be used as objective evidence:

- Epstein-Barr virus, HHV-6, CMV, mycoplasma pneumoniae, or deficiencies of immunoglobulin G (total IgG and subclasses 1, 2, 3, and 4). These immunoglobulin deficiencies are very common in CFS/FMS and can offer objective evidence, so they may be very helpful during the appeals process.

- If you are likely dealing with immune dysfunction or an immune deficiency, I would also consider running a test for pneumonia titers to be able to show low immunity to the pneumonia bacteria.

SSA ruling 12-2p outlines the definition of fibromyalgia and directs examiners to use the 1990 or 2010 American College of Rheumatology's criteria:

- Evidence of chronic widespread pain that has lasted for more than three months that cannot be explained by another illness.
- Tender points in at least eleven of eighteen tender points (old ACR criteria), *or*
- Repeated occurrences of six or more co-occurring symptoms such as cognitive or memory problems, insomnia, depression, anxiety, IBS, headaches, muscle weakness, abdominal pain, dizziness, etc. (For a full list, see www.rheumatology.org. Note: ACR updated its criteria for fibromyalgia in 2016, but SSA continues to use the previous definitions at this time.)

Recommended objective measures based on the SSA ruling 12-2p for fibromyalgia include the following:

- Widespread Pain Index
- Symptom Severity score (see page 171 for these fibromyalgia diagnostic criteria)
- Abnormal lab findings such as an elevated sedimentation rate, which documents inflammation (even though this test is usually low in fibromyalgia)
- Any X-rays or scans that may show some abnormalities

For disabilities that took place much earlier than the date you are applying for benefits, it is possible to use the earlier onset date, but this does provide more of a challenge to get approval. Fortunately, SSA also has a ruling for this type of situation. Please see SSR 18-1p for the full ruling, but here are some highlights. SSA must consider the following when determining the date of onset of your disability:

- Applicant Allegations: statement as to when the disability began.
- Work History: the date the impairment caused work stoppage.

- Medical and Other Evidence: medical records to support diagnosis and condition currently as well as at the time of onset.
- Additionally, SSA is required to make the appropriate inferences grounded in the current condition, the nature of the illness, and the reasonable presumptions that can be made about the course of the illness. In other words, does your current condition based on what we know about the illness make it reasonable to assume that you could have been disabled at the alleged time of onset?
- This is where personal letters can also be helpful if they can support changes in your functional levels that took place at or around a specific time or date.

To summarize for you:

- Use www.disabilitysecrets.com as a resource.
- Search www.ssa.gov for specific rulings mentioned above.
- Make sure your medical records have the necessary objective evidence discussed above.
- Discuss your functional limits with your physicians and ask them to document in your records.
- Apply online at ssa.gov.
- List practitioners that will have medical evidence of your diagnosis and functional limits.
- Be prepared to be denied after your initial review.
- Use specifics from the SSA rulings for your appeal letter.

Below you will find resources to use as part of your claim. Good luck and best wishes for approval of your benefits!

Disability Application Sample Letter

Here is a sample letter collated from letters rewritten for several people. It may be helpful for you, your physician, and your disability attorney to copy the parts that are pertinent to your case.

[Doctor's Letterhead]
Date
To Whom It May Concern:

Jane X, DOB XX-XX-XXXX, is a patient of my office who is being treated for a complex condition that includes fibromyalgia (FMS), chronic fatigue syndrome (CFS), mycotoxin toxicity, and likely a suppressed immune system or immune deficiency disorder. Systemic candida, thyroid receptor resistance, and iron deficiency further complicate her condition. My initial assessment of Ms. X included an extensive review of her medical history. Symptoms initially presented in September 2017 after her inability to recover from ongoing mold exposure. At the time of her visit, Ms. X presented with symptoms of daytime fatigue, headaches, insomnia, multi-joint pain, post-exertion malaise, cognitive dysfunction, dizziness, sensitivities to sound and light, chronic dehydration, and low blood pressures. **Ms. X meets the diagnostic criteria for FMS and CFS** and is suffering from a complex form that includes severe hormonal imbalances and complications from infections.

As with most illnesses, determination of disability and degree/severity are assessed by a combination of history and objective findings, as is the case here. **Ms. X has numerous objective and subjective findings supporting her diagnoses as well as the severity of her illness.** These findings include the following:

Evidence of Fibromyalgia

I. **Meets current ACR (American College of Rheumatology) criteria.** ACR states that a patient satisfies the criteria for fibromyalgia when the following three conditions are met:
   A. WPI greater than or equal to 7 and Symptom Severity score greater than or equal to 5, or WPI 3–6 and SS score greater than or equal to 9.
   WPI score = 10
   SS score = 10
   B. Symptoms have been present at a similar level for at least three months.

    C.   The patient does not have a disorder that would otherwise explain the pain.

II. **Meets the CDC definition of fibromyalgia:**
    A.   Widespread pain
    B.   Abnormal pain processing
    C.   Sleep disturbance
    D.   Fatigue

III. **Satisfies the Social Security Agency's criteria for objective evidence of fibromyalgia:**
    A.   SSR-12p considers objective evidence as:
1. History of widespread pain that has persisted for at least three months—the pain may fluctuate in intensity and may not always be present
2. Repeated manifestations of six or more fibromyalgia symptoms, signs, or co-occurring conditions, especially manifestations of fatigue, cognitive or memory problems ("fibro fog"), waking unrefreshed, depression, anxiety disorder, or irritable bowel syndrome
    B.   See Symptom Severity list with *seventeen* associated FMS symptoms.
    C.   Other conditions have been ruled out.

Evidence of Chronic Fatigue Syndrome

I. **Immune dysfunction:** Testing conducted since Ms. X's claim confirms that she is suffering with an immune deficiency with recurrent infections that have resulted in loss of function. She meets the Impairment Listing 14.07C, Immune Deficiency Disorders. Specifically, the attached laboratory reports indicate Common Variable Immune Deficiency and Specific Antibody Deficiency. Testing confirms the following:
    A.   Appropriate laboratory findings/objective evidence:
1. Low total IgG level
2. Low IgG subtype levels
3. Low pneumonia titers
4. Recurrent infections
    a.   Epstein-Barr virus
    b.   Mycoplasma pneumoniae
5. Recurrent infections with longer than normal recovery period

6. Demonstrates that medical laboratory findings show that a medically determinable impairment is present that could reasonably be expected to produce severe loss of function

II. **Hormonal imbalances**
   A. Thyroid receptor resistance
   B. Suboptimal morning cortisol level, consistent with HPA axis suppression from CFS/FMS
   C. Low antidiuretic hormone

III. **Nutritional deficiencies**
   A. Iron deficiency

IV. **Dysautonomia/low blood pressures**
   A. Kunihisa Miwa and Masatoshi Fujita, "Cardiac Function Fluctuates During Exacerbation and Remission in Young Adults with Chronic Fatigue Syndrome and 'Small Heart,'" *Journal of Cardiology* 54, no. 1 (August 2009): 29–35, https://doi.org/10.1016/j.jjcc.2009.02.008.
   B. Julia L. Newton, Amish Sheth, Jane Shin, et al., "Lower Ambulatory Blood Pressure in Chronic Fatigue Syndrome," *Psychosomatic Medicine* 71, no. 3 (April 2009): 361–365, https://doi.org/10.1097/PSY.0b013e31819ccd2a.

V. **Post-exertional fatigue/malaise**
   A. Hallmark of CFS according to CDC definition
   B. Hallmark of CFS according to Institute of Medicine Report, "Beyond Myalgic Encephalomyelitis/Chronic Fatigue Syndrome: Redefining an Illness," February 10, 2015.
   C. Roy Freeman and Anthony L. Komaroff, "Does the Chronic Fatigue Syndrome Involve the Autonomic Nervous System?" *American Journal of Medicine* 102, no. 4 (April 1997): 357–364, https://doi.org/10.1016/s0002-9343(97)00087-9.

VI. **Satisfies the Social Security Agency's criteria for Chronic Fatigue Syndrome**
   A. SSR-14-1p

1. Defines CFS as a "systemic disorder consisting of a complex set of symptoms that may vary in frequency, duration and severity."

    B.   SSR-14-1p, I.B.1
1. Post-exertional fatigue
2. Impairment in short-term memory or concentration
3. Joint pain
4. Waking unrefreshed
5. Tender neck of axillary lymph nodes

    C.   SSR-14-1p, I.B.2
1. Muscle weakness
2. Disrupted sleep patterns

The CDC describes CFS as "a debilitating and complex disorder characterized by intense fatigue that is not improved by bed rest and that may be worsened by physical activity or mental exertion." They continue the definition by explaining that "people with CFS often function at a substantially lower level of activity than they were capable of before they became ill." CDC studies show that CFS can be as disabling as multiple sclerosis, lupus, rheumatoid arthritis, heart disease, end-stage renal disease, and COPD.

Ms. X meets the criteria of CFS and FMS and these limit her functional ability substantially. However, **case law is absolutely clear that a person eligible for disability insurance benefits does not need to be helpless or completely incapacitated.**

Additionally, Ms. X meets the ADA definition of disabled:

Meets ADA Definition of Disability
I. ADA states that "an individual with a disability is a person who has **a physical or mental impairment that substantially limits one or more major life activities**"
II. **Major life activities** that are limited per ADAAA of 2008
    A.   Pain and fatigue limit Ms. X's ability to sustain prolonged activities such as walking, sitting, and standing.
    B.   Ms. X's condition includes sleep that is disrupted by insomnia and pain associated with FMS.

    C.   Cognitive dysfunction interferes with concentration, focus, organi-
         zation, etc.

III. **Major bodily functions** that are limited per ADAA of 2008
    A.   Immune system
    B.   Endocrine system—suboptimal and unstable hormonal levels

I would also like to note that, above and beyond the restrictions and limitations of Ms. X's experiences due to her medical condition, **the side effects from some of her necessary treatments significantly compromise her ability to function/work**. For example, some medications cause unpredictable diarrhea that make it difficult to manage in any type of work environment. Additionally, several medications on Ms. X's treatment protocol designed to alleviate pain or assist with insomnia also cause severe drowsiness. She can experience next-day sedation from her prescribed sleep aids in attempts to achieve improved sleep quality. **This further limits Ms. X, resulting in the inability to think clearly, concentrate, keep up with any type of workflow, on some occasions drive, and even prepare for the workday.** As you are aware, medication side effects can be as disabling as the illness and are **required to be considered by the insurer, see Hertan v. Unum**.

Ms. X's condition demonstrates that **she is suffering from multiple medical conditions that require her claim to be evaluated based on the combined effects of her impairments in total**. Clearly these additional impairments have increased the severity of her overall condition. This combination results in a decrease in Ms. X's ability to function at home and at any type of employment and increases the severity of her impairment.

With respect to functional limitations, as you should be aware, **the 2015 Institute of Medicine report regarding CFS/SEID greatly details post-exertion malaise (PEM)**. Because Ms. X's functional levels are impacted not only by daily pain and fatigue but also PEM, I will elaborate on these particular limitations. In healthy individuals, pain and fatigue are typically resolved with rest. However, **for individuals with PEM like Ms. X, their symptoms are not alleviated by rest and may require several days or more to resolve. To continue the same level of**

exertion will worsen their symptoms of fatigue and pain each consecutive day. Patients with PEM exhibit abnormal reduction in the VO2max greater than folks without this condition. Compared to age/sex matched normal values, VO2max is lower in patients with PEM than inactive females. Additional days of exertion demonstrate that the VO2max in these patients continues to lower. VO2max refers to the maximum work capacity. Research also shows that when experiencing PEM, maximum work capacity cannot be sustained for more than several minutes and individuals would be unable to sustain routine activities long enough to finish the task. It is critical that when doing exercise testing, the first day's test not be relied on. Rather the test should be repeated twenty-four hours later, and only the second test should be used. This has been documented in the scientific literature as essential in diagnosing and documenting CFS and fibromyalgia.

In other words, **patients with PEM exhibit a drop in VO2max due to metabolic anomalies. Days of consecutive testing provide a measure of functional decrement experienced by patients who report symptoms of PEM.** Additionally, when fatigued, a person with PEM will have an even lower threshold for physical activity. Similar testing of patients with PEM who were challenged cognitively resulted in post-exertion symptom exacerbation following mental effort. It was determined that working environments that present cognitive demands would not be recommended for these individuals. Cognitive demands include tasks such as scheduling, organizing, following directions, decision making, focus, following conversations, etc.

Ms. X's current condition makes it difficult for her to perform household tasks and activities of daily living (ADLs) in addition to employment that would require any type of lifting or carrying as well as any prolonged sitting, standing, or walking. Returning to work also exposes patients to other physical challenges such as commuting, walking from the parking lot, sitting, standing, and reaching that Ms. X cannot physically accomplish and, when attempted, flare her symptoms. Even sedentary tasks would be a challenge and should be avoided. Due to high levels of pain, fatigue, and cognitive dysfunction that substantially limit her activities, Ms. X struggles to complete most deskbound tasks including writing, composing, completing/evaluating paperwork, computer work, reading and composing emails, etc. due to her visual and noise sensitivities. Additionally, her cognitive deficits prohibit Ms. X from being able to organize, concentrate, and make decisions. Communication with coworkers and clients is also compromised due to word-finding difficulties and disrupted thought patterns. Other workplace factors outside the control of a patient with these illnesses include exposure to chemicals, perfumes, dust, mold, and certain temperature variations that can also worsen their condition. **During the course of her treatment, it is imperative that physical and emotional stress be avoided. The stress of finding and keeping any type of employment will not only inhibit any prospect of recovery but also worsen her present condition.**

Ms. X's medical records will show that the above listed multiple health issues that she suffers with have resulted in a loss of function. As noted in the new ruling, 82 FR 5844, effective March 27, 2017, SSD must consider the medical opinion of treating sources in conjunction with the supporting evidence. **In Ms. X's case, the evidence provided is consistent with the medical opinion offered in this report.**

In summary, as highlighted above, **Ms. X meets SSD's criteria for both CFS and FMS** and is severely functionally limited based on these multiple impairments. Her records confirm that she is suffering from multiple medical conditions that require her claim to be evaluated based on the totality of her impairments; complications from possible immune dysfunction, CFS, fibromyalgia, endocrine disorder, and cognitive dysfunction. **It is my firm medical opinion based on the combined effects of Ms. X's impairments that she is not able to fulfill the demands of full-time or part-time employment of any kind.**
I believe that after reviewing Ms. X's claim, you will find the information being presented as reliable, credible, and supported by her current record. However, if after reviewing the claim, if not approved, we request the following information from your agency:

1. The names, credentials, and notes of all reviewers
2. All rules, guidelines, protocols, and criteria referenced or relied upon in making the adverse determination

3. All records, notes, and summaries used in the determination
4. All written reviews conducted by the medical personnel
5. The identity and credentials of all medical personnel who reviewed this claim
6. Any and all other documented information that may have influenced the agency's decision to deny this claim

Thank you for your time and consideration with Ms. X's claim.

Sincerely,
[Doctor's Name]
[Patient Name]

Functional Barriers	
**Note that symptoms are present when at rest but worsen with activity resulting in need to change positions, take a break, rest, etc.	
Symptoms that contribute to the inability to work:	**How symptoms impact work duties:**
Neurological: cognitive dysfunction and brain fog due to fatigue and insomnia; poor concentration and focus; comprehension difficulty *These tasks can sometimes be done in their simplest form but cannot be sustained over periods of time.*	**Inability to:** articulate complex thoughts (and simple thoughts any time over an eight-hour day), process information, make decisions, calculate, meet deadlines, keep a consistent schedule, follow directions, multitask, work at a consistent pace, maintain regular attendance, commit to work duties/goals, follow through
Pain: muscle aches and muscle weakness, flu-like pain	**Limited to:** sitting for 10 to 15 minutes, standing 10 to 15 minutes, walking less than 10 minutes, lifting less than 5 pounds, carrying less than 5 pounds
	Needs to avoid: pushing, pulling, bending, squatting, kneeling, climbing, crouching
	Limited from: driving, using computer, travel away from home *While pain, fatigue, and weakness may be less severe with these limitations, these symptoms are always present during activity while idle.*

Fatigue: severe mental and physical fatigue, poor endurance, and markedly reduced stamina compared to her peers

Inability to: meet deadlines, work fixed schedule, work any schedule that does not allow multiple extended naps/bed rest

Fatigue would result in poor work quality, multiple mistakes, **safety risk**

Limited to: sitting less than 10 to 15 minutes, standing 10 to 15 minutes, walking less than 10 minutes, lifting less than 5 pounds, carrying less than 5 pounds

Needs to avoid: pushing, pulling, bending, squatting, kneeling, climbing, crouching

Limited with: driving, using computer, travel away from home

Sensitivities: chemicals, smells, noise, light, temperature

Inability to work in any environment that does not control and prevent exposure to: perfumes, dusts, molds, soaps, chemicals, poor or too bright indoor and outdoor lighting, varying temperatures

Sleep: insomnia, unrefreshed sleep

Inability to: meet deadlines, work fixed schedule, work any schedule that does not allow multiple extended naps/bed rest

Fatigue would result in poor work quality, multiple mistakes,

Safety risk

Immune deficiency: recurring infections and extended recovery time

Would require: extensive sick time away from work

Limited to: sitting less than 10 to 15 minutes, standing 10 to 15 minutes, walking less than 5 minutes, lifting less than 5 pounds, carrying less than 5 pounds

Needs to avoid: pushing, pulling, bending, squatting, kneeling, climbing, crouching

Limited from: driving, using computer, travel away from home

Limited activities are more limited with infection flares.

continued

Medication effects: sleep and pain remedies cause increased drowsiness, increased fatigue, increased brain fog; anti-infective agents cause toxic die-off reaction; IVIG treatments are time-intensive and require additional time away from work

Would require: extensive time away from work due to increased drowsiness from use of necessary sleep remedies that can cause next-day sedation

Inability to: concentrate, follow directions, comprehend/retain information, meet deadlines, work at normal pace, produce work consistently

Limited with: driving, travel away from home without assistance

Safety risk

Workplace stress: general anxiety, social anxiety *(both secondary to response to condition and underlying issues associated with CFS and Lyme disease)*

Not able to manage: public contact in person or phone, effective communication with customer or clients, adjusting needs of clients, resolving conflicts, decision making, routine or repetitive tasks at consistent pace, detailed or complicated tasks, deadlines, fast-paced tasks or environment

Post-exertional malaise: persistent worsening of main symptoms after even modest exertion that is tolerated by healthy individuals that requires additional rest/recovery

Limited to: sitting less than 10 to 15 minutes, standing 10 to 15 minutes, walking less than 10 minutes, lifting less than 5 pounds, carrying less than 5 pounds

Needs to avoid: pushing, pulling, bending, squatting, kneeling, climbing, crouching

Limited from: driving, using computer, travel away from home

Residual Functional Capacity Form
To be filled out by your physician.
But it can be helpful for you to fill out
a sample noting the details of your case
for your physician, and send it to them.

Residual Functional Capacity Form

Patient: _____Jane X_____ SS# ▮▮▮▮▮▮▮

Date of Birth: ▮▮▮▮▮▮▮▮

Dear Dr.:

Please respond to the following questions regarding your patient's disability. It will be used as medical evidence for a Social Security disability claim or a private long-term disability claim.

Please be specific with regard to your patient's medical ailments and how they affect his or her daily activities both at work and at home:

1. **With regard to your contact with the patient, please describe the frequency and purpose:** Patient since May 2014 followed up every three to four months to introduce new treatments and monitor treatment plan. Due to lack of response to comprehensive protocol, currently follows up every six to twelve months or as needed to coordinate treatments such as IVIG. Works with various practitioners for new ways to address multiple debilitating issues. Assessment and treatment of CFS, immune dysfunction with recurrent infections, chronic pain.

2. **Please describe the patient's symptoms as completely as possible:** Extreme fatigue, weakness, headaches, recurrent infections, nasal congestion, sore throat, intermittent fevers, tender lymph nodes, joint pain, TMJ pain, muscle pain and weakness, nausea, diarrhea, insomnia, frequent rashes/sores, itchy/fiery skin, foot pain, Achilles pain, mouth sores, mouth pain, ear pain, cognitive dysfunction (mental fatigue), and post-exertion malaise and fatigue.

3. **Please state all clinical findings and any medical test results and/ or laboratory results:** Low total IgA, low total IgG, low IgG subclasses, recurrent infections, HHV-6 positive, mycoplasma pneumonia positive, Epstein-Barr positive, chronic sinusitis, pharyngitis, bowel parasites, bowel infections, low blood pressure, thrush, TMJ.

4. **What is your diagnosis of the patient's symptoms and test results?**
Chronic fatigue
Immune dysfunction (CVID) with recurrent infections
Systemic recurrent candida
Fibromyalgia
Orthostatic intolerance/autonomic dysfunction
TMJ
Other chronic pain
Cognitive dysfunction

5. **Please describe any treatment done so far and the results of treatment:** Patient has utilized extensive treatment protocols and has not responded to various clinical approaches to treat multiple underlying factors. Most recently patient has struggled with TMJ treatment with multiple failed attempts at mouthpieces. Additionally, newly developed foot pain that interferes with daily activity is refractory. Current

treatments keep patient from becoming completely bedridden, but some days, patient is forced to spend most of the day in bed or recliner.

6. **What is your prognosis for this patient?** Poor due to the complexity of her illness, the length of time patient has been extremely ill, and the number of treatments tried and failed.

7. **Would you expect the patient's disability or impairment to last one year or more, or has it already lasted one year?**

               X

Yes _____ No _____

8. **Does the disability or impairment prevent the patient from standing for six to eight hours?**

               X

Yes _____ No _____

Can the patient stand at all, and if so, for how long? Standing is limited to about ten minutes due to pain and weakness. Standing for longer periods of time, fifteen to twenty minutes, causes symptoms to worsen substantially.

9. **Does the disability or impairment prevent the patient from sitting upright for six to eight hours?**

               X

Yes _____ No _____

Can the patient sit at all, and if so, for how long? Patient can sit approximately ten to fifteen minutes before neck and shoulder pain worsens, and then she needs to move to a recliner. After time in the recliner, patient then needs to lie down. Patient can only sit in a straight-backed chair. On days when patient tried to push this limit such as her attempts at attending church every other week, patient takes straight-back chair with her to service.

10. **If the patient cannot stand and/or sit upright for six to eight hours, what is the reason?** Patient is limited due to regular fatigue, poor stamina, widespread muscle pain, weakness, TMJ pain, burning

foot pain, and headaches. These regular symptoms that are present when idle prevent her from prolonged sitting and standing. Symptoms worsen when she attempts to sit or stand longer than able. Additionally, intermittent yet frequent symptoms interfere with ability to sit and stand: nausea, infections, sores, itchy/fiery skin.

11. **Does the disability or impairment require the patient to lie down during the day?**

X
Yes   _____ No   _____

If the answer is yes, please explain why: Symptoms of extreme fatigue, exhaustion, weakness, headaches, muscle pain such as neck and shoulder pain, foot pain, TMJ pain, and severe brain fog cause the need for patient to lie down throughout the day and take regular rests, breaks, or naps. Currently requiring regular rest throughout the day. This rest, however, does not alleviate symptoms. Patient required regular use of pain relievers including rotation of heating pad and ice consistently throughout the day in order to keep pain from escalating. Post-exertional malaise and fatigue after performing any activity causes increased need for rests. Days that include leaving the home such as doctor appointments, time with family every few weeks, or time at church every other week results in extreme post-exertional malaise and fatigue and increased need for rest that may last for several days.

12. **How far can the patient walk without stopping?** Patient can walk approximately ten to fifteen minutes. Walking fifteen to twenty minutes results in need to stop due to worsening symptoms and can flare a post-exertional effect.

13. **Please check the frequency with which the patient can perform the following activities:**

Percentage of Time	Never	Rarely 0–30%	Frequently 30–70%	Consistently 70–100%
Reach up above shoulders		X		
Reach down to waist level		X		
Reach down toward floor		X		
Carefully handle objects		X		
Handle with fingers		X		

COMMENTS: Although some of the above activities can be performed, they cannot be sustained for a repeated basis over a period of time. For example, patient can reach down toward the floor during a physical exam but could not sustain this activity due to her medical condition and associated symptoms.

14. **In pounds, how much weight can the patient lift and carry during an eight-hour period?**
< 5 X̲ 5–10 **X̲ 11–20 _____ 21–50 _____ Over 50 _____
Most days patient can lift and carry less than five pounds. Patient can lift up to ten pounds, but is limited with carrying this much weight. Causes a post-exertion effect. During flares, patient cannot lift and carry up to ten pounds.

15. **In pounds, how much weight can the patient lift and carry regularly/daily?**
< 5 X̲ 5–10 _____ 11–20 _____ 21–50 _____ Over 50 _____

16. **Does the patient's disability or impairment prevent him or her from performing certain motions, such as lifting, pulling, holding objects, etc.?** Yes

17. **Please check the frequency with which the patient can perform the following activities:**

Percentage of Time	Never	Rarely 0–30%	Frequently 30–70%	Consistently 70–100%
Bending		X		
Squatting	X			
Kneeling	X			
Crawling	X			

COMMENTS: As before, patient's condition/symptoms impact her ability to perform these activities and prevent her from sustaining these activities. Bending can rarely be performed but not sustained and needs to be avoided as much as possible.

18. **Would the patient's disability or impairment prevent him or her from traveling alone?**

Yes ___X___ No _____

Why? Patient can only drive/manage short limited trips such as a few miles despite physical symptoms being present. Not able to drive for longer distances as it worsens physical and cognitive symptoms. Even has difficulty riding as passenger in car on longer trips due to symptoms. Avoids any travel away from home when symptoms are at their worst or relies on family during symptom flares with limited ability to manage a vehicle. When patient pushes herself to drive farther when absolutely necessary, symptoms escalate to a severe level and require time to recover.

19. **Are there any other factors not addressed in the above questions that you believe may affect the patient's ability to work or function normally in daily life?**
It should be clear after a review of this patient's history that there are multiple contributing issues that make her condition more complex. It should also be clear that her goal has been to recover and return to the workforce, as she has sought help from multiple practitioners with various specialties and continues to search out various avenues for recovery, hence her commitment to therapies such as her therapeutic riding, even though minimal and despite being in pain.

Patient's social life has been greatly affected by illness. Has not been able to attend social events with friends or family or travel to visit family regularly as in the past. Patient's current social life consists of limited planned visits and church services every other week. Patient endures these visits even when symptoms may flare. Patient cannot attend outings or travel as she enjoyed prior to her illness.

Despite careful planning of her minimal time away from home, patient still experiences post-exertion malaise and fatigue and then requires additional time to recover.

20. **If the patient has any complaints of pain, please address the following questions:**
What is the nature of the pain? Neck and shoulder pain, TMJ pain, foot pain, Achilles pain, headaches.
How frequent is the pain? Daily and regular but intensity varies.
How would you describe the level of pain? Most pain symptoms tend to get worse as the day progresses. Pain even when idle runs at about a 5 but varies in intensity. Certain things increase pain more on some days than others, escalating pain to 8 or 9 with the need to get

additional rest and use additional pain therapies. Insomnia worsens daily pain to a higher level as well.

How would you rate the patient's creditability with regards to claims of pain? After specializing in this field for over twenty-five years and conducting an extensive evaluation, I find the patient to be very credible, as her reports of symptoms are consistent with the medical conditions and medical evidence. Patient is also very in tune with her condition and symptoms and gets very frustrated by their presence, especially when her symptoms flare and further limit her abilities.

Is there an objective medical reason for the pain? Fibromyalgia, TMJ, CVID.

21. **Given your experience with the patient, your diagnosis, and the patient's disability or impairment, do you believe he or she could continue or resume work at current or previous employment?**

                                        X
Yes   _____   No   _____

If not, please explain why: Patient is suffering from a multifactorial complex, severe condition that has resulted in severe, frequent daily symptoms. Due to the severity of patient's symptoms of extreme fatigue, weakness, muscle pain, mental fatigue, cognitive dysfunction, and post-exertion malaise, patient is not able to resume any type of work. Patient is severely limited due to her post-exertion effects when activities are attempted. In particular, this heightens her fatigue, pain, and brain fog dramatically, leaving her even less functional for at least a day and at times for several days. Patient requires several hours in the morning before she is able to perform any activity at all and requires frequent or ongoing rests throughout the day.

Patient's nature is to push past her abilities despite dealing with this illness for years, which I've explained is detrimental to her condition. I have advised patient to avoid any extended activities. Any physical activity beyond her ability hinders her condition and ability to recover. Needs to avoid as much physical activity as possible. Therapeutic riding is acceptable because breaks and rest periods are provided to avoid a crash and patient has time to recover after sessions.

Is there other work the patient could do given his or her skills and disability or impairment?

No work of any kind is possible with her loss of function, including non-exertional tasks such as sitting, reaching, repetitive arm and hand movements. Patient also requires frequent rests throughout the day as described above.

22. **How would you expect the patient's diagnosis/disability to change over time?**

    X Disability is not likely to change

    _____ Disability is temporary, from: _____ to: _____

23. **When would you expect the patient to be able to return to work, with and/or without any restrictions?**

    Not able to determine, but based on history, patient is not likely to fully recover. Our hope is that patient will experience enough improvement to reclaim some of her former life.

Please enclose all relevant medical, clinical and laboratory records you have for this patient, and use the space below for any additional comment or information you feel is relevant.

Date Report Completed: _____

Physician Name: _____

Address: _____

Telephone: _____

Specialty: _____

Signature of Physician: _____

Conclusion

Getting a Life You Love:
An Unexpected Gift of the Illness

*E*ver see a mutant movie? Where the character gets some superpower from their illness or spider bite? Seems only fair we should get one too for everything we've been through!

The good news? There is one. It is called authenticity.

This may not seem like such a big deal, but it truly is.

I find that most people have no idea who they really are or what they really want. They go through life doing what everybody else has told them to do, living up to others' expectations.

Until I had the illness, I never even thought about what I wanted. My life was all about "shoulds"—what my parents, religion, school, government, and *everyone else* thought I should be and do.

Talk about what a friend of mine called "getting should on!"

I never even considered what it was that I wanted . . . until CFS and fibromyalgia left me homeless and sleeping in parks, my dreams shattered.

But when I recovered, I realized that not all those things I had been carrying were *my* dreams. As I improved enough to go back to medical school, I chose to pick up the parts of my own life that *felt good* to me, that I was passionate about.

And I left the rest behind.

This created a space for joy and the power to create anything that I chose—including effective treatment for everybody with this illness.

The power to be authentically me . . . which, if you think about it, is quite priceless.

Appendix:
An In-Depth View of Immune Dysfunction in CFS/FMS

The Immunology of Fibromyalgia

by Samuel F. Yanuck, DC, FACFN, FIAMA

CEO, Director of Education, Cogence Immunology

Adjunct Assistant Professor, Program on Integrative Medicine, Department of Physical Medicine and Rehabilitation, University of North Carolina School of Medicine

Clinic Director, The Yanuck Center for Life & Health

Disclosure: Dr. Yanuck is a paid medical advisor for Pure Encapsulations.

A Framework for Understanding Immunity in CFS/FMS

This section will teach you how to improve immunological factors that contribute to FMS. The more of these you can address, the milder your FMS is likely to be. The most important ones are things like inflammation, T cell polarization imbalances, stress chemistry, and other illness processes that patients with FMS are often also dealing with.

The more of these extra burdens you can address and get rid of, the better you'll tend to do. It's one thing to have FMS, but if you've got FMS and four other factors making you more inflamed, or increasing your pain sensitization, or making your fatigue worse, you're more likely to feel symptomatic on any particular day.

You can think of your biology as a meadow. The fibromyalgia is like a ditch in your meadow. If you spend your days at the edge of the ditch, pretty soon you're going to fall in. Those are the bad flare days.

So, what you need to do is to identify factors that can help you move away from the ditch. Some of these will be related to the immune system. Others will be in other areas. Instead of thinking there's one magic thing that will turn your health around, you need to address many factors, each of which gives you some steps away from the ditch. Better blood sugar balance? Ten steps away from the ditch. Better sleep? Another eight steps. Avoiding problematic foods? Another twelve steps. Reduce inflammation? Eighteen more steps. Pretty soon, you're fifty yards from the ditch.

If you're fifty yards from the ditch and you have a couple of nights of poor sleep, or you inadvertently eat something you're reactive to, it might move you fifteen steps toward the ditch, but if you're far enough away, you won't fall in. That's why something might be terrible for you on one occasion, but not bother you much another time. It just depends on your distance from the ditch.

You probably already know what some of the factors are that can make a difference.

The Three Key Focus Points

Inflammation. Inflammation is central to virtually all illness processes. We all have some inflammation going on all the time. That's normal and necessary. It helps us do useful things like fight infection. But, when the level of inflammation gets too high, it can cause problems. As with most things, you want a Goldilocks amount of inflammation. That level of inflammation doesn't give you any symptoms and doesn't damage the tissues.

It's useful to notice that the other problems so common in folks with fibromyalgia are rheumatological problems (arthritis, autoimmune diseases, etc.), psychiatric problems (depression, etc.), cardiovascular problems (heart disease, etc.), and intestinal problems. All of these are driven by inflammation.

Autoimmunity. Inflammation and autoimmune process trigger each other's activation. If you have FMS and also an autoimmune disease, addressing the inflammatory triggers will quiet down the autoimmune process. In turn, addressing the autoimmunity will help quiet down the FMS.

T Cell Polarization Imbalances. When you dig into the ways that inflammation and autoimmunity are generated and how they create problems in fibromyalgia and the other illnesses that tend to go along with fibromyalgia, you find T cells at the heart of a lot of what's going on there. Understanding enough about T cells and how they get out of balance can help you make key changes that lead to real improvement.

How do each of these processes create problems? If you know how the problems are created, it will help you understand what to do about them.

WHAT IS INFLAMMATION?

Two kinds of problems—damage or infection—can cause inflammation in your tissues (muscles, tendons, joints, organs, all the "stuff" of the body). If you sprain your ankle, or if bacteria or viruses come into the tissue, your immune system will send white blood cells into your tissue to deal with it. This is completely normal and is going on in the background all the time for all of us. There are two steps and both need to work. In the first step, neutrophils come in to gobble up the debris from the damage or gobble up the bacteria or viruses. They then call monocytes to come in and gobble the neutrophils and take them out of the tissue. But if that second step doesn't happen effectively, the neutrophils will break apart and their contents will come out and damage the tissue. And since damage to tissue calls more neutrophils to come into the tissue, the cycle repeats. That's inflammation.

How do you restore the balance? Fish oil. Fish oil signals more monocytes to come into the tissue to get rid of neutrophils before they break open. And when there are already enough neutrophils to take care of what's going on, fish oil signals new neutrophils not to come in.

WHAT IS AUTOIMMUNITY?

Autoimmunity is the immune system getting interested in a target that is your own tissue. It could be the thyroid, or the joints, or the lining of the intestine, or another target. It's not the entire organ or tissue, just a group of proteins in that tissue. The immune system is supposed to fight infection, but if the signals get crossed, it can also attack regular tissue.

Different people have different amounts of this target-attacking activity. You can think of it as an argument between the immune system and the target tissue. If you have rheumatoid arthritis, your immune system and your joints are in a disagreement. Your goal is to quiet down that disagreement so that it sits in the background and is as irrelevant as possible. This is like if you and your old friend have a long-standing disagreement about something. You and your friend are very close, but you know that you'll never agree with each other about this topic, so instead of pumping a lot of energy into it, you decide the better approach is to let it be dormant. Don't stir it up. That's the goal with autoimmune disease as well.

So, the goal is to influence the signals in the body chemistry in a way that makes the disease process as quiet as possible. It sits in the background, doing nothing or as close to nothing as possible. How do you influence the body chemistry? By adding healthy food and specific nutritional supplements and related factors (the additions) and by subtracting problematic foods, pesticides and other endocrine-disrupting chemicals, and other noxious substances (the subtractions).

At the center of autoimmune disease is a chemical switch called STAT3. It turns out that the chemical switch at the center of inflammation, called NFkB, turns on STAT3. So, things that make you more inflamed also stir up the autoimmune process. One of the best ways to quiet down autoimmunity is to quiet down inflammation.

WHAT ARE T CELLS AND HOW DO THEY GET OUT OF BALANCE?

T cells are like the police in the immune system. We know about eight types of T helper cells so far. They do specific jobs that are necessary and each type is important, but if the different types get out of balance and get stuck there, it can cause problems. That will create a persistent imbalance in the body, reinforcing illness. Imbalance can occur if the body keeps having a particular kind of problem that causes the signals for one kind of T cell to keep occurring. For example, if you have persistent inflammation in your sinuses, Th2 cells will respond by increasing mucous production. If you have persistent imbalance in your intestinal bacteria (dysbiosis), your immune system will respond by continuing to make Th17 cells, driving chronic inflammation.

Top Ten Immunological Targets in Fibromyalgia

1. REDUCE INFLAMMATION

There are many factors that go into this, some of which are described below. Natural approaches to healing often address factors like food reactions, imbalances in intestinal bacteria, blood sugar problems, stress responses, chronic infections, and a host of other issues that clinicians try to improve in order to help patients with challenging problems. What virtually all of those factors have in common is that, in one way or another, they make inflammation worse. Some key factors from that list are described below.

In addition to addressing those factors directly, the following substances may be useful to address the chemistry of the inflammation itself:

- **High-quality fish oil:** Different people will need different doses. It takes months for the omega-3 fatty acids in fish oil to become incorporated into cell membranes and other structures, so stick with it. What can go wrong? If you've got a lot of oxidative stress in your system, the fish oil can be converted to inflammatory substances called isoprostanes. So, to protect the fish oil, it may be useful to take liposomal glutathione or NAC.
- **Curcumin and resveratrol:** These have been shown in the research to lower the levels of NFkB and STAT3, so they quiet down inflammation and autoimmune processes.
- **Vitamins D and A:** These have also been shown to quiet inflammation and quiet autoimmune process, while also improving immune surveillance against things like viruses.
- **Sulforaphanes:** This broccoli extract has also been shown to be useful in quieting inflammation and autoimmune mechanisms.

2. ADDRESS T CELL POLARIZATION

This is often crucial to success in challenging cases. This is a complex topic that can require skilled attention from a functional medicine clinician skilled in functional immunology. Still, there are a few basics that are often key to

address. We know about eight types of T helper cells. Of the eight, four are useful for us to focus on in our discussion:

Tregs: These are the regulatory T cells that promote immune tolerance. They help us tolerate our own tissues, so autoimmune disease can become quiet. But if you drive them up too much, bacteria and viruses can flourish, since the immune system is quieter.

Th17 Cells: Th17 cells kill bacteria and other pathogens in hollow spaces like the intestines and sinuses. But they also drive the tissue destruction in autoimmunity. There's nothing inherently wrong with them. You might make some if you get a twenty-four-hour intestinal bug, so you can kill the bug. But if you have an intestinal dysbiosis (an imbalance in your normal gut bacteria) that lasts a long time, or if you have a chronic sinus infection, you'll make Th17 cells in abundance all the time. That will drive inflammation and autoimmunity. Even if you don't have an autoimmune disease, Th17 cells create inflammatory tissue destruction. In many chronic illnesses, there is a tendency toward excessive Th17 response.

Th1 Cells: Th1 cells inhibit Th17 cells, so Th1 cells help to quiet the auto-immune tissue destruction that the Th17 cells promote. Th1 cells also drive the process of killing bacteria and viruses. If an infectious agent is small enough for one cell to eat it, a Th1 response is the way to kill it. So, Th1 cells help us with the conundrum of having an autoimmune disease but also hav-ing a chronic infection, since Th1 cells inhibit autoimmune tissue destruc-tion and also inhibit infection. Having enough of these is essential, but their levels start to go down later in life. That's part of the reason that older folks are more susceptible to the flu virus. The ability to sustain a healthy Th1 re-sponse is also diminished by inflammation, stress, candida, mold exposure, pesticide exposure (do you live near a golf course?), ingestion of plastics (the melting plastic particles in the lid of your coffee to-go cup or your plastic net tea bag), and concussions. So, any of those processes can diminish your Th1 response. If that happens, viruses that were dormant in the background can get reactivated, potentially driving illnesses like fibromyalgia.

Immunologists used to think that Th1 cells created autoimmunity. We now know that Th17 cells drive the tissue destruction in the autoimmune process and that Th1 cells inhibit Th17 cells.

Th2 Cells: Th2 cells are useful in killing parasites that get into places like the intestine. Parasites are usually too big for one cell to eat, so the Th2 cells create signals that call bunches of other immune cells to come and attack the parasite. Th2 cells also drive the production of mucous in hollow spaces

like the intestines and sinuses. If you breathe in a bunch of pollen, the Th2 response turns on and you expel the pollen on a river of mucous.

The problem with the Th2 response is that it drives things like excess mucous production, dysfunction of the intestines, and excess histamine production. And because Th2 cells make substances that inhibit Th1 cell activity, too much Th2 response can increase vulnerability to infection. And Th2 cells make antibodies that worsen autoimmunity.

Th2 dominance (having too much Th2 response) is common in people with trouble involving the intestines, sinuses, lungs, vaginal tract, or bladder. Those are all hollow spaces lined with the same kinds of lining tissues.

The Th2 response is increased by inflammation, by stress chemistry, by pollutants and pesticides, and a host of other problems. So, it's common to have too much Th2 response, especially in chronic illnesses like fibromyalgia, where inflammation and stress chemistry are so common.

So, what are the steps that could be important for you to consider?

- **Lower the level of Th2 response.** Th2 response can be quieted down with astragalus, perilla, quercetin, and NAC.
- **Increase Th1 cell response.** Th1 cells can be supported with berberine, baicalin, ginger, and sulforaphanes (a broccoli extract).
- **Lower the level of Th17 response.** Th17 response can be quieted down with curcumin, resveratrol, vitamin D, vitamin A, and sulforaphanes.

3. Avoid the Key Mistake

In some people, if they are Th2 dominant, it can be a mistake to start off by quieting down inflammation. If you take curcumin, resveratrol, fish oil, etc., as your first step, but there are signaling chemicals made by Th2 cells around, the combination of signals can increase inflammation. So, it can be important to lower the Th2 response first, for a week or so, then add in the substances that quiet inflammation. Keep up the Th2-reducing supplements while you're working to lower inflammation.

4. Get a High-Quality Lab Test for Food Sensitivities

Food sensitivities are typically mediated by the antibody IgG. I recommend the ELISA testing method (not ELISA/ACT). Changing your body chemistry is all about additions and subtractions. You can do all the good work you want by adding in healthy foods, nutritional supplements, and other related things. Those are the additions. But if you don't handle the subtractions, by getting rid of the problematic foods, you're not likely to see the improvement you want.

5. Lower Your Histamine Level

For many people, this is essential.

- Histamine has been shown to increase pain sensitivity.
- Histamine stimulates receptors on brain cells called H3 receptors. When this happens, you don't make as much serotonin. Low serotonin is known to increase pain sensitivity.
- H3 receptor stimulation also lowers norepinephrine, so you have more fatigue.
- H3 receptor stimulation lowers the amount of another neurotransmitter called acetylcholine, which helps memory function and is also necessary for the function of the vagus nerve.
- To lower histamine, it's often useful first of all to inhibit Th2 dominance. It's also useful to consider using vitamin C, quercetin, folic acid, and vitamin B6.

6. Improve the Function of Your Vagus Nerve

The vagus nerve starts in the brain. It comes down into the body and has branches that attach to your intestines, liver, spleen, and other organs. The vagus nerve helps you to be calm. And the vagus nerve does all these other things:

- Reduces inflammation in your intestine, which reduces intestinal symptoms and also reduces your inflammation overall.
- Reduces the amount of a chemical called IL-6 that's made by the liver. IL-6 levels are higher in people with FMS.
- Increases the production of digestive enzymes, which helps you break down food into bits too small for your immune system to notice them and reduces food reactions.

- Stimulates the waves of movement in the intestine that move the food downward and promote good digestion. This is a key point, because that downward wave action also keeps the bacteria in the intestine (the microbiome) down in the large intestine (the colon) where they belong. When bacteria get up into the small intestine and ferment the food there, you get gas, bloating, and inflammation in the small intestine, which is called small intestine bacterial overgrowth, or SIBO.

So, how do you improve the vagus nerve?

- Chew your food until it's almost liquid. The sensations from your jaw motion will turn on the area in the brainstem that turns on the vagus nerve.
- Take a nutritional support that helps your brain make acetylcholine, which is the neurotransmitter the vagus nerve uses to send its signals. The substances that support acetylcholine production include choline, alpha-GPC, vitamin B5 (pantothenic acid), and huperzine. But be aware that acetylcholine also helps your muscles contract, so if you support acetylcholine, you might start to get some muscle cramps. You can address that with some magnesium.
- Ask your functional medicine clinician about using a TENS device to do transcutaneous vagal nerve stimulation. That's an approach that involves activating the left side of the vagus nerve. It's quite useful and should only be done with a clinician's supervision.

7. QUIET YOUR STRESS LEVEL

Stressful circumstances in life invite any of us to have a stress response. If you respond to the stressful circumstance by "getting stressed," that's a stress response. So, the stressful circumstance and the stress response are two different things. Just because someone invites you to a party, that doesn't mean you have to go. On the other hand, once the nervous system has gotten used to responding to stress invitations, it can be important to work to shift those response patterns.

If you do get a stress response, your body makes stress response substances. The two main ones are cortisol and adrenaline. These substances, in excess, make inflammation worse. And inflammation in the body drives brain inflammation that can increase the activation of the stress response! So, it's a loop. And when the stress response patterning has been present long enough, it has its own momentum. It's essential to cultivate a daily practice like walking, yoga, or meditation, which helps reorganize your stress response to move your brain toward a calmer neurological state.

The stress response involves very specific changes to chemical signals, including the following:

- Stress increases CRH (corticotrophin-releasing hormone), which has been shown to stimulate mast cells to release IL-6 and substance P, both of which are higher in people with fibromyalgia. IL-6 increases inflammation; substance P stimulates pain sensitivity.
- Stress drives body inflammation, which drives brain inflammation. Brain inflammation drives CRH production, which drives the fight-or-flight response, so you have more stress response. It's a loop.
- When your brain gets inflamed, it makes less serotonin, dopamine, and other substances, which can make you depressed. We already covered the fact that brain inflammation can drive fight-or-flight response, which means anxiety. So, if your body is inflamed and your brain gets inflamed, it's clear in the research that this can make you depressed and anxious. Don't let anyone tell you that you have fibromyalgia "because you're depressed" or "because you're anxious." These psychological factors are present in many patients suffering from illnesses that involve chronic body inflammation that yields brain inflammation that yields depression and/or anxiety.

But that doesn't mean you should ignore depression or anxiety. It's also clear in the research that depression and anxiety can each drive the stress response, driving inflammation, creating another loop.

So, what do you do? Address the inflammation directly. That's one side of the loop. And address the depression and/or anxiety directly with psychotherapy, hypnosis, EMDR, or other appropriate methods. That's the other side of the loop.

It's also useful with chronic stress to consider using adaptogens like Siberian ginseng (also called *Eleutherococcus*) or ashwagandha. Adaptogens reduce how much stress chemistry you make when you're stressed.

Stress is an annoying one. Everybody says to have less stress. You've heard it before, but it's still true. One of the challenging things with chronic illness is to continue to value important strategies even if they're not new or cool. Keep at it. You may also find that addressing the vagus nerve function mentioned above can help you start to make more progress in quieting down your stress response. That can give you some encouragement that helps you sustain this part of your work.

8. Address Your Intestines

The intestine is a very important source of immune system signals. About 70 percent of all your immune responses occur in your intestine, so this can be an important place to pay attention to. There are several ways to do this:

- Get the ELISA food test mentioned above. When you find out the foods to avoid, avoid them 100 percent of the time—not 95 percent. It needs to be complete. No exceptions for your birthday or other special days. Not once a month or once a year. Go to zero on those foods. A good functional medicine clinician skilled in functional immunology can help you navigate this.
- Keep up the diversity of your food. The more diversity you have in your foods, the more diversity you'll have in your microbiome, which will help you reduce inflammation.
- Address the vagus nerve (see above), including chewing your food until it's almost liquid. This is a secret weapon that can pay huge dividends, if you really do it.
- Address any dysbiosis (wrong bacteria growing) that may be present. This typically requires the help of a functional medicine clinician.

If you have chronic intestinal issues, remember that when the intestines get inflamed, it typically shifts the intestinal environment toward Th2 dominance and toward activation of mast cells. Mast cells produce histamine (see the discussion of histamine on pages 272 and 362). Mast cells also produce IL-6, which is elevated in patients with fibromyalgia.

9. Move Your TGF Beta Level into the Normal Range

When you get inflamed, you have to quiet down the inflammation. Tissue damage has to get repaired. The repair involves a kind of subtle version of making a scar. The cells that do this are called fibroblasts, and they are responsible for laying down fibrous tissue as part of the repair process. Too much fibrous tissue formation can make you stiff. The tricky part is that when you lay down scar tissue, it's a little different from the original, so the fibroblasts make a substance that quiets down the immune; thus you don't get an autoimmune response to your own tissues. That substance, TGF beta, promotes the activity of the fibroblasts. That's a loop! In some people, especially when there's a lot of persistent inflammation, that loop can push excess formation of fibrous tissue. So, quieting down TGF beta can be important. One useful way to do that is by raising the level of glutathione, either by taking glutathione itself, or by taking NAC.

High TGF beta levels can drive excessive fibroblast activity, driving the laying down of more fibrous tissue, which can make you stiffer and do other problematic things. It's useful to get a blood test to measure your TGF beta level. If it's high, the best way to bring your TGF beta level down into the normal range is to take liposomal glutathione or NAC.

10. Stick to Your Process

Remember, you're working to get out of the ditch and also to move as far from the ditch as you can, so that the day-to-day variation in function that we all have doesn't affect you, and so that if you run into something that moves you toward the ditch, it doesn't put you into the ditch.

Thank you, Dr. Yanuck, for that overview of a very complex area!

So for those of you interested in the technical information, there you have a summary of what is going on. It ties together how different arms of the inflammation and immune system are interacting. It also gives a number of directions to explore.

A SELECTION OF STUDY REFERENCES AND SOURCE CITATIONS CAN BE found at www.vitality101.com/fftf-selected-references.

Acknowledgments

*S*o many special people helped make this book possible that I cannot possibly list them all. In truth, I have created nothing new; I have simply synthesized the wonderful work done by an army of hardworking and courageous physicians and healers.

I would like to extend my sincerest thanks to, first and foremost, my wife, Laurie, whose insights continue to inspire new ideas in my understanding of chronic fatigue syndrome, fibromyalgia, and healing in general. In addition to being incredibly patient with me while I wrote this book, and planting the seeds for many of the concepts I discuss, she was the first to convince me (translation: pound into my thick manly skull) that I needed to heed my readers and keep this book short and simple. So my special thanks and love to you, Laurie, who, like wives everywhere, often triggers the insights that help their men grow!

Thank you also to:

My staff. Their hard work, compassion, and dedication (and, I must admit, patience with me) are what make my work possible. I want to especially thank my office manager and patient educator, Cheryl Alberto, who is infinitely patient with me no matter how much chaos I create, and makes sure that everything happens correctly, while I am off doing the easy things like writing books; Denise Haire, Sarah Goudie, Sharon Brown, and Stacey Soltis, who keep things flowing smoothly for our patients; and Sherry Gracie, who makes sure that people get their supplements quickly and accurately.

The Anne Arundel Medical Center librarian, Joyce Miller. When I lived in Annapolis, I often wondered when she would politely tell me to stop asking for so many studies. She never did. In fact, she always smiled when I asked her for more. Truly an angel.

Bren Jacobson, Dr. Alan Weiss, and Jain Vaughn, who keep me intellectually, emotionally, and spiritually honest while reminding me to keep my sense of humor.

My wonderful and dedicated publicists, Dean Draznin, Diane Chojnowski, Terri Slater, and the rest of the Dean Draznin gang; and to Richard Crouse, my webmaster, who simply and easily makes everything I ask for happen—over and over again.

These are but a few of my teammates in making effective treatment and health available to everyone. For those I didn't mention, I thank you all!

Special thanks to Megan Newman, my publisher at Avery/Penguin, who has long been a powerful advocate for educating and empowering those with CFS/FMS. And to my superb editors, Hannah Steigmeyer and Nina Shield, who worked with me to make this book the best it could be, as well as copy editor Jennifer Eck. Also to Rudy Shur, my first publisher and a man with an ongoing vision.

My many teachers, the real heroes and heroines in their fields, whose names could fill this book—especially William Crook, Max Boverman, Brugh Joy, Janet Travell, Hugh Riordan, William Jefferies, Neil Nathan, Hal Blatman, Robert Ivker, and Alan Gaby.

The many chronic fatigue syndrome and fibromyalgia support groups. These are easily the best patient support groups I have ever seen.

And finally, God and the universe, for the guidance and infinite blessings I have been given and for using me as an instrument for healing and educating.

Index